THE DIETER'S PHARMACY

THE DIETER'S PHARMACY

The Essential Guide to Drugs That Affect Your Appetite and Body Weight

by
M. Laurence Lieberman, R.Ph.

ST. MARTIN'S PRESS
New York

Design by H. Roberts

Library of Congress Cataloging-in-Publication Data

Lieberman, M. Laurence.
     The dieter's pharmacy : the essential guide to drugs that effect your appetite and body weight / M. Laurence Lieberman.
         p.   cm.
     ISBN 0-312-03818-6 — ISBN (invalid) 0-312-03972-2 (pbk.) — ISBN 0-312-03971-9 (10-copy counter display)
     1. Appetite depressants—Handbooks, manuals, etc. 2. Appetite—Effect of drugs on—Handbooks, manuals, etc.   I. Title.
RM332.3.L54   1990
615'.7—dc20   89-24141

First Edition
10 9 8 7 6 5 4 3 2 1

CONTENTS

ACKNOWLEDGMENTS

Thanks to my wife, Barbara; Ira and Tonie; Leonard and Phyllis; Peter; Allen, Ruth, Lowell, and Jamie; Sheryl; Harry, Cindi, and Marissa; Carl; Sadie; Rae; Dov and Sheri; Brian and Louis; Randi and Michael; Matthew; Murray, Phyllis, and Evan; Darlene and Geof; Loretta. Special thanks to Dr. Carl Neuman, Muffin, and Cha-Cha.

NOTE TO READERS

This book presents general information only. It is not suitable for use as a guide for weight-reduction programs, whether via drug therapy or by other means.

Of course, you should never, under any circumstances, take any prescription drug except at a physician's direction and under his or her supervision, and then only in strict accordance with his or her instructions. Even as to over-the-counter drugs, please read and consider all warning labels, instructions, and recommended dosages. Do not use any over-the-counter drug for any purpose for which it is not intended or for weight loss unless specifically told to by a physician. If in doubt, ask your doctor. The publishers and author of this book do not, and are not equipped to, make any recommendations of any kind as to any drugs.

Neither this nor any other book should be used as a substitute for professional medical care or treatment.

THE DIETER'S PHARMACY

Introduction

Over the last generation, interest in diet and weight reduction has evolved from a mild concern to a national preoccupation. Although changes in the public's awareness of girth control may partially explain this change, the actual "fattening of America" is a very real phenomenon. In 1933, 20 percent of Americans were considered to be 10 percent overweight; by 1949 this figure had risen to 25 percent; in 1973, 33 percent were in this category. Today, with the figure at about 40 percent, an obsession with calorie-counting and youthful appearance has become part of our nation's consciousness.

More than 40 million Americans are considered *obese*, that is, 20 percent or more over their ideal body weight. And more than 80 million need to shed some excess pounds. At least one person in almost half the households of this nation is on a diet. An insight into how Americans view their bodies was revealed in a recent poll: Asked what they feared most in the world, nearly 40 percent of Americans said, "getting fat."

We are also a nation of pill-takers. Many pharmaceuticals taken to treat chronic or acute illness may affect our appetite, our weight, and our body's potential to retain water. In addition, many of these substances can alter our sense of taste, often exerting subtle changes in our eating habits. While people will go to almost any lengths to lose weight, the effect of drugs on this process has been largely overlooked.

With pharmaceuticals accounting for over $26 billion in annual spending in the United States, this represents about 1.7 billion drug prescriptions yearly. Over 30 percent of the population takes some kind of medication at any given time. And with other Americans periodically joining this segment, almost everyone eventually becomes a member of this group.

Being overweight tends to increase one's chances of suffering from certain diseases such as high blood pressure, high cholesterol, various heart problems, diabetes, and poor lung function. Since these conditions require medical care, and since two-thirds of all doctor's office visits result in a drug prescription, a large percentage of the population is both weight-conscious and taking medication.

HOW DRUGS EXERT THEIR EFFECTS

Different drugs can affect our diet goals in different ways. Since the gain or loss of weight is usually dependent on caloric intake, any drug that influences hunger or the esthetics of the eating experience is included in *The Dieter's Pharmacy* if information on that drug is currently available. Some drugs affect taste perceptions, predisposing individuals to alter their consumption of certain foods. While a drug's gastrointestinal side effects may cause loss of appetite, some pharmaceuticals may increase hunger, leading to weight gain. It is not uncommon for drugs to cause metabolic shifts, affecting the way the body deals with calories. Thyroid hormones typify this response, and ephedrine, an over-the-counter weight-loss product, has been found to increase the body's energy expenditure by 10 percent. Water retention is a by-product of some drug therapies, causing swelling of various body parts with accompanying weight gain.

In addition to the incidental effects on weight reported from drugs in general, those medicines whose sole purpose is to promote weight loss are also discussed at length in *The Dieter's Pharmacy*. Various studies have compared these drugs by their relative merits as well as by their potential side effects. Any considerations that preclude their use by some individuals or rate warnings for others help to profile the drugs' similarities and differences.

Side effects occur from all drugs. These may range from minor inconveniences, as is usually the case, to extremely unpleasant or even life-threatening episodes. Although many side effects are listed under each drug entry in *The Dieter's Pharmacy*, they occur variably in each individual. If you experience an unintended reaction to a drug you are taking, check with your doctor if these symptoms become unpleasant or persist.

Many steroid drugs used to treat allergic responses or arthritic conditions can increase hunger, cause the body to retain water, or result in fat accumulation. Certain antipsychotic medications can cause overeating. Lithium, a drug used to treat manic depression, has been reported to induce weight gains of 11 to 22 pounds in 20 to 60 percent of patients. Diuretics, used to rid the body of excess fluid, not only lower body weight through this process, but may also suppress the desire to eat.

OVER-THE-COUNTER DRUGS

Because they are so widely used and readily available without a doctor's prescription, over-the-counter medications that can affect diet goals are included in *The Dieter's Pharmacy*. Nonprescription diet-drug sales have climbed at a rate of more than 20 percent annually. Thompson Medical Company, the leading advertiser of over-the-counter diet preparations and the maker of Appedrine, Prolamine, Control, and Dexatrim, went from sales of $29 million in 1978 to about $1 billion in 1985.

A common pain reliever, ibuprofen (sold as Advil, Nuprin, Medipren, Pamprin-IB, and Trendar), is capable of causing water retention and swelling. L-histidine, an amino acid, has caused decreased appetite, weight loss, and altered taste sensation. The use of mineral oil, a potentially dangerous substance when used in excess, has produced often dramatic weight loss. Niacin and pyridoxine (vitamin B_6), both commonly used vitamins, have been known to cause weight loss. The amino acid L-tryptophan has been used successfully to treat the eating disorders anorexia nervosa and bulimia. Use of vitamin A may cause inhibited appetite and weight loss. Zinc, a common mineral taken as a dietary supplement, has been used to treat altered taste induced by other drugs, to treat anorexia nervosa, and to promote growth in zinc-deficient children.

A BOOK TO COMPLEMENT
YOUR DOCTOR

Although reports claim that 90 percent of Americans consider themselves overweight, with 35 percent desiring to lose at least 15 pounds, a survey of almost 6,000 persons between the ages of 14 and 61 found that only 7 percent of those on an eating program attempted this under a doctor's supervision. This leaves a major segment of the population without a convenient source of information detailing the effects that drugs have on their weight goals. Even when under a doctor's care, the lack of a readily available reference severely restricts the quality of advice given to such patients.

The Dieter's Pharmacy is not intended to undermine the authority of physicians, qualified nutritionists, or diet counselors. It is designed to create an awareness of the many influences drugs exert on our efforts to control our diet and shape our bodies. Their mechanisms of action, as well as their myriad side effects, are often poorly understood even by the medical community.

When seeking to alter the appetite or exert some measure of control over caloric intake, diet books or word of mouth usually serve as a guide. Physicians are consulted in only a small percentage of cases. This effectively restricts access to the authority most competent to assess the effects of medication on weight goals.

The Dieter's Pharmacy will show how almost 150 drugs, including vitamins, pain killers, antidepressants, antipsychotics, oral contraceptives, diuretics, heart medication, high blood pressure drugs, tranquilizers, sleeping pills, antiepileptic drugs, and antibiotics, may affect appetite, body weight, water retention, or taste sensitivity.

HOW DO WE KNOW WHEN
DRUGS AFFECT US?

Since hunger and the assessment of body appearance are such subjective experiences, it is often difficult to evaluate the effects of drugs. Influences may range from the extremely subtle, such as slight loss of appetite, to the overt, such as overeating. Sensory changes, such as unusual or bad taste, diminished taste, loss of taste, and taste distortion, may present nuances difficult for an individual to interpret but readily identifiable if described in a work such as this.

YOUR PERSONAL REFERENCE

With the population aging, and with the need for medications steadily increasing as we age, the effects of drug use on diet goals will affect more people in the future. With body shape and physical appearance a focus of modern existence, this book reveals the influence of pharmaceuticals on the "weight war," offering insights and solutions.

The Dieter's Pharmacy is the first source book to deal with all the drugs, both prescription and over-the-counter, that have been documented to affect the battle of the bulge, and to suggest what can be done to lessen their effects. This may take the form of a change in dosing (such as rescheduling or tapering), dieting strategies, or suggestions about alternative drug therapies. *Caution: Do not attempt to change medications or dosages without consulting your physician.*

The Dieter's Pharmacy covers every major aspect of how drugs affect hunger, body weight, and the body's potential to retain water. It allows you to investigate possible chemical connections between appetite and body weight and drugs taken for a host of illnesses and conditions. It will serve as a unique personal source book describing pharmaceuticals capable of influencing dietary goals.

How to Use This Book

This section serves as a background to "The Drugs" section of *The Dieter's Pharmacy* and tells you how to use the book. Most drugs listed throughout the book will be discussed at length, detailing their known, documented effects on appetite and body weight.

All drugs included in this book are available by prescription only unless otherwise indicated. They should only be used under the supervision of your physician.

The information provided here—regarding what each drug does, its government-approved uses, unofficial uses, when not to use, general side effects, dosage levels, remedies, and reversal of drug effects—is intended as a guide only. It is not all-inclusive and should not be so construed. For more specific information or complete details, consult a qualified medical doctor.

THE DRUG DESCRIPTIONS

Each drug description contains the following information:

Generic Name
This is the designation used by all makers of a drug, regardless of which brand name is advertised to promote the product.

Brand Names
While a drug product often is marketed initially under a single brand name, usually belonging to the drug's innovator, licensing arrangements can allow co-marketing by two or more companies,

each promoting the drug under a different proprietary name.
Once a drug's patent expires, any manufacturer may bring it to
market under its own brand name. In this manner, it is not
uncommon to see dozens of brand names, all versions of the same
chemical entity. These names often differ from one country to
another, creating confusion for international travelers.

Under "brand names," listings include the various names for
each drug as available in the United States, Canada, and Great
Britain. The absence of a brand-name listing for a drug does not
always mean that the product is unavailable. It may be sold by
generic designation only; in the case of new drugs, current information was unavailable at the time of publication.

What This Drug Does

Under this heading you will find the drug's primary use.

How This Drug Affects Body Weight

Details how the drug exerts its influence on diet goals. An
explanation of its mechanism of action offers a background with
which to interpret the clinical observations from medical literature presented for each pharmaceutical.

Government-Approved Uses for This Drug

Highlights the drug's indications as sanctioned by the Food
and Drug Administration (FDA). Many medications have more
than one official use. This information may also be of value in
investigating alternative drugs for the treatment of various conditions when viewed from the perspective of unwanted influences
on appetite and body weight. *This section is intended as a guide
only. Any change in drug therapy should be initiated only under the
care of a medical practitioner.*

Unofficial Uses

Lists experimental uses for the drug, known about by many
physicians but not yet approved by the FDA. (It is often through
pioneering efforts by doctors that these novel drug uses even-
tually are sanctioned.)

When Not to Use This Drug

Highlights those preexisting conditions or circumstances where
a drug should not be prescribed. Although not the norm, these
conditions are frequent enough and present a great enough potential hazard to merit special consideration here.

Side Effects From Use of This Drug

Focuses on the drug's potential adverse effects. These can range from a mild, barely noticeable annoyance to debilitating or life-threatening conditions. All side effects occur variably, depending on each individual as well as the drug taken. This material is presented for general reader interest and should not be considered all-inclusive.

Effects on Appetite and Body Weight as Disclosed by the Drug's Manufacturer

Isolates the dietary side effects for the drug as included in the product's official package-insert literature and the *Physicians' Desk Reference*, a publication widely used by the medical community. By presenting this here, an insight is gained as to what your doctor or other health professionals see when they consult the most accessible sources of drug information.

Detailed Effects on Appetite and Body Weight

Unlike the summary treatment of side effects presented in the section above, the material under this heading provides a more in-depth disclosure of how drugs influence diet goals as researched from unbiased medical literature. Unique to this book, these data are not readily available to doctors, pharmacists, and patients except through time-consuming searching of medical texts and periodicals. For the first time, this diverse information is being brought together in one easily understood section for each drug listed in this work.

Note: A few studies quoted in this book date back to the 1950s or even the 1930s. These are used only when newer studies are unavailable or the information is still relevant.

Dosage Levels at Which Effects Occur

Reveals the minimum daily dosage that has been found to cause the various nutritional side effects of the drug. These may vary according to the specific influences the product is known to exert.

Remedies

This is a guide to helping readers determine how best to balance a drug's therapeutic effects with its influences on dietary goals. This may include a reduction in dosage or the suggestion of alternative drugs where success has been documented by clinical studies. These recommendations should only be attempted under the guidance of your physician.

How Long It Takes Till Reversal of Drug Effects

Details the length of time it takes after withdrawal of a medication for its effects on characteristics such as hunger, taste, and body weight to dissipate. Sometimes this information is drawn from clinical studies, while in other instances it is inferred from the drug's "half-life," the time it takes for 50 percent of a substance to be cleared from the blood or eliminated from the body.

THE DRUGS

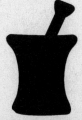

Abused/
Addictive Drugs

ALCOHOL

Brand Names
U.S.A.: *Note*: Besides being widely ingested as a beverage, alcohol is prevalent in many prescription and over-the-counter (otc) liquid medications.
Canada: Marketed by various manufacturers as above.
Great Britain: Marketed by various manufacturers as above.

What This Drug Does
  Peripheral vasodilator.

How This Drug Affects Body Weight
  A standard bottle of 70 proof alcohol provides 1,500 kilocalories, or one-third to one-half a person's daily energy requirement. The problem lies in alcohol's failure to contribute to the body's energy-yielding metabolism in proportion to its intake. It may inhibit one's appetite for other food, as though it had made a normal contribution to the diet.

Government-Approved Uses for This Drug
  None.

Unofficial Uses
  None.

When Not to Use This Drug
  If taking disulfiram or related drugs.

Side Effects From Use of This Drug

Vertigo; flushing; disorientation; sedation; gastrointestinal irritation.

Effects on Appetite and Body Weight as Disclosed by the Drug's Manufacturer

None.

Detailed Effects on Appetite and Body Weight

Weight loss: As a result of alcohol's negative effects on nutrition, it is commonly reported to cause decreased levels of thiamine (vitamin B_1), folic acid, pyridoxine (vitamin B_6), nicotinic acid (niacin), ascorbic acid (vitamin C), calcium, phosphorus, magnesium, and zinc. It comes as no surprise to find that chronic alcohol consumption results in weight loss.

In one report, 31% of a series of 29 hospitalized alcoholics showed decreased body weight.

Dosage Levels at Which Effects Occur

Weight loss: Not available.

Remedies

Weight loss: An approved abstinence program such as Alcoholics Anonymous, combined with a medically supervised program of nutritional supplementation should restore normal body weight.

How Long It Takes Till Reversal of Drug Effects

Ethyl alcohol is metabolized mostly by the liver at a rate of 10 to 20ml. (⅓–⅔ ounces) per hour. Any intake above this rate results in sedation or other signs of alcohol intoxication. Starvation lowers this rate of metabolism.

Sources

Morgan, M.Y. "Alcohol and nutrition." *British Medical Bulletin*, 1982, 38: 21–29.
World, M.J., et al. "Alcohol and body weight." *Alcohol and Alcoholism*, 1984, 19 (1):1–6.

MARIJUANA

Brand Names
U.S.A.: Cesamet (Lilly) [also known as nabilone], Marinol (Roxane) [also known as dronabinol].
Canada: Cesamet (Lilly).
Great Britain: None.

What This Drug Does
Antiemetic.

How This Drug Affects Body Weight
Unknown. Exerts complex effects on the central nervous system.

Government-Approved Uses for This Drug
To control nausea and vomiting due to cancer chemotherapy.

Unofficial Uses
To treat chronic glaucoma (when smoked as a cigarette).

When Not to Use This Drug
If nausea and vomiting are due to any cause other than cancer chemotherapy; in nursing mothers; if allergic to this drug or to any related drug (or sesame oil used in liquid capsule formulation).

Side Effects From Use of This Drug
Drowsiness; elation, easy laughing or other symptoms of a "high"; dizziness; anxiety; impaired thinking and coordination; irritability; depression; weakness; headache; hallucinations; loss of memory; burning or tingling sensations of the skin; visual distortion; confusion; ringing in the ears; nightmares; difficulty in speaking; facial flushing; sweating; fast heartbeat; dizziness upon standing; fainting; dry mouth; diarrhea; muscle pains.
Caution: Marijuana has a high addiction potential and should be avoided especially by those recovering from other addictions. Its use could restimulate addictive cravings and be counterproductive to recovery.
Because marijuana may cause drowsiness and/or changes in

the perception of reality, users should refrain from driving or operating any kind of machinery.

Simultaneous use of alcohol and marijuana can exaggerate the side effects of both substances, causing difficulty in functioning and even physical illness.

Effects on Appetite and Body Weight as Disclosed by the Drug's Manufacturer

Increased or decreased appetite; taste change; facial water retention.

Detailed Effects on Appetite and Body Weight

Increased appetite: Twelve young adult males were evaluated for appetite changes after single doses of marijuana (as the active ingredient tetrahydrocannabinol [THC] added to a flavored, noncaloric soft drink). Hunger increased when compared with other drugs tested. Peak appetite was reached 2.5 hours after receiving the drug.

Weight gain: Casual and heavy users of marijuana were compared with each other and with a control group of nonusers to test the drug's effects on eating and body weight. Both groups of marijuana users showed a significant increase in caloric intake. This was reflected by a 2.8-pound weight gain for casual and a 3.7-pound gain for heavy users over a 21-day period. The control group gained only 0.2 pounds.

In an experiment involving 12 males (aged 20–27) who were given oral marijuana as a gelatin capsule every 4 hours for 3–4 weeks, an average weight gain of almost 8 pounds was recorded.

Dosage Levels at Which Effects Occur

Increased appetite: Reported as low as 27mg. of THC per dose.
Weight gain: In one report, casual users of marijuana received the equivalent of 18–23mg. of THC an average of 13 times per month; heavy users received this on average 42 times monthly.

In the other study, participants received a maximum of 210mg. of THC daily in a sesame-oil gelatin capsule.

Remedies

Increased appetite; weight gain: Substitution of low-calorie foods, beverages, and snacks for normal dietary intake may aid in reversing some drug-induced weight gain.

How Long It Takes Till Reversal of Drug Effects

Increased appetite: Half the dose of marijuana (as the capsule form known as dronabinol [Marinol]) is cleared from the blood in 15–18 hours. Half the dose is eliminated from the body in 1 –1.5 days. As nabilone [Cesamet], duration of action is at least 8 hours. Half the unchanged drug is cleared from the blood in about 2 hours, although its metabolites (products of biotransformation in the liver) are present for longer periods of time.

Weight gain: In one study cited above, body weight began to decrease immediately after discontinuation of marijuana. Within 3–4 days, weight was almost back to pretrial levels.

Sources

Benowitz, N.L., Jones, R.T. "Cardiovascular effects of prolonged delta-9-tetrahydrocannabinol ingestion." *Clinical Pharmacology and Therapeutics*, 1975, 18: 287–97.

Greenberg, I., et al. "Effects of marijuana use on body weight and caloric intake in humans." *Psychopharmacology*, 1976, 49: 79–84.

Hollister, L.E. "Hunger and appetite after single doses of marijuana, alcohol, and dextroamphetamine." *Clinical Pharmacology and Therapeutics*, 1971, 12: 44–49.

METHADONE

Brand Names

U.S.A.: Dolophine (Lilly).
Canada: None.
Great Britain: Physeptone (Wellcome).

What This Drug Does

Narcotic agonist analgesic.

How This Drug Affects Body Weight

Opioid substances, of which methadone is one, are known to affect consummatory behaviors. Appetite and taste sensation are among these.

Government-Approved Uses for This Drug

To relieve severe pain; to temporarily maintain or detoxify narcotics addicts.

Unofficial Uses
None.

When Not to Use This Drug
In diarrhea caused by poisoning (while toxic material is still in the gastrointestinal tract); in premature infants; during labor to deliver a premature infant; if allergic to this drug or to any related drug.

Side Effects From Use of This Drug
Sedation; altered sensations; euphoria; convulsions (at higher doses); low blood pressure; fainting; dizziness on standing; heart-rhythm irregularities; nausea; vomiting; constipation; difficult urination; difficult breathing; various allergic skin responses; physical dependence; reduced libido and/or potency.

Effects on Appetite and Body Weight as Disclosed by the Drug's Manufacturer
Loss of appetite; water retention.

Detailed Effects on Appetite and Body Weight
Warning: Methadone is a highly addictive substance and should be taken only under the direct supervision of a qualified medical doctor. The following reports are for informational purposes only and should not be construed as medical advice.
Increased appetite: Eleven men enrolled in a methadone maintenance program were evaluated for the drug's effect on appetite and taste preference. Six of the 11 reported craving sweets when taking the drug. Average caloric intake for methadone-treated subjects was higher than normal (2,000–13,500 calories per day with a median of 3,070). No weight gain was apparent.
Altered taste: Four of 12 methadone users enrolled in a methadone maintenance program and enlisted for a study reported decreased ability to distinguish foods with salty taste; 42% reported decreased sensitivity to bitter taste, while sweet and sour senses were only slightly impaired.

Dosage Levels at Which Effects Occur
Increased appetite; altered taste: Although specific dosages were not given in the above studies, the usual range of daily maintenance dosage for methadone is 20–120mg.

Remedies

Increased appetite: Substitution of low-calorie foods, beverages, and snacks for normal dietary intake may aid in reversing some drug-induced weight gain.

Altered taste: Methadone-induced taste disturbance may be countered in several ways. Taking the drug with an adequate fluid intake, chewing sugarless gum or using a mouthwash of water and lemon juice, and practicing good oral hygiene may help restore normal taste sensation.

How Long It Takes Till Reversal of Drug Effects

While methadone's duration of action is 4–6 hours, it takes from 22–25 hours for half the drug to be cleared from the blood. These times may increase with chronic methadone use.

Source

Tallman, J., et al. "Effect of chronic methadone use in humans on taste and dietary preference." *Federation Proceedings of the Federation of American Society for Experimental Biology*, 1984, 43: 1058A.

NICOTINE

Brand Names

U.S.A.: Nicorette (Lakeside).
Canada: Nicorette (Dow).
Great Britain: Nicorette (Lundbeck).

What This Drug Does

Nicotine substitute.

How This Drug Affects Body Weight

Several theories have sought to explain how nicotine and cigarette-smoking affect body weight. Some studies have concluded that calories from the diet are less efficiently stored as fat in smokers. This may be due to an inhibiting influence that nicotine is thought to exert on insulin. Insulin promotes the storage of blood glucose as fat.

Smoking may affect the consumption of specific foods. Nicotine's ability to alter glucose availability to the body may create a preference for sweets.

Nicotine may increase the body's metabolic rate, burning up more calories than normal. Smokers appear, on average, to weigh less than nonsmokers. Smoking may act as a substitute for eating. The tendency for smokers to light up at the end of a meal may be replaced by a second or third helping of dessert in those who have kicked the habit.

Smoking may alter one's sense of taste and smell through the direct effect of nicotine on the oropharyngeal cavity (part of the throat).

Government-Approved Uses for This Drug
As a temporary aid to stop cigarette-smoking.

Unofficial Uses
None.

When Not to Use This Drug
In nonsmokers; in those with certain heart problems; if pregnant or trying to become pregnant; if allergic to nicotine.

Side Effects From Use of This Drug
Excess salivation; insomnia; dizziness; light-headedness; irritability; headache; gastrointestinal distress; nausea; vomiting; constipation; sore mouth or throat; jaw muscle ache; hiccups; dry mouth; flushing; sneezing; cough; euphoria; gas pains; heart irregularities; nicotine intoxication.

Effects on Appetite and Body Weight as Disclosed by the Drug's Manufacturer
Loss of appetite; laxative effect.

Detailed Effects on Appetite and Body Weight
Altered taste: In a questionnaire survey of 79 smokers and 77 nonsmokers, some significant differences in taste preference emerged. Half the smokers preferred bland food while almost 80% of nonsmokers had this preference. In gauging nicotine's influence on dietary fat intake, heavy smokers consumed significantly more meat and eggs than nonsmokers, while nonsmokers obtained more fat in the form of cakes, sweets, and chocolate. Total fat intake did not statistically differ between the two groups.

In an 18-month study of 175 cigarette smokers who were enrolled in a program to stop smoking, cigarettes were found to affect the taste sensation of bitter substances. Those who successfully quit claimed they could better distinguish bitter tastes within 2–3 days. Ex-smokers expressed a preference for bland and salty foods, while those who continued to smoke favored sweet and salty foods.

In a study of 43 volunteers (28 smokers and 15 nonsmokers), the effects of nicotine were seen to decrease preference for sweet foods. Smokers who were allowed to continue with their nicotine habit chose fewer sweet foods than nonsmokers or smokers who were deprived of cigarettes.

In a study of 17 adult males, changes in taste sensitivity were measured after use of smokeless tobacco (snuff and chewing tobacco). Eight subjects were regular users, indulging for 10 hours per week for at least 18 months, and 9 were nonusers. Taste thresholds were tested immediately after 5 minutes of tobacco use and again after 12 hours of abstinence (in the case of users). Users showed a 2- to 4-fold increase in taste recognition thresholds after 12 hours. Short-term use had little effect on users but did elevate thresholds for nonusers. It is concluded that long-term smokeless tobacco use decreases taste sensitivity.

Weight changes: Although generally conceded that smokers weigh less on average than nonsmokers, the assumption that smokers eat less food may be wrong. Ample data suggest that smokers may really consume more than nonsmokers but do not store calories as efficiently. Smokers who gain weight after quitting may just be continuing their normal caloric intake but with a more efficient system for storing calories as fat.

The average weight gained after cessation of smoking, as culled from most studies, is about 10 pounds. Weight gain usually continues until the weight of ex-smokers is about the same as those who never indulged.

In a study of over 600 men aged 40–54 who smoked cigarettes since age 20, weight gain was highest when 20 or more cigarettes were smoked daily.

In a large-scale, long-term Welsh study of 10,482 men, those over 40 years old who never smoked were an average of 13 pounds heavier than smokers.

In a study of more than 57,000 women who quit smoking, it was found that after kicking the habit, light smokers (up to 10 cigarettes a day) gained about 5 pounds; moderate smokers

(11–30 cigarettes daily) gained about 15 pounds; heavy smokers (over 41 cigarettes daily) gained about 30 pounds. The study found that weight gained after quitting is permanent. Those who are former smokers remain heavier for at least 25 years after they quit than those who continue smoking.

In a 5-year survey of 1,749 adult male smokers, several interesting facts emerged. Lean ex-smokers tended on average to gain weight while stout ex-smokers tended to lose. Ex-smokers with the largest daily tar consumption prior to quitting gained the most weight.

A recent study has yielded intriguing new insight as to why smokers weigh less on average than nonsmokers. While previous investigators have shown that smokers burn more calories than nonsmokers when at rest, this new study presents evidence that this effect more than doubles when smoking is done simultaneously with light activity. When the data were extrapolated over an 8-hour period, smokers at rest burned an extra 31 calories over the rate for nonsmokers. During light exercise this figure worked out to an extra 69-calorie expenditure over that of nonsmokers.

The study also suggests an explanation for the variable weight gains seen in ex-smokers. Those who did their smoking while mostly at rest, such as during coffee breaks or when relaxing after work, gained weight at a different rate than those who smoked during times of physical activity. Total daily nicotine consumption of the two groups was equal and it was not specified which group of ex-smokers gained more weight.

Dosage Levels at Which Effects Occur
Altered taste: Unknown.
Weight changes: Most weight changes occur when nicotine is discontinued. Highest gains are seen when the habit exceeded 40 cigarettes daily.

Remedies
Altered taste: Although nicotine-induced taste disturbance may be difficult to counter except by giving up cigarettes, adequate fluid intake, chewing sugarless gum or using a mouthwash of water and lemon juice, and practicing good oral hygiene may help restore normal taste sensation.
Weight changes: Substitution of low-calorie foods, beverages,

and snacks for normal dietary intake may aid in reversing some weight gain induced by giving up nicotine.

How Long It Takes Till Reversal of Drug Effects

Nicotine's effects are of short duration, probably no more than 1 hour. Since the nature of nicotine addiction is to require constant dosage, effects tend to be cumulative.

Sources

Birch, D. "Control: Cigarettes and calories." *Canadian Nurse*, 1975, 71(3): 33–35.

Blitzer, P.H., et al. "The effect of cessation of smoking on body weight in 57,032 women: Cross-sectional and longitudinal analyses." *Journal of Chronic Diseases*, 1977, 30: 415–29.

Bosse, R., et al. "Predictors of weight change following smoking cessation." *International Journal of Addictive Behavior*, 1980, 15: 969–91.

Grunberg, N.E. "The effect of nicotine and cigarette smoking on food consumption and taste preferences." *Addictive Behaviors*, 1982, 7: 317–31.

Grunberg, N.E. "Nicotine, cigarette smoking, and body weight." *British Journal of Addiction*, 1985, 80(4): 369–77.

Grunberg, N.E. "Nicotine as a psychoactive drug: Appetite regulation." *Psychopharmacology Bulletin*, 1986, 22(3): 875–81.

Howell, R.W. "Obesity and smoking habits." *British Medical Journal*, 1971, 4(5787): 625.

Khosla, T., Lowe, C.R. "Obesity and smoking habits." *British Medical Journal*, 1971, 4(5778): 10–13.

Mela, D.J. "Smokeless tobacco and taste sensitivity." *New England Journal of Medicine*, 1987, 316(18): 1165–66.

Perkins, K.A., et al. "The effect of nicotine on energy expenditure during light physical activity." *New England Journal of Medicine*, 1989, 320(14): 898–903.

Perrin, M.J., et al. "Smoking and food preferences." *British Medical Journal*, 1961, 1: 387–88.

Peterson, D.L., et al. "Smoking and taste perception." *Archives of Environmental Health*, 1968, 16: 219.

Rabkin, S. "Relationship between weight change and the reduction or cessation of cigarette smoking." *International Journal of Obesity*, 1984, 8(6): 665–73.

Tsai. A.V., et al. "Smoking and its effects on body weight and the systems of caloric regulation." *American Journal of Clinical Nutrition*, 1982, 35(2): 366–80.

Anabolic Steroids

METHANDROSTENOLONE

Brand Names
U.S.A.: Dianabol (Ciba-Geigy; withdrawn from the market in 1982). Marketed as "methandrostenolone" by various manufacturers.
Canada: Marketed as "methandrostenolone" by various manufacturers.
Great Britain: Marketed as "methandienone" by various manufacturers.

What This Drug Does
Anabolic steroid.

How This Drug Affects Body Weight
Weight gain in those taking methandrostenolone may be due to the drug's anabolic (tissue-building) effects. In debilitated patients, anabolic steroids can induce a sense of well-being. This may encourage the patient to eat more and gain weight.

Government-Approved Uses for This Drug
To prevent bone loss due to old age and menopause.

Unofficial Uses
To increase muscle mass and improve strength and power in competitive athletes; as an appetite stimulant in young children.

When Not to Use This Drug

In males with prostate or breast cancer; in certain males with enlarged prostate; in some females with breast cancer; in presence of pituitary insufficiency; in certain heart disease due to high cholesterol levels; in certain kidney dysfunction; if pregnant; in infants; in nursing mothers; if allergic to this drug or to any related drug.

Side Effects From Use of This Drug

Acne and oily skin (in females); nausea; vomiting; gastroenteritis; diarrhea; irritable bladder; jaundice (reversible); flushing and sweating (in females); changes in libido; inhibited secretion of gonadotropin (a hormone that regulates the sex glands); high blood calcium levels.

In preadolescent males: Phallic (penis) enlargement; increased frequency of erections; hirsutism (adult male-type hair growth).

In adult males: Inhibition of testicular function with oligospermia (lowered sperm count); gynecomastia (enlargement of the male breasts); testicular atrophy; chronic priapism (prolonged, often painful erection unrelated to sexual desire); decrease in seminal volume; impotence.

In females: Hirsutism (male-type hair growth); hoarseness or deepening of the voice; clitoral enlargement; menstrual irregularities.

Effects on Appetite and Body Weight as Disclosed by the Drug's Manufacturer

Change in appetite; weight gain; water retention.

Detailed Effects on Appetite and Body Weight

Weight gain: In a study from India, 28 healthy males aged 18–28 desiring to gain weight were divided into two equal groups. Half were given methandrostenolone for 4–8 weeks and the others a placebo. All subjects had tried vitamins, tonics, nutritional supplements, and exercise to no avail. At the end of the trial, those taking active medication showed an average weight gain of 4.54 pounds versus about a 2-pound average gain for those on placebo. Nine of 14 in the methandrostenolone group reported increased appetite, and among those the average weight gain was 6.3 pounds. In a follow-up done on 8 of the subjects 3.5 months after the drug was withdrawn, only 3 maintained the weight increase.

An Australian study of 20 athletes taking anabolic steroids over an 18-month period showed weight gains of from 1.5–13.2% of their total body weight, with an average of 5.7%.

A report of 8 males given methandrostenolone for about 1 month showed an average weight gain of 0.66 pounds. However, an increase in lean body mass (nonfat) of 4.4 pounds was seen. This is significant because, although total body weight did not alter dramatically, there was a shift in the composition of total body mass.

In two separate studies by the same author, a total of 18 males were given methandrostenolone for an average of 42 days. A mean weight gain of 7.7 pounds was seen, with lean body mass increasing by 11–12 pounds.

An unusual case study describes a 26-year-old man taking methandrostenolone to increase his strength and mass as a professional body builder. Using a dose about 10 times greater than that recommended for the drug's legitimate use, he saw a weight gain of about 28 pounds in 2 years accompanied by spectacular muscular development.

Dosage Levels at Which Effects Occur
Weight gain: Reported as low as 5mg. daily. The usual daily dosage range of methandrostenolone is 2.5–5mg. Athletes using it to build muscle mass and increase performance have taken as much as 100mg. daily.

Remedies
Weight gain: Not applicable.

How Long It Takes Till Reversal of Drug Effects
Weight gain: In the Indian study cited above, only 3 of 8 subjects maintained weight gains 3.5 months after discontinuation of methandrostenolone.

Sources
Doshi, J.C., et al. "Methandienone—an anabolic agent in underweight healthy subjects." *Indian Journal of Medical Sciences*, 1966, 20(10): 673–76.

Forbes, G.B. "The effect of anabolic steroids on lean body mass: The dose response curve." *Metabolism, Clinical and Experimental*, 1985, 34(6): 571–73.

Tahminjis, A.J. "The use of anabolic steroids by athletes to increase body weight and strength." *Medical Journal of Australia*, 1976, 1: 991–93.

NANDROLONE

Brand Names
U.S.A.: Anabolin (Alto), Anabolin L.A. (Alto), Androlone (Keene), Androlone-D 100 (Keene), Deca-Durabolin (Organon), Decolone (Kay), Decolone-100 (Kay), Durabolin (Organon), Hybolin Decanoate (Hyrex), Hybolin Improved (Hyrex), Nandrobolic (Forest), Nandrobolic L.A. (Forest), Neo-Durabolic (Hauck).
Canada: Deca-Durabolin Decanoate (Organon), Durabolin phenpropionate (Organon).
Great Britain: Deca-Durabolin (Organon), Durabolin (Organon).

What This Drug Does
Anabolic steroid.

How This Drug Affects Body Weight
Weight gain in those taking nandrolone may be due to the drug's anabolic (tissue-building) effects. In debilitated patients, anabolic steroids can promote a sense of well-being. This may induce the patient to eat more and gain weight.

Government-Approved Uses for This Drug
To control certain breast cancers (phenpropionate form of the drug is used); to treat anemia due to kidney dysfunction (decanoate form of the drug).

Unofficial Uses
To increase muscle mass and improve strength and power in competitive athletes.

When Not to Use This Drug
In males with prostate or breast cancer; in certain males with enlarged prostate; in some females with breast cancer; in pituitary insufficiency; in certain heart disease due to high cholesterol levels; in certain kidney dysfunction; if pregnant; in infants; in nursing mothers; if allergic to this drug or to any related drug.

Side Effects From Use of This Drug

In males and females: Nausea; vomiting; gastroenteritis; diarrhea; irritable bladder; high blood calcium levels; jaundice (reversible); changes in libido; inhibition of gonadotropin secretion (gonadotropin is the hormone needed to stimulate the body's reproductive mechanisms; in males, this affects sperm production, while in females it is vital to normal menstrual cycling and mature egg production).

In preadolescent males: Phallic (penis) enlargement; increased frequency of erections; hirsutism (adult male-type hair growth).

In adult males: Inhibition of testicular function with oligospermia (lowered sperm count); gynecomastia (enlargement of the male breasts); testicular atrophy; chronic priapism (prolonged, often painful erection unrelated to sexual desire); decrease in seminal volume; impotence.

In females: Acne and oily skin; flushing and sweating; hirsutism (male-type hair growth); hoarseness or deepening of the voice; clitoral enlargement; menstrual irregularities.

Effects on Appetite and Body Weight as Disclosed by the Drug's Manufacturer

Change in appetite; weight gain; water retention; ankle swelling.

Detailed Effects on Appetite and Body Weight

Weight gain: Two case reports describe a 10-year-old and 14-year-old girl. The older patient went from 115 pounds to 75 pounds in 2 months; this occurred after she became upset at the sight of an obese girl in summer camp. Intramuscular injections of nandrolone given every 2 weeks gave dramatic results. After 1 month of drug treatment, she started eating, and after 3 months, her weight had gone to 135 pounds.

In the second case, involving the 10-year-old, severe disturbance followed an incident in which her pet duckling was killed by a dog. After she went from 75 pounds to 50 pounds, nandrolone was administered by intramuscular injection. Given every 2 weeks, the drug caused her to begin eating within 1 month and after 3 months she weighed 80 pounds.

Another case by the same researchers as above describes a 14-year-old girl with anorexia nervosa who had dropped from 134 pounds to 50 pounds and resembled "pictures of prisoners re-

leased from Bergen-Belsen (a Nazi concentration camp) . . ."
Since all other methods of encouraging the patient to eat had
failed, nandrolone was given by injection. Two weeks later, with
no improvement seen (in fact the girl had lost even more weight),
a second injection was administered. Two weeks after this, the
patient began to eat but "felt very unhappy about it." Within 3
months, she had regained all the lost weight and now worried
about becoming overweight.

In a study of 4 males given nandrolone weekly for 3 weeks,
average weight gain was 3.5 pounds.

Dosage Levels at Which Effects Occur
Weight gain: In children, the dosage given in the above studies
was 25mg. every 2 weeks by intramuscular injection. In the adult
study, the dose was 75mg. weekly by intramuscular injection for
3 weeks.

Remedies
Weight gain: Not applicable.

How Long It Takes Till Reversal of Drug Effects
Nandrolone is manufactured in 2 forms; decanoate and phenpropionate. Given as intramuscular injections, the decanoate has
a duration of action of 3–4 weeks, while the phenpropionate lasts
1–2 weeks.

Sources
Forbes, G.B. "The effect of anabolic steroids on lean body mass: The dose
response curve." *Metabolism, Clinical end Experimental*, 1985, 34(6): 571–
73.

Tec, L. "Durabolin in anorexia nervosa." *American Journal of Psychiatry*, 1963,
120(3): 282.

Tec, L. "Anorexia nervosa: Follow-up on a special method of treatment."
American Journal of Psychiatry, 1971, 127: 1702.

NORETHANDROLONE

Brand Names
U.S.A.: None.
Canada: Nilevar (Searle).
Great Britain: Nilevar (Searle).

What This Drug Does
Anabolic steroid.

How This Drug Affects Body Weight
Weight gain in those taking norethandrolone may be due to the drug's anabolic (tissue-building) effects. In debilitated patients, anabolic steroids can promote a sense of well-being. This may induce the patient to eat more and gain weight.

Government-Approved Uses for This Drug
None in the U.S.A. In other countries it is approved to treat osteoporosis; to treat some aplastic anemias; to promote weight gain in those with protein- and bone-wasting conditions.

Unofficial Uses
To increase muscle mass and improve strength and power in competitive athletes; to treat male infertility.

When Not to Use This Drug
In males with prostate or breast cancer; in certain males with enlarged prostate; in some females with breast cancer; in pituitary insufficiency; in certain heart disease due to high cholesterol levels; in certain kidney dysfunction; if pregnant; in infants; in nursing mothers; if allergic to this drug or to any related drug.

Side Effects From Use of This Drug
In males and females: Nausea; vomiting; gastroenteritis; diarrhea; irritable bladder; high blood calcium levels; jaundice (reversible); changes in libido; inhibition of gonadotropin secretion (gonadotropin is the hormone needed to stimulate the body's reproductive mechanisms; in males, this affects sperm production, while in females it is vital to normal menstrual cycling and mature egg production).
In preadolescent males: Phallic (penis) enlargement; increased frequency of erections; hirsutism (adult male-type hair growth).
In adult males: Inhibition of testicular function with oligospermia (lowered sperm count); gynecomastia (enlargement of the male breasts); testicular atrophy; chronic priapism (prolonged, often painful erection unrelated to sexual desire); decrease in seminal volume; impotence.
In females: Acne and oily skin; flushing and sweating; hirsutism (male-type hair growth); hoarseness or deepening of the voice; clitoral enlargement; menstrual irregularities.

Effects on Appetite and Body Weight as Disclosed by the Drug's Manufacturer
Change in appetite; weight gain; water retention; ankle swelling.

Detailed Effects on Appetite and Body Weight
Weight gain: In a group of 25 underweight but otherwise healthy subjects, administration of norethandrolone for 12 weeks resulted in an average weight gain of 5.5 pounds. In a follow-up 6 months after the drug was withdrawn, 76% of subjects had maintained their increased weight.

Dosage Levels at Which Effects Occur
Weight gain: Reported at a daily dose of 25mg. given for 12 weeks.

Remedies
Weight gain: Not applicable.

How Long It Takes Till Reversal of Drug Effects
Weight gain: In the study cited above, 76% of subjects had still maintained all weight gained 6 months after withdrawal of norethandrolone.

Source
Watson, R.N., et al. "A six-month evaluation of an anabolic drug, nor-ethandrolone, in underweight persons." *American Journal of Medicine*, 1959, 26: 240.

OXANDROLONE

Brand Names
U.S.A.: Anavar (Searle).
Canada: None.
Great Britain: None.

What This Drug Does
Anabolic steroid.

How This Drug Affects Body Weight
Weight gain in those taking oxandrolone may be due to the drug's anabolic (tissue-building) effects. In debilitated patients,

anabolic steroids can promote a sense of well-being. This may induce the patient to eat more and gain weight.

Government-Approved Uses for This Drug
To promote weight gain; to relieve bone pain in osteoporosis (bone loss); to offset protein breakdown associated with chronic use of corticosteroids.

Unofficial Uses
To increase muscle mass and improve strength and power in competitive athletes.

When Not to Use This Drug
In males with prostate or breast cancer; in certain males with enlarged prostate; in some females with breast cancer; in pituitary insufficiency; in certain heart disease due to high cholesterol levels; in certain kidney dysfunction; if pregnant; in infants; in nursing mothers; if allergic to this drug or to any related drug.

Side Effects From Use of This Drug
Nausea; vomiting; gastroenteritis; diarrhea; irritable bladder; jaundice (reversible); high blood calcium levels.
In preadolescent males: Phallic (penis) enlargement; increased frequency of erections.
In adult males: Inhibition of testicular function with oligospermia (lowered sperm count); gynecomastia (enlargement of the male breasts).
In females: Acne and oily skin; hirsutism (male-type hair growth); flushing and sweating; hoarseness or deepening of the voice; clitoral enlargement; menstrual irregularities.
In males and females: Changes in libido; inhibited secretion of gonadotropin (a hormone that regulates the sex glands).

Effects on Appetite and Body Weight as Disclosed by the Drug's Manufacturer
Change in appetite; weight gain; water retention.

Detailed Effects on Appetite and Body Weight
Weight gain: In a study of 9 subjects (3 females and 6 males) given oxandrolone for an average of 2 weeks, a mean increase in lean (nonfat) body mass of 2.2 pounds was recorded.

A case report of a professional body builder describes a competitor who took oxandrolone for 140 days while undergoing an intensive weight-training program. He showed a total gain of over 21 pounds, but his increase in lean body mass was over 42 pounds.

Dosage Levels at Which Effects Occur
Weight gain: Reported as low as 10mg. daily.

Remedies
Weight gain: Not applicable.

How Long It Takes Till Reversal of Drug Effects
Unknown.

Source
Forbes, G.B. "The effect of anabolic steriods on lean body mass: The dose response curve." *Metabolism, Clinical and Experimental*, 1985, 34(6): 571–73.

Antiarthritic/Anti-Inflammatory Drugs

IBUPROFEN

Brand Names
U.S.A.: †Advil (Whitehall), †Coda.Med (Jeffrey Martin), †Haltran (Upjohn) †Ibuprin (Thompson), †Ibuprohm (OHM), †Ifen (Everett), †Medipren (McNeil), ‡Motrin (Upjohn), †Motrin IB (Upjohn), †Nuprin (Bristol-Meyers), †Pamprin-IB (Chattem), †Profen (Private Formulations), ‡Rufen (Boots), †Trendar (Whitehall).
Canada: Amersol (Horner), Apo-Ibuprofen (Apotex), Motrin (Upjohn), Novoprofen (Novopharm).
Great Britain: Apsifen (Approved Prescription Services), Brufen (Boots), Ebufac (DDSA), Ibu-Slo (Rona).

What This Drug Does
Anti-inflammatory.

How This Drug Affects Body Weight
Inhibits prostaglandin synthesis. Prostaglandins are hormone or hormone-like substances found primarily in semen and menstrual fluid. They may be involved in blood-pressure control and other body processes. Ibuprofen's tendency to cause water retention in the body may be due to its effect on salt and water metabolism in the kidneys. It may also exert an enhancing effect

---

†Denotes over-the-counter availability in the U.S.A.
‡Denotes prescription-only status in the U.S.A.

on ADH (antidiuretic hormone). ADH decreases urine production by causing water to be soaked up by the kidneys and retained in the body.

Government-Approved Uses for This Drug

To relieve symptoms of rheumatoid arthritis and osteoarthritis; to relieve pain; to treat painful menstruation; to reduce fever.

Unofficial Uses

To treat juvenile rheumatoid arthritis; to treat symptoms of sunburn; to prevent migraine headaches; to treat tension headache.

When Not to Use This Drug

If breast-feeding; if pregnant; if allergic to this drug or to any related drug (i.e., aspirin).

Side Effects From Use of This Drug

Nausea; stomach upset or pain; heartburn; diarrhea (1–3%) or constipation (1–3%); vomiting; dizziness; headache; nervousness; ringing in the ears; ulcer or bleeding of the stomach or duodenum; liver dysfunction (jaundice, hepatitis); inflammation of the pancreas; mental depression; confusion; hallucinations; burning sensations of the skin; hearing loss; blurred vision and other eye problems; various skin reactions and other allergic responses; hair loss; various blood abnormalities; nosebleed; low blood sugar; various heart problems; kidney dysfunction; dry eyes and mouth; ulcerated gums; inflammation of the nasal membranes; gynecomastia (enlargement of the male breasts); menorrhagia (abnormally heavy or long menstruation).

Effects on Appetite and Body Weight as Disclosed by the Drug's Manufacturer

Water retention and swelling; decreased appetite.

Detailed Effects on Appetite and Body Weight

Water retention and swelling: One of ibuprofen's more popular uses is to relieve premenstrual or menstrual cramps and pain. It is precisely at this time of the month that women find water retention by the body to be greatest. Ibuprofen's potential to exacerbate this condition should be kept in mind.

In a 5-year British study of 191 patients over 65 years old and using ibuprofen, 4% were found to retain water as a side effect.

In those under 65 years of age, this incidence dropped to less than 1%.

An 8-week Dutch investigation showed 5% of patients receiving ibuprofen for 4 weeks complaining of swelling from water retention.

One case report describes a 71-year-old male taking ibuprofen for back pain. At a routine doctor's visit on the seventeenth day of medication, no abnormality was evident. Six days later, the patient's ankles became swollen and 4 days after this he was admitted to the hospital. Examination revealed a water-weight gain of 6.75 pounds since the previous office visit. Withdrawal of ibuprofen and administration of a diuretic effected a 3-pound weight loss within the first 3 days. Within 10 days, the patient's weight was back to normal. Six months later, without further use of ibuprofen or diuretics, no swelling was evident.

Dosage Levels at Which Effects Occur
Water retention and swelling: May occur within a range of 400–1,600mg. daily. *Do not take more than 1,200 mg. daily without consulting your physician.*

Remedies
Water retention and swelling: Diuretics, such as furosemide (Lasix) or hydrochlorothiazide (HydroDiuril, Esidrix) should help rid the body of excess fluid. In the case of the 71-year-old man cited above, a total of 80mg. of furosemide given over a 3-day period reversed swelling. This should only be attempted under the supervision of a doctor.

How Long It Takes Till Reversal of Drug Effects
Water retention and swelling: When accompanied by use of the diuretic furosemide, the 71-year-old man cited in the case above returned to normal within 10 days of discontinuing ibuprofen.

Sources
Buckler, J.W., et al. "The tolerance and acceptability of ibuprofen in the elderly patient." *Current Medical Research and Opinion*, 1975, 3: 558–62.

deBlecourt, J.J. "A comparative study of ibuprofen ('Bufen') and indomethacin in uncomplicated arthrosis." *Current Medical Research and Opinion*, 1975, 3: 477–80.

Kantor, T.G. "Ibuprofen." *Annals of Internal Medicine*, 1979, 91: 877–82.

Scholley, R.T., et al. "Edema associated with ibuprofen therapy." *Journal of the American Medical Association*, 1977, 237(16): 1716–17.

NAPROXEN

Brand Names
U.S.A: Anaprox (Syntex), Naprosyn (Syntex).
Canada: Anaprox (Syntex), Apo-Naproxen (Apotex), Naprosyn (Syntex), Novonaprox (Novopharm).
Great Britain: Naprosyn (Syntex), Synflex (Syntex).

What This Drug Does
Nonsteroidal anti-inflammatory (NSAID).

How This Drug Affects Body Weight
Inhibits prostaglandin synthesis. Prostaglandins are hormone or hormone-like substances found primarily in semen and menstrual fluid. They may be involved in blood-pressure control and other body processes. Naproxen's tendency to cause water retention in the body may be due to its effect on salt and water metabolism in the kidneys. It may also exert an enhancing effect on ADH (antidiuretic hormone). ADH decreases urine production by causing water to be soaked up by the kidneys and retained in the body.

Government-Approved Uses for This Drug
To relieve pain; to treat painful menstruation; to treat rheumatoid arthritis and osteoarthritis; to treat gout.

Unofficial Uses
To treat juvenile rheumatoid arthritis; to treat symptoms of sunburn; to prevent migraine headache.

When Not to Use This Drug
If breast-feeding; if allergic to this drug, to aspirin, or to any other related drug.

Side Effects From Use of This Drug
Prolonged bleeding time; headache; drowsiness; dizziness; stomach upset; blood in the stool; nausea; kidney toxicity;

elevated liver enzymes; skin rash or itching; menstrual disorders.

Effects on Appetite and Body Weight as Disclosed by the Drug's Manufacturer

Edema; increased or decreased appetite; weight gain or loss.

Detailed Effects on Appetite and Body Weight

Detailed manufacturer's disclosure: Although naproxen's official literature lists water retention, appetite changes, and weight change as potential side effects, more detailed information from independent sources is unavailable.

Water retention is known to occur in 3–9% of those taking this medication.

Dosage Levels at Which Effects Occur

May occur within the normal daily dosage range of 500–1,000mg.

Remedies

Weight gain: Substitution of low-calorie foods, beverages, and snacks for normal dietary intake may aid in reversing some naproxen-induced weight gain.

Decreased appetite; weight loss: The maintenance of adequate fluid intake and the avoidance of excessive alcohol use may aid in restoring normal appetite.

Water retention: Use of a diuretic may help rid the body of excess water. This should only be attempted under the supervision of a doctor.

How Long It Takes Till Reversal of Drug Effects:

Naproxen's duration of action may last up to 7 hours.

Sources

Olin, B.R. (ed.) *Facts and Comparisons*. St. Louis: Facts and Comparisons, 1988.

Physicians' Desk Reference. Oradell, NJ: Medical Economics, 1988.

USP DI. Rockville, MD: The United States Pharmacopeial Convention, Inc., 1989.

PENICILLAMINE

Brand Names
U.S.A.: Cuprimine (MSD), Depen (Wallace).
Canada: Cupramine (MSD), Depen (Horner).
Great Britain: Cupramine (MSD), Distamine (Dista), Pendramine (E. Merck).

What This Drug Does
Antiarthritic.

How This Drug Affects Body Weight
Penicillamine acts as a chelating agent, removing excess metals such as copper, zinc, iron, mercury, lead, and arsenic from the blood. Zinc deficiency has been linked to alterations in taste, and penicillamine use may contribute to this phenomenon. It is also speculated that the drug may act by inhibiting nerve impulses from the taste buds.

Government-Approved Uses for This Drug
To treat rheumatoid arthritis; to treat Wilson's disease (an abnormality of copper metabolism); to treat certain urinary stone formation.

Unofficial Uses
To treat biliary cirrhosis (a condition where bile flow through the liver is restricted); to treat scleroderma (a disease affecting the blood vessels and connective tissue and characterized by hardened skin on the face and hands).

When Not to Use This Drug
If there is a history of kidney dysfunction; if pregnant; if breastfeeding; if allergic to this drug or to any related drug.

Side Effects From Use of This Drug
Warning: This is a potentially dangerous drug and strict medical supervision during its use is essential. Among this drug's many side effects are: various blood abnormalities; ringing in the ears; skin wrinkling and various other skin reactions; vitamin B_6 deficiency; stomach pain; nausea; vomiting; occasional

diarrhea; mouth irritation; liver dysfunction; inflammation of the pancreas; kidney dysfunction; hair loss; myasthenia gravis (a condition of chronic tiredness and muscle weakness).

Effects on Appetite and Body Weight as Disclosed by the Drug's Manufacturer

Loss of appetite; blunting, diminution, or total loss of taste perception.

Detailed Effects on Appetite and Body Weight

Altered taste: Seven of 20 patients treated with penicillamine reported taste changes. These effects were most often noted within 3–6 weeks of starting the drug; in one case this occurred in 3 days. The first sign of abnormality was a salty or metallic taste. Most subjects reported ice cream or chocolate to be tasteless, and in one case all chocolate tasted bitter. Patients could not distinguish fish or meat. Fruits and vegetables were also reported to be tasteless.

Among 73 patients given penicillamine, 23 complained of decreased taste acuity. All reported onset at 4–6 weeks after starting the drug, usually after the dose of penicillamine was increased above 1,000mg. daily. Reports included a metallic or salty taste. Chocolate and ice cream were judged to be flavorless, and distinguishing between various foods by taste alone was impossible.

A case report describes a patient who, within 2 months of taking penicillamine, noted a decreased ability to taste various foods. The patient responded favorably to the addition of zinc to the diet, but within 1 week of its withdrawal, altered taste returned.

A researcher reports that in 1962, when penicillamine was first used to treat rheumatoid arthritis, about 25% of patients complained of some loss of taste sensation. Four patients reported complete loss of taste; they needed increasing amounts of salt, sugar, and spices in their food, and certain foods could no longer be identified by taste alone. Two patients had to discontinue the drug, with complete return to normal occurring within 8–10 weeks. The other 2 continued using penicillamine and taste also normalized within the same time period. Further investigations have revealed taste loss to occur in about 4% of those using penicillamine in the treatment of Wilson's disease, while about 30% of those receiving it for other uses report this phenomenon.

Dosage Levels At Which Effects Occur
Altered taste: Reported as low as 250mg. daily.

Remedies
Altered taste: Two methods have been suggested to treat taste alterations as a result of penicillamine use. The first is dietary zinc supplements. In one case, a dose of 60mg. daily normalized taste sensation after 2 months of continuous usage.

The second method is the use of copper sulfate. In one report, 60mg. daily reversed altered taste within 4 weeks, even though penicillamine was not discontinued. Other researchers have suggested copper sulfate in doses of 5–15mg. daily.

How Long It Takes Till Reversal of Drug Effects
Altered taste: Various reports describe reversal within 4–10 weeks after withdrawal of penicillamine. Another researcher claims onset of altered taste usually occurs within the first 6 weeks of penicillamine use, while normal taste may return within 6 months, even when penicillamine use is continued.

Sources
Henkin, R.I., et al. "Decreased taste sensitivity after d-penicillamine reversed by copper administration." *Lancet*, 1967, 2(7529): 1268–71.

Henkin, R.I., Bradley, D.F. "Hypogeusia corrected by Ni + + and Zn + + ." *Life Science*, 1970, 9: 701–9.

Jaffe, I.A. "Effects of penicillamine on the kidney and on taste." *Postgraduate Medical Journal* (Suppl.), 1968, 44(suppl.): 15–18.

Keiser, H.R., et al. "Loss of taste during therapy with penicillamine." *Journal of the American Medical Association*, 1968, 203: 381–83.

MacFarlane, M.D. "Penicillamine and zinc." *Lancet*, 1974, 2: 962.

PIROXICAM

Brand Names
U.S.A.: Feldene (Pfizer).
Canada: Feldene (Pfizer).
Great Britain: Feldene (Pfizer), Larapam (Lagap).

What This Drug Does
Anti-inflammatory.

How This Drug Affects Body Weight
Inhibits prostaglandin synthesis. Prostaglandins are hormone or hormone-like substances found primarily in semen and menstrual fluid. They may be involved in blood-pressure control and other body processes. Piroxicam's tendency to cause water retention in the body may be due to its effect on salt and water metabolism in the kidneys. It may also exert an enhancing effect on ADH (antidiuretic hormone). ADH decreases urine production by causing water to be soaked up by the kidneys and retained in the body.

Government-Approved Uses for This Drug
To relieve symptoms of rheumatoid arthritis and osteoarthritis.

Unofficial Uses
None.

When Not to Use This Drug
If breast-feeding; if allergic to this drug or to any related drug.

Side Effects From Use of This Drug
Nausea; stomach upset or pain; indigestion; diarrhea or constipation (both occur in more than 1% of cases); nausea; vomiting; dizziness; headache; nervousness; ringing in the ears; hearing loss; ulcer or bleeding of the stomach or duodenum; liver dysfunction (jaundice, hepatitis); inflammation of the pancreas; mental depression; confusion; hallucinations; burning sensations of the skin; blurred vision and other eye problems; various skin reactions and other allergic responses; hair loss; various blood abnormalities; nosebleed; low blood sugar; various heart problems; kidney dysfunction.

Effects on Appetite and Body Weight as Disclosed by the Drug's Manufacturer
Edema; anorexia; weight increase or decrease.

Detailed Effects on Appetite and Body Weight
Detailed manufacturer's disclosure: Although piroxicam's official literature lists water retention, appetite loss, and weight change as potential side effects, more detailed information from independent sources is unavailable.

Water retention and loss of appetite are known to occur in 1 –3% of those taking this medication. Weight changes occur in less than 1% of cases.

Dosage Levels at Which Effects Occur
May occur at the usual daily dose of 20mg.

Remedies
Water retention: Use of a diuretic may help rid the body of excess water. This should only be attempted under the supervision of a doctor.
Weight gain: Substitution of low-calorie foods, beverages, and snacks for normal dietary intake may aid in reversing some naproxen-induced weight gain.
Loss of appetite; weight loss: The maintenance of adequate fluid intake and the avoidance of excessive alcohol use may aid in restoring normal appetite.

How Long It Takes Till Reversal of Drug Effects
While half the dose of piroxicam is cleared from the blood within 30–86 hours, its duration of action ranges from 48–72 hours.

Sources
Olin, B.R. (ed.). *Facts and Comparisons*. St. Louis: Facts and Comparisons, 1988.
Physicians' Desk Reference. Oradell, NJ: Medical Economics, 1988.
USP DI. Rockville, MD: The United States Pharmacopeial Convention, Inc., 1989.

SULINDAC

Brand Names
U.S.A: Clinoril (MSD).
Canada: Clinoril (Frosst).
Great Britain: Clinoril (MSD).

What This Drug Does
Anti-inflammatory.

How This Drug Affects Body Weight

Inhibits prostaglandin synthesis. Prostaglandins are hormone or hormone-like substances found primarily in semen and menstrual fluid. They may be involved in blood-pressure control and other body processes. Sulindac's tendency to cause water retention in the body may be due to its effect on salt and water metabolism in the kidneys. It may also exert an enhancing effect on ADH (antidiuretic hormone). ADH decreases urine production by causing water to be soaked up by the kidneys and retained in the body.

Government-Approved Uses for This Drug

To treat symptoms of various arthritic diseases.

Unofficial Uses

None.

When Not to Use This Drug

If breast-feeding; if allergic to this drug or to any related drug.

Side Effects From Use of This Drug

Nausea; stomach upset or pain; heartburn; diarrhea; vomiting; constipation; dizziness; headache; nervousness; ringing in the ears; ulcer or bleeding of the stomach or duodenum; liver dysfunction (jaundice, hepatitis); inflammation of the pancreas; mental depression; confusion; hallucinations; burning sensations of the skin; hearing loss; blurred vision and other eye problems; various skin reactions and other allergic responses; hair loss; various blood abnormalities; nosebleed; low blood sugar; various heart problems; kidney dysfunction; dry eyes and mouth; ulcerated gums; inflammation of the nasal membranes; vaginal bleeding; gynecomastia (enlargement of the male breast, often accompanied by tenderness).

Effects on Appetite and Body Weight as Disclosed by the Drug's Manufacturer

Anorexia; edema; metallic or bitter taste.

Detailed Effects on Appetite and Body Weight

Detailed manufacturer's disclosure: Although sulindac's official literature lists loss of appetite, water retention, and altered taste as potential side effects, more detailed information from independent sources is unavailable.

Loss of appetite and water retention are known to occur in 1–3% of those taking this medication. Metallic or bitter taste occurs in less than 1% of cases.

Dosage Levels at Which Effects Occur
May occur within the usual daily dosage range of 300–400mg.

Remedies
Loss of appetite: The maintenance of adequate fluid intake and the avoidance of excessive alcohol use may aid in restoring normal appetite.

Water retention: Use of a diuretic may help rid the body of excess water. This should only be attempted under the supervision of a doctor.

Taste change: Sulindac-induced taste disturbance may be countered in several ways. Taking the drug with an adequate fluid intake, chewing sugarless gum or using a mouthwash of water and lemon juice, and practicing good oral hygiene may help restore normal taste sensation.

How Long It Takes Till Reversal of Drug Effects
Although half the dose of sulindac is cleared from the blood in 7.8 hours, its duration of action may persist up to 12 hours.

Sources
Olin, B.R. (ed.). *Facts and Comparisons*. St. Louis: Facts and Comparisons, 1988.

Physicians' Desk Reference. Oradell, NJ: Medical Economics, 1988.

USP DI. Rockville, MD: The United States Pharmacopeial Convention, Inc., 1989.

Antiasthma Drugs

ALBUTEROL

Brand Names
U.S.A.: Proventil (Schering), Ventolin (Glaxo).
Canada: Novosalmol (Novopharm), Ventolin (Allen & Hanburys).
Great Britain: Aerolin (Riker), Asmaven (Approved Prescription Services), Cobutolin (Cox), Salbulin (Riker), Ventide (Allen & Hanburys), Ventodisks (Allen & Hanburys), Ventolin (Allen & Hanburys), Volmax (Duncan, Flockhart).

What This Drug Does
  Bronchodilator.

How This Drug Affects Body Weight
  Unknown. It relaxes smooth muscle in the lungs which allows freer breathing in those with asthma, bronchitis, or emphysema. It also exerts a stimulatory effect on the central nervous system, an effect seen in drugs used to lose weight, such as amphetamine and related substances.

Government-Approved Uses for This Drug
  To relieve bronchospasm in those with certain obstructive airway disease; to prevent exercise-induced bronchospasm.

Unofficial Uses
  None.

When Not to Use This Drug
In children under 2 years of age; in certain types of heart disease; if allergic to this drug or to any related drug.

Side Effects From Use of This Drug
Nervousness; tremor; headache; heart-rhythm irregularities; insomnia; nausea; vomiting; weakness; dizziness; drowsiness; flushing; difficulty urinating; high blood pressure.

Effects on Appetite and Body Weight as Disclosed by the Drug's Manufacturer
Anorexia; unusual or bad taste.

Detailed Effects on Appetite and Body Weight
Detailed manufacturer's disclosure: Although albuterol's official literature lists loss of appetite and taste changes as potential side effects, more detailed information from independent sources is unavailable.

Dosage Levels at Which Effects Occur
May occur within the usual daily dosage range of 6–16mg.

Remedies
Loss of appetite: The maintenance of adequate fluid intake and the avoidance of excessive alcohol use may aid in restoring normal appetite.
Taste change: Albuterol-induced taste disturbance may be countered in several ways. Taking the drug with an adequate fluid intake, chewing sugarless gum or using a mouthwash of water and lemon juice, and practicing good oral hygiene may help restore normal taste sensation.

How Long It Takes Till Reversal of Drug Effects
When taken as a tablet or syrup, albuterol's duration of action is 4–8 hours; when used as an inhalator, its actions last 3–4 hours.

Sources
Olin, B.R. (ed.). *Facts and Comparisons*. St. Louis: Facts and Comparisons, 1988.
Physicians' Desk Reference. Oradell, NJ: Medical Economics, 1988.
USP DI. Rockville, MD: The United States Pharmacopeial Convention, Inc., 1989.

THEOPHYLLINE

Brand Names
U.S.A.: Accubron (Merrell Dow), Bronkodyl (Winthrop-Breon), Constant-T (Geigy), Duraphyl (Forest), Elixicon (Berlex), Elixophyllin (Berlex), LaBID (Norwich Eaton), Quibron (Mead Johnson), Respbid (Boehringer Ingelheim), Slo-bid (Rorer), Slo-Phyllin (Rorer), Somophyllin (Fisons), Sustaire (Pfipharmecs), Theo-24 (Searle), Theobid (Glaxo), Theochron (Forest), Theo-Dur (Key), Theophyll (McNeil), Theolair (Riker), Theovent (Schering), Uniphyl (Perdue Frederick).
Canada: Elixophyllin (Berlex), PMS Theophylline (Pharmascience), Pulmophylline (Riva), Quibron-T/SR (Bristol), Respbid (Boehringer Ingelheim), Slo-Bid (Rorer), Somophyllin (Fisons), Theochron (Kingswood), Theo-Dur (Astra), Theolair (Riker), Theo-SR (Rhône-Poulenc), Uniphyl (Perdue Frederick).
Great Britain: Biophylline (Delandale), Labophylline (Laboratories for Applied Biology), Lasma (Pharmax), Nuelin (Riker), Pro-Vent (Calmic), Slo-Phyllin (Lipha), Theo-Dur (Astra), Uniphyllin (Napp).

What This Drug Does
Bronchodilator.

How This Drug Affects Body Weight
It relaxes smooth muscle in the lungs which allows freer breathing in those with asthma, bronchitis, or emphysema. It also has a stimulatory effect on the central nervous system, an effect seen in drugs used to lose weight, such as amphetamine and related substances.

Government-Approved Uses for This Drug
To relieve and/or prevent bronchospasm associated with asthma, bronchitis, and emphysema.

Unofficial Uses
None.

When Not to Use This Drug

In infants under 6 months; in children under 6 years (for the long-acting dosage form); if allergic to this drug or to any related drug.

Side Effects From Use of This Drug

Nausea; vomiting; diarrhea; irritability; dizziness; headache; insomnia; various mental disturbances; heart-rhythm irregularities; breathing difficulties; increased urination.

Effects on Appetite and Body Weight as Disclosed by the Drug's Manufacturer

Anorexia.

Detailed Effects on Appetite and Body Weight

Detailed manufacturer's disclosure: Although theophylline's official literature lists loss of appetite as a potential side effect, more detailed information from independent sources is unavailable.

Dosage Levels at Which Effects Occur

Due to the various dosage forms (long- and short-acting) of theophylline available, specific dosing information may be misleading. Laboratory blood analysis is necessary to keep theophylline serum concentrations at an ideal therapeutic level of 20mcg. per milliliter or lower.

Remedies

Loss of appetite: The maintenance of adequate fluid intake and the avoidance of excessive alcohol use may aid in restoring normal appetite.

How Long It Takes Till Reversal of Drug Effects

Half the dose of theophylline is eliminated from the body in 7–9 hours in nonsmoking adults; 4–5 hours in smokers (1–2 packs per day); 3–5 hours in children.

Sources

Olin, B.R. (ed.). *Facts and Comparisons*. St. Louis: Facts and Comparisons, 1988.

Physicians' Desk Reference. Oradell, NJ: Medical Economics, 1988.

USP DI. Rockville, MD: The United States Pharmacopeial Convention, Inc., 1989.

Antibiotics

AMPICILLIN

Brand Names
U.S.A.: Amcap (Circle), Amcill (Parke-Davis), D-Amp (Dunhall), Omnipen (Wyeth), Pfizerpen-A (Pfipharmecs), Polycillin (Bristol), Principen (Squibb), *Principen w/Probenecid (Squibb), *Polycillin-PRB (Bristol), Supen (Reid-Provident), Totacillin (Beecham).
Canada: Amcill (Parke-Davis), Ampicin (Bristol), Ampilean (Organon), Novo-Ampicillin (Novopharm), Penbritin (Ayerst).

Great Britain:
Amfipen (Brocades), Ampiclox (Beecham), *Magnapen (Beecham), Penbritin (Beecham), Pentrexyl (Bristol-Meyers), Vidopen (Berk).

What This Drug Does
Antibiotic.

How This Drug Works
Ampicillin, a drug of the penicillin family, may yield penicillamine during metabolic degradation by the liver. Penicillamine, itself a drug used to treat arthritis, is known to cause taste abnormalities.

*Combination drug.

Government-Approved Uses for This Drug
To treat various infections caused by a variety of microorganisms.

Unofficial Uses
None.

When Not to Use This Drug
If allergic to this drug, to any form of penicillin or cephalosporin, or to any other related drug.

Side Effects From Use of This Drug
Nausea; vomiting; stomach upset; gas; diarrhea; various skin rashes; white blood cell suppression; possible superinfection.

Effects on Appetite and Body Weight as Disclosed by the Drug's Manufacturer
Abnormal taste sensation.

Detailed Effects on Appetite and Body Weight
Altered taste: Although no studies have been carried out specifically to measure its incidence, long-term use of ampicillin has been observed to exert a deleterious effect on taste acuity.

Dosage Levels at Which Effects Occur
Altered taste: May occur within the usual daily dosage range of 1,000–4,000mg.

Remedies
Ampicillin-induced taste disturbance may be countered in several ways. Taking the drug with an adequate fluid intake, chewing sugarless gum or using a mouthwash of water and lemon juice, and practicing good oral hygiene may help restore normal taste sensation.

How Long It Takes Till Reversal of Drug Effects
Although half the dose of ampicillin is eliminated from the body in about 1 hour, its duration of action may persist for 3–6 hours in patients with normal kidney function.

Source
Jaffe, I.A. "Ampicillin rashes." *Lancet*, 1970, 1: 245.

CEFACLOR

Brand Names
U.S.A.: Ceclor (Lilly).
Canada: Ceclor (Lilly).
Great Britain: Distaclor (Dista).

What This Drug Does
Antibiotic.

How This Drug Affects Body Weight
Unknown. Probably causes stomach upset by altering the normal bacterial environment in the gastrointestinal tract.

Government-Approved Uses for This Drug
To treat various infections caused by a variety of microorganisms.

Unofficial Uses
To treat certain cases of urinary tract infection.

When Not to Use This Drug
If allergic to this drug or to any related drug.

Side Effects From Use of This Drug
Dizziness; headache; nausea; vomiting; diarrhea; various skin reactions; possible superinfection; various blood abnormalities.

Effects on Appetite and Body Weight as Disclosed by the Drug's Manufacturer
Anorexia.

Detailed Effects on Appetite and Body Weight
Detailed manufacturer's disclosure: Although cefaclor's official literature lists loss of appetite as a potential side effect, more detailed information from independent sources is unavailable.

In addition to eradicating its target bacteria, cefaclor may also kill desirable organisms residing in the digestive tract. These are essential for the maintenance of normal bowel function, and their depletion is thought to be responsible for appetite loss experienced when taking this drug.

Dosage Levels at Which Effects Occur
May occur within the usual dosage range of 250–500mg. taken every 8 hours.

Remedies
Loss of appetite: The maintenance of adequate fluid intake and the avoidance of excessive alcohol use may aid in restoring normal appetite.

The addition of yogurt to the diet or taking lactobacillus acidophilus supplements (as tablets, capsules, or granules) may restore a normal gastrointestinal environment.

How Long It Takes Till Reversal of Drug Effects
Half the dose of cefaclor is cleared from the blood in 36–54 minutes.

Sources
Olin, B.R. (ed.). *Facts and Comparisons*. St. Louis: Facts and Comparisons, 1988.
Physicians' Desk Reference. Oradell, NJ: Medical Economics, 1988.
USP DI. Rockville, MD: The United States Pharmacopeial Convention, Inc., 1989.

CEFADROXIL

Brand Names
U.S.A.: Duricef (Mead Johnson), Ultracef (Bristol).
Canada: Duricef (Bristol).
Great Britain: Baxan (Bristol-Meyers).

What This Drug Does
Antibiotic.

How This Drug Affects Body Weight
Unknown. Probably causes stomach upset by altering the normal bacterial environment in the gastrointestinal tract.

Government-Approved Uses for This Drug
To treat various infections caused by a variety of microorganisms.

Unofficial Uses
None.

When Not to Use This Drug
If allergic to this drug or to any related drug.

Side Effects From Use of This Drug
Dizziness; headache; nausea; vomiting; diarrhea; stomach up-set; various skin reactions; possible superinfection; various blood abnormalities.

Effects on Appetite and Body Weight as Disclosed by the Drug's Manufacturer
Anorexia.

Detailed Effects on Appetite and Body Weight
Detailed manufacturer's disclosure: Although cefadroxil's official literature lists loss of appetite as a potential side effect, more detailed information from independent sources is unavailable.

In addition to eradicating its target bacteria, cefadroxil may also kill desirable organisms residing in the digestive tract. These are essential for the maintenance of normal bowel function, and their depletion is thought to be responsible for appetite loss experienced when taking this drug.

Dosage Levels at Which Effects Occur
May occur within the usual dosage range of 500–2,000mg.

Remedies
Loss of appetite: The maintenance of adequate fluid intake and the avoidance of excessive alcohol use may aid in restoring normal appetite.

The addition of yogurt to the diet or taking lactobacillus acidophilus supplements (as tablets, capsules, or granules) may restore a normal gastrointestinal environment.

How Long it Takes Till Reversal of Drug Effects
Half the dose of cefadroxil is cleared from the blood in 72–90 minutes.

Sources
Olin, B.R. (ed.). *Facts and Comparisons*. St. Louis: Facts and Comparisons, 1988.

Physicians' Desk Reference. Oradell, NJ: Medical Economics, 1988.

USP DI. Rockville, MD: The United States Pharmacopeial Convention, Inc., 1989.

CEPHALEXIN

Brand Names
U.S.A.: Keflet (Dista), Keflex (Dista), Keftab (Dista).
Canada: Ceporex (Glaxo), Keflex (Lilly), Novolexin (Novo-pharm).
Great Britain: Ceporex (Glaxo), Keflex (Lilly).

What This Drug Does
Antibiotic.

How This Drug Affects Body Weight
Unknown. Probably causes stomach upset by altering the normal bacterial environment in the gastrointestinal tract.

Government-Approved Uses for This Drug
To treat various infections caused by a variety of microorganisms.

Unofficial Uses
None.

When Not to Use This Drug
If allergic to this drug or to any related drug.

Side Effects From Use of This Drug
Dizziness; headache; nausea; vomiting; diarrhea; stomach upset; various skin reactions; possible superinfection; various blood abnormalities.

Effects on Appetite and Body Weight as Disclosed by the Drug's Manufacturer
Anorexia.

Detailed Effects on Appetite and Body Weight
Detailed manufacturer's disclosure: Although cephalexin's official literature lists loss of appetite as a potential side effect, more detailed information from independent sources is unavailable.

In addition to eradicating its target bacteria, cephalexin may also kill desirable organisms residing in the digestive tract. These are essential for the maintenance of normal bowel function, and their depletion is thought to be responsible for appetite loss experienced when taking this drug.

Dosage Levels at Which Effects Occur
May occur within the usual dosage range of 250–1,000mg. taken every 6 hours.

Remedies
Loss of appetite: The maintenance of adequate fluid intake and the avoidance of excessive alcohol use may aid in restoring normal appetite.

The addition of yogurt to the diet or taking lactobacillus acidophilus supplements (as tablets, capsules, or granules) may restore a normal gastrointestinal environment.

How Long It Takes Till Reversal of Drug Effects
Half the dose of cephalexin is cleared from the blood in 36–54 minutes.

Sources
Olin, B.R. (ed.). *Facts and Comparisons*. St. Louis: Facts and Comparisons, 1988.
Physicians' Desk Reference. Oradell, NJ: Medical Economics, 1988.
USP DI. Rockville, MD: The United States Pharmacopeial Convention, Inc., 1989.

CHLORHEXIDINE GLUCONATE

Brand Names
U.S.A.: Peridex (Procter & Gamble).
Canada: Hibidil (Ayerst), Hibitane (Ayerst), Rouhex-G (Rougier).
Great Britain: Corsodyl (ICI), *Eludril Mouthwash (Concept Pharm.), Hibidil (ICI).

What This Drug Does
Mouthwash used to treat various gum diseases.

How This Drug Affects Body Weight
Acts as an antimicrobial agent to decrease the amounts of various bacteria in the mouth.

*Combination drug.

Government-Approved Uses for This Drug
To treat redness and swelling of the gums.

Unofficial Uses
None.

When Not to Use This Drug
If allergic to this drug or to any related drug.

Side Effects From Use of This Drug
Increased staining of the teeth and mouth; increased oral calculus (mineral deposit) formation; minor mouth irritation; superficial loss of top layer of skin in the mouth (mostly among children); inflammation of the salivary glands.

Effects on Appetite and Body Weight as Disclosed by the Drug's Manufacturer
Altered taste perception.

Detailed Effects on Appetite and Body Weight
Altered taste: In a case report describing a severe allergic reaction to chlorhexidine in a 28-year-old female, the authors document the drug's potential to cause altered taste. Its effect on taste sensation is characterized as a bitter aftertaste varying from several minutes' duration to several hours'. No long-term effects are manifest after discontinuation of chlorhexidine.

Dosage Levels at Which Effects Occur
Altered taste: May occur at the usual dosage of 15ml. twice daily (used as a mouthwash for 30 seconds).

Remedies
Altered taste: None.

How Long It Takes Till Reversal of Drug Effects
Altered taste: Discontinuation of chlorhexidine use should result in a return to normal taste sensation within a few minutes to several hours.

Source
Yaacob, H., Jalil, R. "An unusual hypersensitivity reaction to chlorhexidine." *Journal of Oral Medicine*, 1986, 41(3): 145–46.

CHLORTETRACYCLINE

Brand Names
U.S.A.: Aureomycin (Lederle) [topical ointment], Aureomycin Ophthalmic (Lederle) [ophthalmic ointment]. No oral form of chlortetracycline is marketed in the U.S.
Canada: *Aureocort (Lederle) [tropical ointment], Aureomycin (Lederle) [topical ointment]. No oral form of chlortetracycline is marketed in Canada.
Great Britain: Aureomycin (Lederle).

What This Drug Does
Antibiotic.

How This Drug Affects Body Weight
Chlortetracycline binds to bacteria and other susceptible microorganisms, preventing their reproduction. This drug, as well as other antibiotics, alters the bacterial flora of the gastrointestinal tract. Gut bacteria influence the synthesis or utilization of vitamins and other essential nutrients. This may influence diet goals by increasing or decreasing the supply of nutrients available from food.

Government-Approved Uses for This Drug
As an antibacterial for topical and ophthalmic use.
Note: In Great Britain, chlortetracycline is also marketed as an oral antibiotic to treat infections due to a broad range of microorganisms.

Unofficial Uses
None.

When Not to Use This Drug
During pregnancy; if a nursing mother; if allergic to this drug or to any related drug.

Side Effects From Use of This Drug
When taken orally, chlortetracycline may cause nausea; vomiting; diarrhea; irritation of the tongue; black tongue (a fungal

*Combination drug.

infection); superinfection due to yeast overgrowth affecting the mouth, intestinal tract, rectum, and vagina; various skin reactions including sensitivity to sunlight; kidney dysfunction; various allergic responses; various blood abnormalities; tooth discoloration or malformation in children under 9 years of age (including infants and unborn); inflammatory lesions (with monilial overgrowth) in the anogenital region.

Effects on Appetite and Body Weight as Disclosed by the Drug's Manufacturer

Loss of appetite.

Detailed Effects on Appetite and Body Weight

Because the two drugs mentioned below (chlortetracycline and oxytetracycline) are so closely related to their better-known prototype, tetracycline, effects on body weight may also apply to tetracycline.

Weight loss: In a series of case reports describing the effects of antibiotics on undernourished men, chlortetracycline caused weight loss.

Weight gain: In a group of 19 patients suffering from liver disease and given chlortetracycline and oxytetracycline (another close analog of tetracycline), 11 (58%) reported weight gains ranging from 3–20 pounds in 1–2 months. Because there was increased fat deposition in the liver, it has been speculated that this was paralleled by increased fat deposits in other tissue.

Dosage Levels at Which Effects Occur

Weight loss: Reported as low as 2,500mg. daily (chlortetracycline).

Weight gain: Reported as low as 2,000mg. daily (chlortetracycline).

Remedies

Weight loss: A decrease in daily dosage could help alleviate chlortetracycline's effects on body weight. But this must be carefully balanced against maintaining adequate therapeutic blood levels.

A switch to a different agent in the same therapeutic category could accomplish similar benefits while minimizing undesirable dietary influences. Consult your physician.

Weight gain: Substitution of low-calorie foods, beverages, and snacks for normal dietary intake may aid in reversing some chlortetracycline-induced weight gain.

How Long It Takes Till Reversal of Drug Effects
Weight loss: Half the dose of chlortetracycline is cleared from the blood in 2.3–5.6 hours.
Weight gain: In the study cited above, most of those who reported weight gain while on chlortetracycline continued to gain for a few weeks after withdrawal of the medication. After this time, most gradually returned to their predrug body weight, although a few maintained the increased weight indefinitely.

Sources
Gabuzda, G.J., et al. "Some effects of antibiotics on nutrition in man." *Archives of Internal Medicine*, 1958, 101: 476–513.
Sborov, V.M., Sutherland, D.A. "Fatty liver following aureomycin and terramycin therapy in chronic hepatic disease." *Gastroenterology*, 1951, 18: 598–605.

ERYTHROMYCIN

Brand Names
U.S.A.: E.E.S. (Abbott), E-Mycin (Boots), Eryc (Parke-Davis), Erypar (Parke-Davis), Ery-Tab (Abbott), Erythrocin Stearate (Abbott), Ethril (Squibb), Ilotycin (Dista), Ilosone (Dista), P.C.E. (Abbott), Pediamycin (Ross), Pfizer-E (Pfizer), Wyamycin S (Wyeth).
Canada: Apo-Erythro (Apotex), E-Mycin (Upjohn), ERYC (Parke-Davis), Erythromid (Abbott), Ilotycin (Lilly).
Great Britain: Erycen (Berk), Erymax (Parke-Davis), Erythromid (Abbott), Retcin (DDSA).

What This Drug Does
Antibiotic.

How This Drug Affects Body Weight
Unknown. Probably causes stomach upset by altering the normal bacterial environment in the gastrointestinal tract.

Government-Approved Uses for This Drug
To treat various infections caused by a variety of microorganisms.

Unofficial Uses
To treat certain infectious diarrheas; to treat certain venereal disease; to treat chancroid; prior to certain colorectal surgery to facilitate normal healing.

When Not to Use This Drug
In presence of liver disease (estolate and ethylsuccinate forms of erythromycin only); if allergic to this drug or to any related drug.

Side Effects From Use of This Drug
Stomach upset; cramping; nausea; vomiting; diarrhea; various skin reactions; possible superinfection.

Effects on Appetite and Body Weight as Disclosed by the Drug's Manufacturer
Anorexia.

Detailed Effects on Appetite and Body Weight
Detailed manufacturer's disclosure: Although erythromycin's official literature lists loss of appetite as a potential side effect, more detailed information from independent sources is unavailable.

In addition to eradicating its target bacteria, erythromycin may also kill desirable organisms residing in the digestive tract. These are essential for the maintenance of normal bowel function, and their depletion is thought to be responsible for appetite loss experienced when taking this drug.

Dosage Levels at Which Effects Occur
May occur within the usual dose range of 250–500mg. taken every 6 hours.

Remedies
Loss of appetite: The maintenance of adequate fluid intake and the avoidance of excessive alcohol use may aid in restoring normal appetite.

The addition of yogurt to the diet or taking lactobacillus acidophilus supplements (as tablets, capsules, or granules) may restore a normal gastrointestinal environment.

How Long it Takes Till Reversal of Drug Effects
Half the dose of erythromycin is cleared from the blood in about 1.4 hours.

Sources

Olin, B.R. (ed.). *Facts and Comparisons*. St. Louis: Facts and Comparisons, 1988.
Physicians' Desk Reference. Oradell, NJ: Medical Economics, 1988.
USP DI. Rockville, MD: The United States Pharmacopeial Convention, Inc., 1989.

GRISEOFULVIN

Brand Names
U.S.A.: Fulvicin P/G (Schering), Fulvicin-U/F (Schering), Grifulvin V (Ortho), Grisactin (Ayerst), Grisactin Ultra (Ayerst), Gris-PEG (Herbert).
Canada: Fulvicin P/G (Schering), Fulvicin U/F (Schering), Grisovin-FP (Glaxo).
Great Britain: Fulcin (ICI), Grisovin (Glaxo).

What This Drug Does
Antifungal.

How This Drug Affects Body Weight
It has been speculated that free electrons in the griseofulvin molecule might form chemical bonds with a protein component of the taste-bud membrane. This may alter the membrane's conformation and function.

Government-Approved Uses for This Drug
To treat fungus infections.

Unofficial Uses
None.

When Not to Use This Drug
If there are disturbances in porphyrin (biological pigments) metabolism; in certain liver problems; if pregnant; if allergic to this drug or to any related drug.

Side Effects From Use of This Drug
Various skin reactions; oral thrush (a yeast infection of the mouth); stomach upset; nausea; vomiting; diarrhea; headache; dizziness; fatigue; mental confusion; sensitivity to sunlight; burning sensations of the hands and feet.

Effects on Appetite and Body Weight as Disclosed by the Drug's Manufacturer
None.

Detailed Effects on Appetite and Body Weight
Altered taste: A 31-year-old male taking griseofulvin for 25 days experienced no untoward effects. One week after the drug was discontinued it was restarted. Three weeks later taste disturbance was noted, with the patient complaining of a "monotonous, singular taste" as well as "tastlessness to all foods and flavors." No peculiar taste was noticed when not eating. After griseofulvin was withdrawn, taste sensation gradually returned to normal.

Dosage Levels at Which Effects Occur
Altered taste: Reported to occur at 375–750mg. daily in divided doses.

Remedies
Altered taste: Griseofulvin-induced taste disturbance may be countered in several ways. Taking the drug with an adequate fluid intake, chewing sugarless gum or using a mouthwash of water and lemon juice, and practicing good oral hygiene may help restore normal taste sensation.

How Long It Takes Till Reversal of Drug Effects
Altered taste: In the case cited above, normal taste returned 1 week after discontinuation of griseofulvin.

Source
Fogan, L., Henkin, R.I, "Griseofulvin and dysgeusia: Implications?" *Annals of Internal Medicine*, 1971, 74: 795–96.

METRONIDAZOLE

Brand Names
U.S.A.: Flagyl (Searle), Metric 21 (Fielding), Metryl (Lemmon), Protostat (Ortho), Satric (Savage).
Canada: Flagyl (Rhône-Poulenc), Neo-Tric (Neolab), Novonidazol (Novopharm).
Great Britain: Flagyl (May & Baker), Flagyl-S (May & Baker), Vaginyl (DDSA).

What This Drug Does
Antibiotic.

How This Drug Affects Body Weight
Unknown. Kills susceptible anaerobic (able to live without air) bacteria and protozoa in the intestines and in other parts of the body.

Government-Approved Uses for This Drug
To treat various bacterial, amoebic, and protozoan infections.

Unofficial Uses
To prevent infections during gynecologic, abdominal, and colonic surgery; to treat hepatic encephalopathy (brain disease due to liver dysfunction); to render resistant tumors more susceptible to radiation therapy; to treat Gardnerella vaginalis (a bacterial vaginal infection).

When Not to Use This Drug
During the first 3 months of pregnancy; if taking alcohol at the same time; if breast-feeding; if allergic to this drug or to any related drug.

Side Effects From Use of This Drug
Nausea; headache; vomiting; constipation or diarrhea (more common); stomach upset; abdominal cramps; convulsive seizures; numbness or burning sensations of an extremity; irritation of the mouth and tongue; low white blood cell count; dizziness; loss of coordination; mental depression; insomnia; irritability; weakness; various skin reactions; flushing; nasal congestion; dry mouth; fever; kidney dysfunction; dryness of the vagina or vulva; vaginal candidiasis; dyspareunia (painful intercourse in females); decrease in libido; proctitis (anal irritation).

Effects on Appetite and Body Weight as Disclosed by the Drug's Manufacturer
Loss of appetite; sharp, unpleasant metallic taste; change in taste of alcoholic beverages.

Detailed Effects on Appetite and Body Weight
Altered taste: A long-term study of 21 sufferers of Crohn's disease (an intestinal ailment) who were treated with metronidazole showed 12 (57%) reporting a metallic taste.

In a follow-up investigation of 26 patients given long-term (more than 3 months) metronidazole for Crohn's disease, 24 (92%) complained of a metallic taste.

In a 24-week study of 20 patients treated with metronidazole and placebo (12 weeks of each), 6 complained of unpleasant taste when taking the active medication.

Loss of appetite: In the same study of 21 patients with Crohn's disease as described above, 3 (14%) complained of appetite loss.

In a 24-week study of 20 patients who received 12 weeks of metronidazole and 12 weeks of placebo, 6 reported appetite loss when taking the active drug.

Eight out of 15 patients treated with metronidazole for 7 days complained of a loss of appetite.

Dosage Levels at Which Effects Occur

Altered taste: Reported as low as 20mg. per kilogram of body weight daily. [In a 150-pound adult, this would translate to 1,364 mg. daily; at 100 pounds, the daily dose would be 909mg.]

Loss of appetite: Reported as low as 600mg. daily.

Remedies

Altered taste: Metronidazole-induced taste disturbance may be countered in several ways. Taking the drug with an adequate fluid intake, chewing sugarless gum or using a mouthwash of water and lemon juice, and practicing good oral hygiene may help restore normal taste sensation.

Loss of appetite: The maintenance of adequate fluid intake and the avoidance of excessive alcohol use may aid in reversing appetite loss.

How Long It Takes Till Reversal of Drug Effects

Half the dose of metronidazole is eliminated from the body within 6.2–11.5 hours.

Sources

Bernstein, L.H., et al. "Healing of Perineal Crohn's Disease with metronidazole." *Gastroenterology*, 1980, 79: 357–65.

Brandt, L.J., et al. "Metronidazole therapy for Perineal Crohn's Disease: A follow-up study." *Gastroenterology*, 1982, 83: 383–87.

Jones, D.I. "The effect of metronidazole on exophthalmos in man." *Journal of Endocrinology*, 1968, 41(4): 609–10.

Khambatta, R.B. "Metronidazole in giardiasis." *Annals of Tropical Medicine and Parasitology*, 1971, 65(4): 487–89.

OXYTETRACYCLINE

Brand Names
U.S.A.: E.P. Mycin (Edwards), Oxymycin (Forest), Terramycin (Pfizer), Uri-Tet (American Urologicals).
Canada: None.
Great Britain Abbocin (Abbott), Berkmycen (Berk), Chemocycline (Consolidated Chemicals), Galenomycin (Galen), Imperacin (ICI), Oxymed (Unimed), Oxymycin (DDSA), *Terra-Bron (Pfizer), Terramycin (Pfizer), Unimycin (Unigreg) (Vestric).

What This Drug Does
Antibiotic.

How This Drug Affects Body Weight
Oxytetracycline binds to bacteria and other susceptible microorganisms, preventing their reproduction. This drug, as well as other antibiotics, alters the bacterial flora of the gastrointestinal tract. Gut bacteria influence the synthesis or utilization of vitamins and other essential nutrients. This may influence diet goals by increasing or decreasing the supply of nutrients available from food.

Government-Approved Uses for This Drug
As an antibiotic to treat infections due to a broad range of microorganisms.

Unofficial Uses
None.

When Not to Use This Drug
During pregnancy; if a nursing mother; if allergic to this drug or to any related drug.

Side Effects From Use of This Drug
Nausea; vomiting; diarrhea; irritation of the tongue; black tongue (a fungal infection); superinfection due to yeast overgrowth affecting the mouth, intestinal tract, rectum, and va-

*Combination drug.

gina; various skin reactions including sensitivity to sunlight; kidney dysfunction; various allergic responses; various blood abnormalities; tooth discoloration or malformation in children under 9 years of age (including infants and unborn); inflammatory lesions (with monilial overgrowth) in the anogenital region.

Effects on Appetite and Body Weight as Disclosed by the Drug's Manufacturer
Loss of appetite.

Detailed Effects on Appetite and Body Weight
Weight loss: In a series of case reports describing the effects of antibiotics on undernourished men, oxytetracycline caused weight loss.

Weight gain: In a group of 19 patients suffering from liver disease and given oxytetracycline and chlortetracycline (another close analog of tetracycline), 11 (58%) reported weight gains ranging from 3–20 pounds in 1–2 months. Because there was increased fat deposition in the liver, it has been speculated that this was paralleled by increased fat deposits in other tissue.

Note: Because the two drugs mentioned above (chlortetracycline and oxytetracycline) are so closely related to their better-known prototype, tetracycline, effects on body weight may also apply to tetracycline.

Dosage Levels at Which Effects Occur
Weight loss: Reported as low as 2,500mg. daily (oxytetracycline).
Weight gain: Reported as low as 2,000mg. daily (chlortetracycline).

Remedies
Weight loss: A decrease in daily dosage could help alleviate oxytetracycline's effects on body weight. But this must be carefully balanced against maintaining adequate therapeutic blood levels.

A switch to a different agent in the same therapeutic category could accomplish similar benefits while minimizing undesirable dietary influences. Consult your physician.
Weight gain: Substitution of low-calorie foods, beverages, and

snacks for normal dietary intake may aid in reversing some oxytetracycline-induced weight gain.

How Long It Takes Till Reversal of Drug Effects

Weight loss: Half the dose of oxytetracycline is cleared from the blood in 6–10 hours.

Weight gain: In the study cited above, most of those who reported weight gain while on oxytetracycline continued to gain for a few weeks after withdrawal of the medication. After this time, most gradually returned to their predrug body weight, although a few maintained the increased weight indefinitely.

Sources

Gabuzda, G.J., et al. "Some effects of antibiotics on nutrition in man." *Archives of Internal Medicine* 1958, 101: 476–513.

Sborov, V.M., Sutherland, D.A. "Fatty liver following aureomycin and terramycin therapy in chronic hepatic disease." *Gastroenterology* 1951, 18: 598–605.

TETRACYCLINE

Brand Names

U.S.A.: Achromycin V (Lederle), Biocycline (National/Barre), Bristacycline (Bristol), Cycline-250 (Scrip), Cyclinex (Holloway), Cyclopar (Parke-Davis), Deltamycin (Trimen), *Mysteclin-F (Squibb), Nor-Tet (Vortech), Panmycin (Upjohn), Retet (Reid-Rowell), Robitet (Robins), Sumycin (Squibb), Tetra-C (Century), Tetracap (Circle), Tetrachel (Rachelle), Tetracyn (Pfizer), Tetracyn IM (Roerig), Tetralan (Lannett), Tetram (Dunhall), Tetramed (Zenith), *Tetrastatin (Pfipharmecs), Tetrex (Bristol).

Canada: Achromycin (Lederle), Cefracycline (Frosst), Medicycline (Medic), Neo-Tetrine (Neolab), Novotetra (Novopharm), Tetracyn (Pfizer), Tetralean (Organon), Tetrex (Bristol).

Great Britain Achromycin (Lederle), Achromycin V (Lederle), *Chymocyclar (Armour), Co-Caps Tetracycline (Co-Caps), *Detelco (Lederle), Economycin (DDSA), *Mysteclin (Squibb), Sustamycin (MCP), *Tetrabid-Organon (Organon), Tetrachel (Berk), Tetracyn (Pfizer).

*Combination drug.

What This Drug Does
Antibiotic.

How This Drug Affects Body Weight
Tetracycline binds to bacteria and other susceptible microorganisms, preventing their reproduction. This drug, as well as other antibiotics, alters the bacterial flora of the gastrointestinal tract. Gut bacteria influence the synthesis or utilization of vitamins and other essential nutrients. This may influence diet goals by increasing or decreasing the supply of nutrients available from food.

Government-Approved Uses for This Drug
As an antibiotic to treat infections due to a broad range of microorganisms.

Unofficial Uses
As a sclerosing agent (swells and hardens tissue) to treat malignant pleural effusion.

When Not to Use This Drug
During pregnancy; if a nursing mother; if allergic to this drug or to any related drug.

Side Effects From Use of This Drug
Nausea; vomiting; diarrhea; irritation of the tongue; black tongue (a fungal infection); superinfection due to yeast overgrowth affecting the mouth, intestinal tract, rectum, and vagina; various skin reactions including sensitivity to sunlight; kidney dysfunction; various allergic responses; various blood abnormalities; tooth discoloration or malformation in children under 9 years of age (including infants and unborn); inflammatory lesions (with monilial overgrowth) in the anogenital region.

Effects on Appetite and Body Weight as Disclosed by the Drug's Manufacturer
Loss of appetite:

Detailed Effects on Appetite and Body Weight
Weight loss: In a series of case reports describing the effects of antibiotics on undernourished men, chlortetracycline (a close analog of tetracycline) caused weight loss.
Weight gain: In a group of 19 patients suffering from liver dis-

ease and given chlortetracycline and oxytetracycline (close analogs of tetracycline), 11 (58%) reported weight gains ranging from 3–20 pounds in 1–2 months. Because there was increased fat deposition in the liver, it has been speculated that this was paralleled by increased fat deposits in other tissue.

Note: Because the two drugs mentioned above (chlortetracycline and oxytetracycline) are so closely related to their better-known prototype, tetracycline, effects on body weight may also apply to tetracycline.

Dosage Levels at Which Effects Occur
Weight loss: Reported as low as 2,500mg. daily (chlortetracycline).
Weight gain: Reported as low as 2,000mg. daily (chlortetracycline).

Remedies
Weight loss: A decrease in daily dosage could help alleviate tetracycline's effects on body weight. But this must be carefully balanced against maintaining adequate therapeutic blood levels.

A switch to a different agent in the same therapeutic category could accomplish similar benefits while minimizing undesirable dietary influences. Consult your physician.
Weight gain: Substitution of low-calorie foods, beverages, and snacks for normal dietary intake may aid in reversing some tetracycline-induced weight gain.

How Long It Takes Till Reversal of Drug Effects
Weight loss: Half the dose of tetracycline is cleared from the blood in 6–10 hours.
Weight gain: In the study cited above, most of those who reported weight gain while on tetracycline continued to gain for a few weeks after withdrawal of the medication. After this time, most gradually returned to their predrug body weight, although a few maintained the increased weight indefinitely.

Sources
Gabuzda, G.J., et al. "Some effects of antibiotics on nutrition in man." *Archives of Internal Medicine*, 1958, 101: 476–513.
Sborov, V.M., Sutherland, D.A. "Fatty liver following aureomycin and terramycin therapy in chronic hepatic disease." *Gastroenterology*, 1951, 18: 598–605.

Anticancer Drugs

INTERFERON

Brand Names
U.S.A.: Intron A (Schering), Roferon-A (Roche).
Canada: None.
Great Britain: Marketed as "interferon" by Searle and Wellcome.

What This Drug Does
   Anticancer drug.

How This Drug Affects Body Weight
   Unknown. Interferon stops tumor cells from multiplying and has an effect on the body's immune response.

Government-Approved Uses for This Drug
   To treat hairy cell leukemia; to treat AIDS-related Kaposi's Sarcoma.

Unofficial Uses
   Alpha interferons are being investigated for use in treating many neoplastic diseases and viral infections.

When Not to Use This Drug
   If allergic to this drug or to any related drug.

Side Effects From Use of This Drug
   Flu-like symptoms (fever, fatigue, muscle pain, headache, and chills); dizziness; mental confusion; numbness and tingling;

depression; visual disturbance; sleeping difficulties; poor coordination; hallucinations; seizures; various mental aberrations; loss of libido; impotence (temporary); low (4–6%) or high (less than 3%) blood pressure; chest pain; various heart abnormalities; fainting; various skin reactions; sweating; breathing difficulties.

Effects on Appetite and Body Weight as Disclosed by the Drug's Manufacturer
Loss of appetite; water retention; weight loss; taste changes.

Detailed Effects on Appetite and Body Weight
Loss of appetite: In a study of 10 females given interferon for up to 12 weeks to treat breast cancer, loss of appetite was noted after 1 week. Four of the 10 refused food altogether for periods as long as 7 days, showing weight loss of more than 10% of their pretrial body weight.

Dosage Levels at Which Effects Occur
Loss of appetite: For Roferon-A, may occur within the usual dosage range of 3 million I.U. 3 times weekly to 36 million I.U. daily.

Remedies
For Intron A, may occur within the usual dosage range of 2–30 million I.U. per square meter of body area 3 times weekly.
Loss of appetite: The maintenance of adequate fluid intake and the avoidance of excessive alcohol use may aid in reversing appetite loss.

How Long It Takes Till Reversal of Drug Effects
Loss of appetite: In the study cited above, all patients reported normal appetite 7–10 days after discontinuation of interferon.

Source
Smedley, H., et al. "Neurological effects of recombinant human interferon." *British Medical Journal*, 1983, 286: 262–64.

MEGESTROL

Brand Names
U.S.A.: Megace (Mead Johnson), Pallace (Bristol).
Canada: Megace (Bristol).

Great Britain: Volidan (Duncan, Flockhart; was produced under this brand name but has since been withdrawn from the market). Marketed as "megastrol" by various manufacturers.

What This Drug Does
Anticancer drug.

How This Drug Affects Body Weight
Weight gain in those taking megestrol may be due to the drug's anabolic (tissue-building) effects. Weakness and fatigue, often associated with the underlying cancer being treated, may cause decreased physical activity and subsequent increases in body weight.

Government-Approved Uses for This Drug
To treat cancer of the breast or uterus.

Unofficial Uses
None.

When Not to Use This Drug
As a diagnostic test for pregnancy; during the first 4 months of pregnancy; if allergic to this drug or to any related drug.

Side Effects From Use of This Drug
Carpal-tunnel syndrome (a painful defect of the wrist and hand caused by pressure on the middle nerve in the carpal tunnel); hair loss; thrombophlebitis (vein swelling, often accompanied by a blood clot).

Effects on Appetite and Body Weight as Disclosed by the Drug's Manufacturer
None.

Detailed Effects on Appetite and Body Weight
Increased appetite; weight gain: In a study of 33 patients suffering from various cancers, loss of appetite associated with the disease was treated with megestrol; 27% of patients gained more than 5 pounds.

In an investigation of the effects of high-dose megestrol use, 27 of 28 patients with advanced breast cancer who were treated with the drug gained from 2–44.2 pounds over a median time of 18 weeks.

Of 160 postmenopausal women treated with megestrol for breast cancer, 10% reported a weight gain of more than 5% of their total body weight after 6 weeks. This gain did not appear to be related to any water retention.

In a group of 48 women with breast cancer treated with megestrol for 4–6 weeks, 70% experienced a median weight gain of 4.4 pounds.

A study of 124 females with breast cancer and treated with megestrol showed 14.5% exhibiting weight gains of 10% or more over their initial body weight.

Dosage Levels at Which Effects Occur
Increased appetite; weight gain: Reported as low as 60mg. daily.

Remedies
Increased appetite; weight gain: Substitution of low-calorie foods, beverages, and snacks for normal dietary intake may aid in reversing some drug-induced weight gain. The author of one study cited above suggests a diet of 1,200 calories per day.

How Long It Takes Till Reversal of Drug Effects
Increased appetite; weight gain: Varies with disease and patient response.

Sources
Alexleva-Figusch, J., et al. "Progestin therapy in advanced breast cancer: Megestrol acetate—an evaluation of 160 treated cases." *Cancer*, 1980, 46: 2369–72.

Gregory, E.J., et al. "Megestrol acetate therapy for advanced breast cancer." *Journal of Clinical Oncology*, 1985, 3: 155–60.

Ross, M.B., et al. "Treatment of advanced breast cancer with megestrol acetate after therapy with tamoxifen." *Cancer*, 1982, 49: 415–17.

Tchekmedyian, N.S., et al. "Appetite stimulation with megestrol acetate in cachectic cancer patients." *Seminars in Oncology*, 1986, 13 (suppl. 4): 37–43.

METHOTREXATE

Brand Names
U.S.A.: Folex (Adria), Mexate (Bristol), Rheumatrex Dose Pack (Lederle).
Canada: Amethopterin (Horner; Lederle).
Great Britain: Emtexate (Nordic).

What This Drug Does
Anticancer drug.

How This Drug Affects Body Weight
Damages the lining of the intestinal tract, causing impaired absorption of food from the small intestine.

Government-Approved Uses for This Drug
To treat various cancers; to treat severe psoriasis; to treat certain rheumatoid arthritis.

Unofficial Uses
None.

When Not to Use This Drug
In severe liver or kidney disorders; with various blood abnormalities; if pregnant; if breast-feeding; if allergic to this drug or to any related drug.

Side Effects From Use of This Drug
Mouth ulceration; inflammation of the gums; various blood abnormalities; nausea; vomiting; diarrhea; abdominal upset; fatigue; drowsiness; fever and chills; dizziness; lowered resistance to infection; various skin reactions including rash, itching, increased sensitivity to sunlight; hair loss; various liver problems; abnormal kidney function; lowered sperm count; irregular menstruation; infertility; various lung problems; headache; blurred vision.

Effects on Appetite and Body Weight as Disclosed by the Drug's Manufacturer
Loss of appetite.

Detailed Effects on Appetite and Body Weight
Food malabsorption: In a test of 18 children being treated for acute lymphoblastic leukemia, use of methotrexate was shown to cause interference with intestinal absorption of nutrients. This could cause potential problems in utilizing food and other drugs taken by mouth. Timing of methotrexate doses seemed to affect how severely the subjects reacted.

Dosage Levels at Which Effects Occur
Food malabsorption: Reported to occur up to a cumulative dose of 300mg. per square meter of body area.

Remedies

Food malabsorption: Those children tested 7 days after the last methotrexate dose showed more severe malabsorption than a group tested after 14 days. Intervals of more than 7 days between methotrexate doses may be required for normal food absorption.

How Long It Takes Till Reversal of Drug Effects

Food malabsorption: It may take up to 12 hours for half the dose of methotrexate to be cleared from the blood.

Source

Craft, A.W., et al. "Methotrexate-induced malabsorption in children with acute lymphoblastic leukemia." *British Medical Journal*, 1977, 2: 1511–12.

Antidepressants

AMITRIPTYLINE

Brand Names
U.S.A.: Amitid (Squibb), Amitril (Parke-Davis), Elavil (MSD), Emitrip (Major), Endep (Roche), Enovil (Hauck), *Etrafon (Schering), *Limbitrol (Roche), *Triavil (MSD).
Canada: Apo-Amitriptyline (Apotex), Elavil (MSD), *Elavil Plus (MSD), *Etrafon (Schering), Levate (ICN), Meravil (Medic), Novotriptyn (Novopharm), *Triavil (MSD).

Great Britain
Domical (Berk), Elavil (DDSA), Lentizol (Warner), *Limbitrol (Roche), Saroten (Warner), *Triptafen-DA (Allen & Hanburys), *Triptafen-Forte (Allen & Hanburys), *Triptafen-Minor (Allen & Hanburys), Triptizol (Morson).

What This Drug Does
Antidepressant.

How This Drug Affects Body Weight
Amitriptyline may cause increased body-weight set point (an equilibrium between appetite and body weight), producing increased appetite and decreased satiety until a new increased body weight is reached.

Government-Approved Uses for This Drug
To relieve depression.

*Combination drug.

Unofficial uses: To control chronic pain; to prevent onset of cluster and migraine headaches; to treat hiccups.

When Not to Use This Drug

During recovery from certain heart conditions; if taking or have taken within the last 14 days any monoamine oxidase inhibitor drug; in children under 12 years; if allergic to this drug or to any related drug.

Side Effects From Use of This Drug

Fast heartbeat; other heart rhythm irregularities; disorientation; anxiety; insomnia; dry mouth; blurred vision; skin rash; sedation; nausea; stomach upset; vomiting; dizziness; headache; diarrhea or constipation (more common); testicular swelling; gynecomastia (enlargement of the male breasts); galactorrhea (breast-milk flow unrelated to childbirth or nursing) in the female; increased or decreased libido (reported with equal frequency).

Effects on Appetite and Body Weight as Disclosed by the Drug's Manufacturer

Anorexia; increase or decrease in weight; water retention; peculiar taste.

Detailed Effects on Appetite and Body Weight

Weight gain: Three females in their forties, all suffering from depression, were treated with amitriptyline. All responded to the drug but gained 2.7–9 pounds above their normal body weight. Dieting did not seem to help.

In a series of large-scale tests, amitriptyline was evaluated over a period of at least 21 days. Short-term studies showed on average a 3-pound weight increase, while longer studies revealed almost 9-pound gains.

Fifty-one female depressives aged 26 to 60 were given amitriptyline for 3 months. During this time, most gained an average of 8.8 pounds and those remaining on the drug continued to gain weight steadily, averaging an additional 5 pounds in 3 months. This study showed that continuing treatment with amitriptyline after recovery from depressive illness may result in significant unwanted weight gain. In addition, the drug also caused a dose-related craving for carbohydrate foods within 1–2 months of its use.

One physician reported that almost all 30 female patients given amitriptyline developed a large and often voracious appetite, preferring foods rich in carbohydrates. This was accompanied by weight gain, in some cases totaling almost 28 pounds in 4–5 weeks. Most of the increased weight was added as fat deposits in the abdomen and around the waist, hips, and thighs. Breasts often became enlarged and tender.

In a study of 25 patients taking amitriptyline (13 females and 12 males), for more than 6 months on average, steady weight gain was noted on the order of 2.9 pounds average per month, with 72% of subjects gaining 5 pounds or more in total; 44% of the patients discontinued treatment with the drug due to this phenomenon. Among those receiving higher doses of amitriptyline (75–150mg. daily), weight gain was found to average almost 4 pounds per month. A large percentage of patients had cravings for sweets, with about one-third reporting overeating.

Treatment of anorexia nervosa and bulimia: Because many victims of anorexia nervosa (a mental problem causing long-term refusal to eat) display signs of depression, antidepressant medications, such as amitriptyline, are used in its treatment.

One case report describes a 20-year-old female who had dropped in body weight from about 102 pounds to 62 pounds. After hospitalization and behavior-modification therapy, she gained 23 pounds in 2 months. When discharged and left on her own, she dropped to 79 pounds within 2 months. At this point, she was started on amitriptyline and within 8 days her appetite increased and she gained 2.2 pounds. As an outpatient, she was maintained on the drug and gained 2.2 pounds per week over the next 7 weeks. At 108 pounds, she claimed to feel hungry all the time despite consumption of large amounts of high-calorie foods. At 115.5 pounds, amitriptyline was stopped but weight gain continued. The patient stabilized at 131 pounds. To sum up, this patient went from 60% of her ideal body weight while suffering from anorexia nervosa to more than 25% over her ideal weight with use of amitriptyline.

In another study of 6 patients (5 females aged 11–17 and 1 male aged 17 years), all showed weight loss greater than 20%. All were started on amitriptyline with weight gains starting between the sixth and twelfth day of treatment. All subjects gained between 6 and 37 pounds over periods from 32 to 200 days.

A case report describes a 20-year-old female college senior with a habit of going rapidly from store to store in an eating binge of doughnuts, pizza, ice cream, chocolate, and fruit until uncomfortably full. She would then find a quiet, secluded place to vomit. This sometimes occurred daily. Her weight had gone from 140 pounds in her sophomore year to 105 pounds as a senior. After several drug treatments tried by her physician proved ineffective, amitriptyline was started. After the first week, she reported vomiting only twice. During the second week, with an increased drug dose, she reported no desire to vomit, although concerns about weight gain made her anxious. After 4 months of amitriptyline use, she had gained a total of 11 pounds and was of normal weight. When amitriptyline was finally discontinued after a tapering of the dose, bulimia symptoms returned the next day. Reintroduction of amitriptyline halted these symptoms within 2 days.

An 8-week study of 32 female bulimics given amitriptyline showed considerable improvement in eating behavior. A 72.1% decrease in the number of binge-eating episodes per week and a 78.6% decrease in the incidence of weekly vomiting were the most significant results of the study.

Dosage Levels at Which Effects Occur
Weight gain: Reported as low as 4mg. daily with the average dose at about 56–75mg. daily.
Treatment of anorexia nervosa and bulimia: 75–150mg. daily.

Remedies
Weight gain: A decrease in daily dosage may help alleviate amitriptyline's adverse dietary influences. But this must be balanced against maintaining adequate therapeutic blood levels.

Substitution of low-calorie foods, beverages, and snacks for normal dietary intake may aid in reversing some drug-induced weight gain.

Switching to mianserin, another antidepressant drug available in Great Britain, has led to weight loss to pretreatment levels in 6–12 weeks.

Bupropion has been used in place of amitriptyline with minimal weight changes (a 1- to 2-pound weight loss) as noted in a 1-month study. Some patients lost as much as 5 pounds.

How Long It Takes Till Reversal of Drug Effects
Weight gain: In one study, an average 6-pound weight loss was reported 5 months after withdrawal of amitriptyline.

Half this drug's dose is cleared from the blood within 17–40 hours.

Sources
Arenillas, L. "Amitriptyline and body weight." *Lancet*, 1964, 1: 432–33.

Berken, G.H., et al. "Weight gain. A side effect of tricyclic antidepressants." *Journal of Affective Disorders*, 1984, 7(2): 133–38.

Brown, J.D. "Drugs causing weight gain." *British Medical Journal*, 1974, 1: 168.

Harto-Truax, N., et al. "Effects of bupropion on body weight." *Journal of Clinical Psychiatry*, 1983, 44(5 pt. 2): 183–86.

Kendler, K.S. "Amitriptyline-induced obesity in anorexia nervosa: a case report." *American Journal of Psychiatry*, 1978, 135: 1107.

Mitchell, J.E., Groat, R. "A placebo-controlled, double-blind trial of amitriptyline in bulimia." *Journal of Clinical Psychopharmacology*, 1984, 4: 186–93.

Moore, D.C. "Amitriptyline therapy in anorexia nervosa." *American Journal of Psychiatry*, 1977, 134: 1303–4.

Needleman, H.L., Waber, D. "Amitriptyline therapy in patients with anorexia nervosa." *Lancet*, 1976, 2: 580.

Paykel, E.S., et al. "Amitriptyline, weight gain and carbohydrate craving: a side effect." *British Journal of Psychiatry*, 1973, 123: 501–7.

Williams, W. "Possible use of mianserin in cases of unacceptable weight gain due to tricyclic antidepressant therapy." *Medical Journal of Australia*, Feb. 9, 1980, 1(3): 132–33.

BUPROPION

Brand Names
U.S.A.: Wellbutrin (Burroughs Wellcome).
Canada: None.
Great Britain: None.

What This Drug Does
Antidepressant.

How This Drug Affects Body Weight
Bupropion is an antidepressant structurally related to amphetamine. This could account for its appetite-suppressing effects. The drug may also increase dopamine concentrations in

the brain. Dopamine is a chemical transmitter in the nervous system thought to depress the appetite.

Government-Approved Uses for This Drug
To treat depression.

Unofficial Uses
None.

When Not to Use This Drug
In convulsive disorders; if taken within 14 days of any mono-amine oxidase inhibitor drug; in those with bulimia or anorexia nervosa; in nursing mothers; if allergic to this drug or to any related drug.

Side Effects From Use of This Drug
Dry mouth; dizziness; fainting; tremor; increased body move-ments; excitement; confusion; euphoria; agitation; insomnia; blurred vision; hearing disturbance; headache; high blood pres-sure; constipation; nausea; vomiting; stomach upset; various skin reactions; fever/chills; fast heartbeat; brain-wave abnormalities; sweating; seizures; increased or decreased libido; impotence; menstrual irregularities; gynecomastia (enlargement of the male breasts); increased urination; sweating; irritation of the mouth; flu-like symptoms.

Effects on Appetite and Body Weight as Disclosed by the Drug's Manufacturer
Loss of appetite; increased appetite; weight gain or loss; altered taste; water retention.

Detailed Effects on Appetite and Body Weight
Bupropion presents a different clinical profile from most other antidepressant medications. While most tend to cause weight gains (often substantial), bupropion appears to induce this to a much lesser degree. In fact, bupropion has been frequently cited as possessing mild appetite suppressant properties. Weight loss totaling 1–2 pounds in a 1-month treatment period is not un-common.

Decreased appetite; weight loss: A large-scale study reported 23% of those who were overweight and taking bupropion lost at least 5 pounds. The most usual scenario is for bupropion to effect an average weight loss of 1–2 pounds in about 20% of cases.

Greatest loss was seen in those who were overweight before treatment.

In clinical trials of more than 1,200 patients, bupropion caused anorexia or decreased appetite in 1.8%.

A 6–13 week study of 183 depressed patients was reported in which some received amitriptyline and others bupropion. Of the bupropion group (73 patients), 45% reported decreased appetite or anorexia.

In a study examining the effects of bupropion on 11 schizophrenics, 5 patients receiving only bupropion reported a mean weight loss of 17.8 pounds over an average of 15.5 months.

The official drug literature published by bupropion's manufacturer, Burroughs Wellcome, describes clinical trials showing weight loss greater than 5 pounds seen in 28% of patients. This is said to be double the incidence of weight loss seen with tricyclic antidepressants, the most common type of drug used to treat depression.

Weight gain: In clinical trials of bupropion totaling more than 1,200 patients, weight gain was seen in 1.4%. After 6 months of treatment, the average weight gain was only 1% over the baseline value at the start of the trial. This compares very favorably with amitriptyline, another antidepressant, which caused an average gain of more than 6% over baseline weight.

In clinical trials reported by the drug's manufacturer, Burroughs Wellcome, 9.4% of patients are said to have gained weight versus a 34.5% incidence in those receiving tricyclic antidepressants, the most common type of drug used to treat depression.

A 6–13 week study of 183 depressed patients was reported in which some received amitriptyline and others bupropion. Of the bupropion group (73 patients), 18% claimed increased hunger. During withdrawal of bupropion, 19% reported increased appetite.

Dosage Levels at Which Effects Occur
Decreased appetite; weight loss: Reported as low as 50mg. daily.
Weight gain: Reported as low as 300mg. daily.

Remedies
Decreased appetite; weight loss: The maintenance of adequate

fluid intake and the avoidance of excessive alcohol use may aid in reversing appetite loss.

Weight gain: Substitution of low-calorie foods, beverages, and snacks for normal dietary intake may aid in reversing some drug-induced weight gain.

How Long It Takes Till Reversal of Drug Effects
Half the dose of bupropion is eliminated from the body in 10–21 hours.

Sources
Chouinard, G. "Bupropion and amitriptyline in the treatment of depressed patients." *Journal of Clinical Psychiatry*, 1983, 44(5 pt. 2), 121–29.
Dufresne, R.L., et al. "Bupropion hydrochloride." *Drug Intelligence and Clinical Pharmacy*, 1984, 18(12): 957–64.
Harto-Truax, N., et al. "Effects of bupropion on body weight." *Journal of Clinical Psychiatry*, 1983, 44(5 pt. 2), 183–86.
Prien, R.F., et al. "Antidepressant drug therapy: The role of the new antidepressants." *Hospital and Community Psychiatry*, 1985, 36(5): 513–16.
Wright, G., et al. "Bupropion in the long-term treatment of cyclic mood disorders: Mood stabilizing effects." *Journal of Clinical Psychiatry*, 1985, 46(1): 22–25.

CLOMIPRAMINE

Brand Names
U.S.A.: Anafranil (Ciba-Geigy).
Note: Clomipramine is currently available only through an Investigational New Drug (IND) Application which must be filed with the U.S. Food and Drug Administration.
Canada: Anafranil (Geigy).
Great Britain: Anafranil (Geigy).

What This Drug Does
Antidepressant.

How This Drug Affects Body Weight
The hypothalamus (a portion of the brain) is sensitive to changes in body weight. Clomipramine, which acts at the hypothalamic level, appears to influence hunger, appetite, and food intake according to the initial body weight of the patient. Clomipramine

may also act by augmenting insulin release in the body by direct action on the pancreas (where insulin is produced). An increased blood level of insulin is accompanied by increased hunger.

Government-Approved Uses for This Drug
Clomipramine's manufacturer, Ciba-Geigy, has received FDA approval to investigate the drug's use in the treatment of obsessive-compulusive disorders. Trials are now being conducted at 20 research centers around the U.S. and the manufacturer hopes to have marketing approval in the near future.

The drug is approved for treatment of depression in Canada and Great Britain.

Unofficial Uses
To treat obsessive-compulsive disorder.

When Not to Use This Drug
During recovery from certain heart conditions; if taking or have taken within the last 14 days any monoamine oxidase inhibitor drug; in children under 12 years; if allergic to this drug or to any related drug.

Side Effects From Use of This Drug
Fast heartbeat; other heart irregularities; disorientation; anxiety; insomnia; dry mouth; blurred vision; skin rash; sedation; nausea; stomach upset; vomiting; dizziness; headache; diarrhea or constipation (more common); changes in libido; delayed ejaculation.

Effects on Appetite and Body Weight as Disclosed by the Drug's Manufacturer
Weight changes; loss of appetite.

Detailed Effects on Appetite and Body Weight
Treatment of anorexia nervosa: Sixteen female anorexics in a British study were split into two groups, one given clomipramine and the other a placebo. Because hyperactivity is a symptom of anorexia nervosa, all patients were required to stay in bed for the duration of the study. This was done to maximize the affects of caloric intake (each received 2,600 calories per day). After 11 weeks, both groups had attained their target weight, with those receiving placebo actually showing greater weight gains. However, those taking the active medication reported greater feelings

of hunger and tended to better maintain their weight gains after leaving the drug trial.

Dosage Levels at Which Effects Occur
Treatment of anorexia nervosa: Reported effective at 50mg. daily.

Remedies
Not applicable.

How Long It Takes Till Reversal of Drug Effects
Half the dose of clomipramine is cleared from the blood within 17–28 hours. In some depressed individuals, this has been found to take up to 3.5 days.

Source
Lacey, J.H., Crisp, A.H. "Hunger, food intake and weight: The impact of clomipramine on a refeeding anorexia nervosa population." *Postgraduate Medical Journal*, 1980, 56(suppl. 1): 79–85.

DESIPRAMINE

Brand Names
U.S.A.: Norpramin (Merrell Dow), Pertofrane (USV).
Canada: Norpramin (Merrell), Pertofrane (Geigy).
Great Britain: Pertofran (Geigy).

What This Drug Does
Antidepressant.

How This Drug Affects Body Weight
Probably restores appetite by relieving depression.

Government-Approved Uses for This Drug
To relieve depression.

Unofficial Uses
To treat attention-deficit disorders; to facilitate cocaine withdrawal.

When Not to Use This Drug
If taking or have taken within 2 weeks any monoamine oxidase inhibitor drug; during recovery from myocardial infarction (dam-

age to the heart muscle due to loss of its blood supply); in children; if allergic to this drug or to any related drug.

Side Effects From Use of This Drug

Drowsiness; dizziness or dizziness upon standing; tremors; weakness; confusion; headache; nervousness; fast heartbeat; high blood pressure; blurred vision; ringing in the ears; gynecomastia (enlargement of the breasts) in males; breast enlargement and galactorrhea (breast-milk flow unrelated to childbirth or nursing) in females; increased or decreased libido (reported with equal frequency); impotence; testicular swelling.

Effects on Appetite and Body Weight as Disclosed by the Drug's Manufacturer

Loss of appetite; peculiar taste; weight gain or loss.

Detailed Effects on Appetite and Body Weight

Treatment of bulimia: Twenty-nine sufferers of bulimia were recruited for a 6-week study of the effects of desipramine on binge eating and purging behavior. While those given a placebo were found to increase binging frequency by 19%, patients given desipramine decreased this activity by 84%. When those given a placebo were then crossed over to active medication, binging activity dropped by 91%. Fifteen of 22 patients (68%) attained complete freedom from binging-purging activity.

Several case reports describe female bulimics responding favorably to desipramine treatment. One woman went from 7 binges per week to none, while another decreased from 7 to 1. A third patient dropped from 14 to 7.

Dosage Levels at Which Effects Occur

Treatment of bulimia: Successful treatment has been reported at from 125–350mg. daily.

Remedies

Not applicable.

How Long It Takes Till Reversal of Drug Effects

From 12 to 76 hours are needed for half this drug to be cleared from the blood.

Sources

Brotman, A.W., et al. "Antidepressant treatment of bulimia: The relationship between binging and depressive symptomology." *Journal of Clinical Psychiatry*, 1984, 45: 7–9.

Hughes, P.L., et al. "Treating bulimia with desipramine: A placebo-controlled double-blind study." *Archives of General Psychiatry*, 1986, 43(1): 182–86.

DOXEPIN

Brand Names
U.S.A.: Adapin (Pennwalt), Sinequan (Roerig).
Canada: Sinequan (Pfizer), Triadapin (Pennwalt).
Great Britain: Sinequan (Pfizer).

What This Drug Does
Antidepressant.

How This Drug Affects Body Weight
May increase levels of the chemical transmitters norepinephrine and serotonin by blocking their removal by the nervous system. This is thought to elevate mood and improve depression.

Government-Approved Uses for This Drug
To treat depression in patients with manic-depressive illness; to treat anxiety.

Unofficial USes
None.

When Not to Use This Drug
If taking or have taken within 2 weeks any monoamine oxidase inhibitor drug; during recovery from myocardial infarction (damage to the heart muscle due to loss of its blood supply); in glaucoma; if there is a tendency to urinary retention; in children; if allergic to this drug or to any related drug.

Side Effects From Use of This Drug
Drowsiness; dizziness or dizziness upon standing; tremors; weakness; confusion; headache; nervousness; fast heartbeat; high blood pressure; blurred vision; ringing in the ears; gynecomastia (enlargement of the breasts) in males; breast enlargement and galactorrhea (breast-milk flow unrelated to childbirth or nursing) in females; increased or decreased libido (reported with equal frequency); impotence; testicular swelling.

Effects on Appetite and Body Weight as Disclosed by the Drug's Manufacturer
Loss of appetite; taste disturbance; weight gain.

Detailed Effects on Appetite and Body Weight
Weight gain: In a study group of 31 depressed patients treated with doxepin, an average weight gain of 4.3 pounds over a 6-week period was recorded.

In an 8-week study of 15 patients taking doxepin, researchers reported an average weight increase of 6.5 pounds.

Dosage Levels at Which Effects Occur
Weight gain: Reported as low as 55mg. daily.

Remedies
Weight gain: Substitution of low-calorie foods, beverages, and snacks for normal dietary intake may aid in reversing some drug-induced weight gain.

A decrease in daily dosage could help alleviate doxepin's effects on body weight. But this must be carefully balanced against maintaining adequate therapeutic blood levels.

A switch to a different agent in the same therapeutic category could accomplish similar benefits while minimizing undesirable dietary influences. Consult your physician.

How Long It Takes Till Reversal of Drug Effects
Weight gain: Doxepin and its metabolites (products of biotransformation in the liver) are excreted within 72 hours.

Sources
d'Elia, G., et al. "A double-blind comparison between doxepin and diazepam in the treatment of anxiety." *Acta Psychiatrica Scandinavica* (Suppl.), 1974 (Suppl. 255): 35–46.
Haskell, D.S., et al. "Doxepin or diazepam for anxious and anxious-depressed outpatients." *Journal of Clinical Psychiatry*, 1978, 39: 135–39.

FLUOXETINE

Brand Names
U.S.A.: Prozac (Dista).
Canada: None.

Great Britain: None.

What This Drug Does
Antidepressant.

How This Drug Affects Body Weight
Inhibits the removal of the chemical messenger serotonin by the nervous system, increasing its concentration in the brain. Serotonin is thought to be an appetite inhibitor, especially of carbohydrates.

Government-Approved Uses for This Drug
As an antidepressant.

Unofficial Uses
None.

When Not to Use This Drug
If allergic to this drug or to any related drug.

Side Effects From Use of This Drug
Nausea; vomiting; nervousness; headache; insomnia; anxiety; muscle tremor; drowsiness; fatigue; dry mouth; excessive sweating; diarrhea (12.3%) or constipation (4.5%); dizziness; light-headedness; weakness; upset stomach; abdominal pain; gas; various skin reactions; upper respiratory infections; flu-like symptoms; viral infection; nasal congestion; sore throat; difficult breathing; heart palpitations; joint or muscle pain; frequent urination; painful menstruation; sexual dysfunction; decreased libido; visual disturbance.

Effects on Appetite and Body Weight as Disclosed by the Drug's Manufacturer
Loss of appetite; increased appetite; weight loss; weight gain; taste change; facial swelling.

Detailed Effects on Appetite and Body Weight
Weight loss: Because many patients treated with fluoxetine often exhibit moderate weight loss, the drug is currently under investigation as a possible treatment for obesity.

In a large-scale study of 150 subjects, most of whom were female and more than 20 pounds overweight, fluoxetine was compared with benzphetamine (an amphetamine-related drug) and placebo for their effects on weight loss. The average starting weight of the subjects was 203.6 pounds. After 8 weeks, those taking fluoxetine lost an average of 10.63 pounds. In early animal studies, fluoxetine was shown to alter food preference away from carbohydrates to protein meals. In this human trial, patients who craved carbohydrates lost more weight than the others.

Fluoxetine's manufacturer, Dista, in its official package-insert literature, lists the drug's potential to cause significant weight loss, especially among underweight and depressed patients. They quote a controlled clinical drug trial in which about 9% of patients experienced loss of appetite. This incidence was 6 times greater than in those given a placebo. Among patients taking the active drug, 13% recorded a weight loss of more than 5% of their total body weight.

In a 6-week fluoxetine drug trial involving 22 patients, 14 (about 65%) lost an average of less than 1.4 pounds. Although not a significant loss of weight, these short-term results may translate to much greater losses with long-term fluoxetine use.

In a study of 20 overweight type II diabetics, half were given fluoxetine and half placebo. After 8 weeks, the fluoxetine group showed an average 6-pound weight loss while the others showed no change.

In a 5-week study of 16 patients treated with fluoxetine, an average decrease in body weight of 3.85 pounds was recorded.

Loss of appetite: Of 78 elderly patients treated with fluoxetine for depression, about 15% reported loss of appetite during the 6-week period. In a similar study of 28 elderly depressives treated with the drug for 48 weeks, about 10% had a similar complaint. This is consistent with the 8.7% incidence reported by the drug's manufacturer.

Treatment of bulimia: In a trial of 10 bulimics given fluoxetine, 8 were cured within a few days to several weeks, with the ninth patient showing partial improvement. In follow-up periods of up to a year or more, this improvement was maintained.

Dosage Levels at Which Effects Occur

Weight loss: Reported as low as 40mg. daily.
Loss of appetite: Reported as low as 20mg. daily.
Treatment of bulimia: Unknown. Usual daily dosage range is 20–80mg.

Remedies

Loss of appetite: The maintenance of adequate fluid intake and the avoidance of excessive alcohol use may aid in reversing appetite loss.

How Long It Takes Till Reversal of Drug Effects

While half the dose of fluoxetine is eliminated from the body in 2–3 days, the half-life of its active metabolite (product of biotransformation in the liver) is 7–9 days. The drug's effects may linger for several weeks after it is discontinued.

Sources

Bremner, J.D. "Fluoxetine in depressed patients: A comparison with imipramine." *Journal of Clinical Psychiatry*, 1984, 45(10): 414–49.

Feighner, J.P., Cohn, J.B. "Double-blind comparative trials of fluoxetine and doxepin in geriatric patients with major depressive disorder." *Journal of Clinical Psychiatry*, 1985, 46(3 pt. 2): 20–25.

Ferguson, M.D. "Fluoxetine-induced weight loss in overweight, nondepressed subjects." *American Journal of Psychiatry*, 1986, 143(11): 1496.

"Fluoxetine HC1 (Prozac by Dista)." *Drug Newsletter*, 1988, 7(2): 16.

"Fluoxetine may possess weight control potential." *Pharmacy Times*, 1987, 53(9): 63.

Levine, S., et al. "A comparative trial of a new antidepressant, fluoxetine." *British Journal of Psychiatry*, 1987, 150: 653–55.

IMIPRAMINE

Brand Names

U.S.A.: Antipress (Lemmon), Imavate (Robins), Janimine (Abbott), Presamine (USV), SK-Pramine (SKF), Tipramine (Major), Tofranil (Geigy).
Canada: Apo-Imipramine (Apotex), Impril (ICN), Novopramine (Novopharm), Tofranil (Geigy).
Great Britain: Berkomine (Berk), Praminil (DDSA), Tofranil (Geigy).

What This Drug Does

Antidepressant.

How This Drug Affects Body Weight

Imipramine may cause a higher body-weight set point (an equilibrium between appetite and body weight). This could promote increased appetite and decreased satiety until a new heavier body weight is reached.

Government-Approved Uses for This Drug

To relieve depression; to treat bed-wetting in children over 6 years old.

Unofficial Uses

To control chronic pain; to treat retrograde (reverse) ejaculation.

When Not to Use This Drug

In certain heart disease; within 14 days of taking any monoamine oxidase inhibitor drug; if breast-feeding; if allergic to this drug or to any related drug.

Side Effects From Use of This Drug

Dry mouth; blurred vision and other eye problems; diarrhea or constipation (more common); difficulty in urinating; paralysis of the small intestine; mental disorientation; confusion, anxiety, or hallucinations; dizziness upon standing; tremors; high blood pressure; various heart problems including fast heartbeat and heart-rhythm irregularities; numbness, tingling, and burning sensations of the extremities; loss of coordination; ringing in the ears; Parkinson-like symptoms (fixed mask-like facial expression; trembling hands, legs, and arms; stiff arm and leg movements); various skin reactions including sensitivity to sunlight; bone-marrow and blood abnormalities; nausea; vomiting; stomach upset; irritation of the tongue or mouth; black tongue (a fungal infection); altered blood-sugar levels; liver dysfunction (jaundice or hepatitis); sweating; flushing; drowsiness; headache; hair loss; gynecomastia (enlargement of the breasts) in males; breast enlargement and galactorrhea (breast-milk flow unrelated to childbirth or nursing) in females; increased or decreased libido (reported with equal frequency); impotence; testicular swelling.

Effects on Appetite and Body Weight as Disclosed by the Drug's Manufacturer

Loss of appetite; peculiar taste; loss or gain in weight.

Detailed Effects on Appetite and Body Weight

Weight gain: In a study of 5 female patients taking imipramine for more than 10 months on average, a mean weight gain of 3 pounds was seen. The average monthly weight gain was 1.3 pounds, with 40% reporting a total gain of 5 pounds or more. Many of the subjects described a craving for sweets and about one-third reported overeating.

Treatment of bulimia: Of 22 bulimics who were engaged in a 6-week imipramine study, 19 completed the trial. Of these, 9 were treated with imipramine and 10 with a placebo. Of those receiving the active drug, 4 reported a more than 75% decrease in binge eating, while 4 claimed a more than 50% decline; 1 remained unchanged. In a follow-up conducted from 1–8 months after completion of the study, 90% still had a moderate or marked decrease in binge eating with continued antidepressant treatment.

Dosage Levels at Which Effects Occur
Weight gain: Reported at 200mg. daily.
Treatment of bulimia: Reported effective at an average daily dose of 41mg. (range 10–80mg.).

Remedies
Weight gain: Substitution of low-calorie foods, beverages, and snacks for normal dietary intake may aid in reversing some imipramine-induced weight gain.

How Long It Takes Till Reversal of Drug Effects
Half the dose of imipramine is cleared from the blood within 6 hours to 1 day.
Weight gain: In the study cited above, a follow-up conducted 5 months after discontinuation of imipramine showed an average 6-pound weight loss.

Sources
Berkin, G.H., et al. "Weight gain. A side effect of tricyclic antidepressants." *Journal of Affective Disorders*, 1984, 7(2): 133–38.
Pope, H.G., et al. "Bulimia treated with imipramine: A placebo-controlled double-blind study." *American Journal of Psychiatry*, 1983, 140: 554–58.
White, J.H., Schnaultz, N.L. "Successful treatment of anorexia nervosa with imipramine." *Diseases of the Nervous System*, 1977, 38(7): 567–68.

ISOCARBOXAZID

Brand Names
U.S.A.: Marplan (Roche).
Canada: Marplan (Roche).
Great Britain: None.

What This Drug Does
Antidepressant.

How This Drug Affects Body Weight
As an inhibitor of monoamine oxidase (an enzyme responsible for the decomposition and inactivation of various chemical transmitters in the body), isocarboxazid increases the concentration of the body's natural epinephrine, norepinephrine, and serotonin in nervous system storage sites. It has been speculated that serotonin, a naturally occurring substance found in the brain and intestines, may influence the subjective appreciation of hunger.

Government-Approved Uses for This Drug
To treat depression.

Unofficial Uses
To treat bulimia; to treat premature ejaculation.

When Not to Use This Drug
In severe impairment of liver or kidney function; in congestive heart failure; in pheochromacytoma (adrenal gland tumor); if taking any sympathomimetic drug (such as amphetamines, methyldopa, levodopa, dopamine, tryptophan, epinephrine, norepinephrine); if eating foods with high concentrations of tryptophan or tyramine; if ingesting excessive caffeine; when taking most antidepressants; when taking central nervous system depressants; if allergic to this drug or to any related drug.
CAUTION: There are many drugs, foods, and conditions that are incompatible with isocarboxazid use. Food groups to be avoided include certain cheese and dairy products, certain meat and fish, red wine and certain undistilled alcoholic beverages, certain fruits

and vegetables, chocolate, and caffeine-containing colas, coffee, and teas. Consult your physician.

Side Effects From Use of This Drug

Dizziness or dizziness upon standing; vertigo; weakness; headache; muscle tremors and twitching; mania; insomnia; confusion; impaired memory; fatigue; heart-rhythm irregularities; high blood pressure; blurred vision; dry mouth; nausea; diarrhea or constipation (reported with equal frequency); rash; sweating; sexual disturbances.

Effects on Appetite and Body Weight as Disclosed by the Drug's Manufacturer

Loss of appetite; water retention; body-weight changes.

Detailed Effects on Appetite and Body Weight

Weight loss: One study found isocarboxazid to reverse weight gain and reduce or abolish overeating in depressive patients who predominantly display these symptoms. Sixteen of 20 of these patients who took the drug showed weight loss. A rapid, early, and almost complete decrease in overeating occurred in these patients within 1–2 weeks. Weight loss was seen within 2–4 weeks. These results have been claimed short-term only. Evidence does not yet support long-term use of isocarboxazid for this purpose.

Treatment of bulimia: In a 12-week trial involving 29 bulimic patients given isocarboxazid, an average decrease in binging episodes from 7 to 2.8 occurred within 6 weeks.

Dosage Levels at Which Effects Occur

Weight loss: Short-term success has been claimed with a starting dose of 20mg. daily increased to 40mg. by day 5. The dosage range used has been 20–80mg. daily.

Treatment of bulimia: Reported at 60mg. daily.

Remedies

Weight loss: A decrease in daily dosage may help alleviate isocarboxazid's adverse dietary influences. But this must be balanced against maintaining adequate therapeutic blood levels.

A switch to a different agent in the same therapeutic category could accomplish similar benefits while minimizing adverse influences on body weight. Examples of these drugs are phenelzine (Nardil) and tranylcypromine (Parnate).

How Long It Takes Till Reversal of Drug Effects
Weight loss: In one case, isocarboxazid's effects were reversed after 20 days abstinence from the drug.

In most cases, isocarboxazid's effects may last up to 2 weeks after withdrawal of the drug.

Sources
Davidson, J., et. al. "Loss of appetite associated with the MAOI isocarboxazid." *Journal of Clinical Psychopharmacology*, 1982, 2(4): 263–66.
Kennedy, S., et al. "Isocarboxazid in the treatment of bulimia." *American Journal of Psychiatry*, 1986, 143: 1495–96.
Smith, C.H., Bidlack, W.R. "Dietary concerns associated with the use of medications." *Journal of the American Dietary Association*, 1984, 84: 901–14.

MAPROTILINE

Brand Names
U.S.A.: Ludiomil (Ciba).
Canada: Ludiomil (Ciba).
Great Britain: Ludiomil (Ciba).

What This Drug Does
Antidepressant.

How This Drug Affects Body Weight
Maprotiline may cause a higher body-weight set point (an equilibrium between appetite and body weight). This could promote increased appetite and decreased satiety until a new heavier body weight is reached.

Government-Approved Uses for This Drug
As an antidepressant; to relieve anxiety associated with depression.

Unofficial Uses
None.

When Not to Use This Drug
In known or suspected seizure disorders; if taking or have taken within the last 14 days any monoamine oxidase inhibitor drug; if allergic to this drug or to any related drug.

Side Effects From Use of This Drug

Drowsiness; dizziness or dizziness upon standing; seizures; tremors; weakness; confusion; headache; nervousness; fast heartbeat; high blood pressure; blurred vision; dilated pupils; ringing in the ears; dry mouth; constipation; nausea; vomiting; loss of intestinal movement; skin rash and itching; sweating; various allergic reactions; increased or decreased libido (reported with equal frequency); impotence; galactorrhea (breast-milk flow unrelated to childbirth or nursing); breast enlargement in females; gynecomastia (enlargement of the male breasts); testicular swelling.

Effects on Appetite and Body Weight as Disclosed by the Drug's Manufacturer

Loss of appetite; bitter taste; weight loss or gain.

Detailed Effects on Appetite and Body Weight

Weight gain: A case report of a 65-year-old female describes a patient suffering from depression of 2 years' duration. She exhibited a decreased appetite and a weight loss of 8 pounds. After 1 month of maprotiline therapy, she reported significant mood elevation. She also simultaneously developed a voracious appetite and craving for sweets. This resulted in a weight gain of 18 pounds in 4 weeks. After discontinuing maprotiline, recurring depression necessitated a return to the drug about 1 year later. This time, after 2 months of therapy, she gained 22 pounds, with an additional gain of 10 pounds in the third month. Maprotiline was again withdrawn and at a 6-month follow-up she had lost 22 pounds but still remained 10 pounds heavier than her premedication level.

A 70-year-old man suffering from depression for about 3 months was started on maprotiline. When seen 3 weeks later, he reported a craving for sweets and a weight gain of 8 pounds. When switched to a different antidepressant drug, he lost 5 pounds within 2 weeks and his craving for sweets disappeared.

Dosage Levels at Which Effects Occur

Weight gain: Reported as low as 75mg. daily.

Remedies

Weight gain: In one case described above, switching to a different antidepressant, trazadone, eliminated sweetness craving and partially reversed weight gain.

How Long It Takes Till Reversal of Drug Effects
Weight gain: In one case cited above, the patient lost 22 of the 32 pounds gained while on maprotiline 6 months after its withdrawal. In the other instance, the patient lost 5 of 8 extra pounds 2 weeks after being switched to an alternative drug.

Source
Nakra, B.R., Grossberg, G.T. "Carbohydrate craving and weight gain with maprotiline." *Psychosomatics*, 1986, 27(5): 376, 381.

NORTRIPTYLINE

Brand Names
U.S.A.: Aventyl (Lilly), Pamelor (Sandoz).
Canada: Aventyl (Lilly).
Great Britain: Allergron (Dista), Aventyl (Lilly), *Motipress (Squibb), *Motival (Squibb).

What This Drug Does
Antidepressant.

How This Drug Affects Body Weight
Nortriptyline may cause a higher body-weight set point (an equilibrium between appetite and body weight). This could promote increased appetite and decreased satiety until a new heavier body weight is reached.

Government-Approved Uses for This Drug
To relieve depression.

Unofficial Uses
None.

When Not to Use This Drug
If taking or have taken within the last 14 days any monoamine oxidase inhibitor drug; in certain heart conditions; in children; if allergic to this drug or to any related drug.

*Combination drug.

Side Effects From Use of This Drug

Drowsiness; dizziness; seizures; tremors; weakness; confusion; headache; nervousness; fast heartbeat; high blood pressure; blurred vision; ringing in the ears; dilated pupils; dry mouth; constipation; nausea; vomiting; intestinal paralysis; difficult urination; skin rash; sweating; various allergic responses; gynecomastia (enlargement of the male breasts); female breast enlargement and galactorrhea (breast-milk flow unrelated to childbirth or nursing); increased or decreased libido (reported with equal frequency); impotence; testicular swelling.

Effects on Appetite and Body Weight as Disclosed by the Drug's Manufacturer

Loss of appetite; peculiar taste; weight gain or loss.

Detailed Effects on Appetite and Body Weight

Weight gain: In a study of 10 patients (7 females and 3 males) taking nortriptyline for an average of over 5 months, mean weight gain was 9 pounds. This worked out to an average gain of 2.2 pounds per month. Six (60%) of the subjects gained 5 pounds or more in total and 7 (70%) discontinued the drug due to the unwanted weight gains. A majority of the patients reported a craving for sweets, with overeating occurring in about one-third of cases.

Dosage Levels at Which Effects Occur

Weight gain: Reported to occur at an average daily dosage of 37mg. (range 15–50mg.).

Remedies

Weight gain: Substitution of low-calorie foods, beverages, and snacks for normal dietary intake may aid in reversing some drug-induced weight gain.

How Long It Takes Till Reversal of Drug Effects

Weight gain: In the study described above, there was an average weight loss of 6 pounds 5 months after withdrawal of nortriptyline.

Half the dose of nortriptyline is cleared from the blood within 15–93 hours.

Source

Berken, G.H., et al. "Weight gain: A side-effect of tricyclic antidepressants." *Journal of Affective Disorders*, 1984, 7 (2): 133–38.

ANTIDEPRESSANTS / **101**

PHENELZINE

Brand Names
U.S.A.: Nardil (Parke-Davis).
Canada: Nardil (Parke-Davis).
Great Britain: Nardil (Warner).

What This Drug Does
Antidepressant.

How This Drug Affects Body Weight
Phenelzine is an inhibitor of monoamine oxidase, an enzyme responsible for the breakdown and inactivation of various chemical transmitters in the body. Phenelzine increases the concentration of the body's natural epinephrine, norepinephrine, and serotonin in nervous system storage sites. It has been speculated that serotonin, a naturally occurring substance found in the brain and intestines, may influence the subjective appreciation of hunger.

Government-Approved Uses for This Drug
As an antidepressant.

Unofficial Uses
To treat bulimia (an eating disorder); to treat tension headache; to treat premature ejaculation.

When Not to Use This Drug
In pheochromocytoma (adrenal gland tumor); in congestive heart failure; if there is a history of liver disease or abnormal liver-function tests; in children under 16 years of age; if taking any sympathomimetic drug (such as amphetamines, methyldopa, levodopa, dopamine, tryptophan, epinephrine, norepinephrine); if taking drugs that depress the central nervous system; if eating foods with high concentrations of tryptophan or tyramine; if ingesting excessive caffeine; at least 10 days before spinal anesthesia; if allergic to this drug or to any related drug.
CAUTION: There are many drugs, foods, and conditions that are incompatible with phenelzine use. Food groups to be avoided

include certain cheese and dairy products, certain meat and fish, red wine and certain undistilled alcoholic beverages, certain fruits and vegetables, chocolate, and caffeine-containing colas, coffee, and teas. Consult your physician.

Side Effects From Use of This Drug

Dizziness or dizziness upon standing; vertigo; headache; muscle twitching or tremor; mania; insomnia; mental confusion; impaired memory; drowsiness; weakness; fatigue; high blood pressure; heart-rhythm irregularities; dry mouth; nausea; constipation; sweating; sexual disturbances.

Effects on Appetite and Body Weight as Disclosed by the Drug's Manufacturer

Loss of appetite; weight changes; water retention.

Detailed Effects on Appetite and Body Weight

Water retention: In a series of 22 patients receiving phenelzine for depression, severe water retention of the ankles was noted in 4 of them; all 4 were women over 50. Another earlier study showed this phenomenon occurring in 10% of subjects taking phenelzine.

A case report describes a 64-year-old male admitted to the hospital with leg edema (water swelling) of 10 weeks' duration. He had been taking, among other drugs, phenelzine for 16 weeks. Since no physical cause could be determined as the source of the swelling, phenelzine was discontinued and a diuretic administered. In 6 weeks, edema was gone and the patient lost almost 27 pounds of water weight.

Treatment of bulimia: Bulimia, a syndrome of binge eating and purging, seems to affect mostly women. In one study of 10 such females between 18 and 37 years of age, 8 showed a dramatic reduction in weekly binging when treated with phenelzine for 4–8 weeks. Binging episodes went from a pretreatment high of 28 per week down to an average of 1.

In a 10-week study of 20 bulimic women, 9 of whom received phenelzine and 11 a placebo, 56% of those on active medication quit binging altogether and the remaining 44% decreased binge frequency by at least half. In the placebo group, no subjects stopped binging and only 2 showed a decrease of 50% or more.

A case report describes a 37-year-old female with a 10-year

history of binge eating followed by self-induced vomiting. This progressed to the point where she was spending up to $300 a week on food and was binging and vomiting 3–4 times daily. Treatment with phenelzine produced a marked improvement after 3 weeks. During 10 months of drug therapy, she only binged and vomited 3 times.

Dosage Levels at Which Effects Occur
Water retention: Reported as low as 90mg. daily.
Treatment of bulimia: Reported effective as low as 30mg. daily.

Remedies
Water retention: In one case cited above, withdrawal of phenelzine and addition of the diuretic furosemide, 40mg. daily, reversed water retention.

How Long It Takes Till Reversal of Drug Effects
Water retention: In one case cited above, phenelzine-induced water retention was reversed 6 weeks after its withdrawal and administration of furosemide, a diuretic. In another case, the condition did not respond to diuretics, but improved only after discontinuation of phenelzine or a reduction of its dose.

Sources
Dunleavy, D.L.F "Phenelzine and oedema." *British Medical Journal*, 1977, 1(6072): 1353.

Goonewardene, A., Toghill, P.J. "Gross oedema occurring during treatment for depression." *British Medical Journal*, 1977, 1(6065): 879–80.

Rees, L., Davies, B. "A controlled trial of phenelzine ('Nardil') in the treatment of severe depressive illness." *Journal of Mental Science*, 1961, 107: 560.

Stewart, J.W., et al. "An open trial of MAO inhibitors in bulimia." *Journal of Clinical Psychiatry*, 1984, 45(5): 217–19.

Walsh, B.T., et al. "Treatment of bulimia with monoamine oxidase inhibitors." *American Journal of Psychiatry*, 1982, 139: 1629–30.

Walsh, B.T., et al. "Treatment of bulimia with phenelzine: A double-blind, placebo-controlled study." *Archives of General Psychiatry*, 1984, 41: 1105–9.

TRAZODONE

Brand Names
U.S.A.: Desyrel (Mead Johnson).

Canada: None.
Great Britain: Molipaxin (Roussel).

What This Drug Does
Antidepressant.

How This Drug Affects Body Weight
Trazodone may work by inhibiting the removal of serotonin in the brain. Serotonin, a neurotransmitter in the body, acts to decrease appetite. By raising serotonin levels, trazodone may act as an appetite suppressant.

Government-Approved Uses for This Drug
To treat depression.

Unoffical Uses
To treat tension headache.

When Not to Use This Drug
If allergic to this drug or to any related drug.

Side Effects From Use of This Drug
Drowsiness; dizziness or dizziness upon standing; nervousness; confusion; muscle tremors; weakness; fast heartbeat; blurred vision; ringing in the ears; dry mouth; constipation; nausea; vomiting; difficulty in urinating; skin rash; sweating; decreased or increased libido (reported with equal frequency); impotence; early menses; missed periods; retrograde ejaculation (backward ejaculation into the urinary bladder); priapism (prolonged, often painful erection unrelated to sexual desire).

Effects on Appetite and Body Weight as Disclosed by the Drug's Manufacturer
Increased or decreased appetite; weight gain or loss; water retention; bad taste in mouth.

Detailed Effects on Appetite and Body Weight
Treatment of bulimia: Of a total of 12 trials using trazodone to treat bulimia, half resulted in moderate to marked improvement (from over 50% to more than a 75% decrease in binge eating frequency). The authors of this series speculate that, due to certain preclassification of their patients, trazodone's value may be even greater, approximating success rates

seen with tricyclic antidepressants (such as imipramine, desipramine, amitriptyline).

Several case reports of bulimics treated with trazodone have claimed encouraging success rates. One case describes a female with a pretrial binging frequency of 12 episodes per week. After trazodone treatment, she reported no binging at all for a follow-up period of 3 months. Another woman who binged at a rate of 3 times weekly reported total cessation of this behavior after trazodone treatment during a 3-month follow-up. In yet another case, a woman with a pretreatment binging frequency of 15 per week dropped to 3 per week with trazodone use, but the medication had to be withdrawn due to adverse side effects.

Dosage Levels at Which Effects Occur
Treatment of bulimia: Reported successful within a range of 150–300mg. daily.

Remedies
Treatment of bulimia: Not applicable.

How Long It Takes Till Reversal of Drug Effects
Trazodone's effects may persist for up to 12 hours after its withdrawal, with traces detectable in the urine and feces long after that time.

Sources
Brotman, A.W., et al. "Antidepressant treatment of bulimia: The relationship between bingeing and depressive symptomology." *Journal of Clinical Psychiatry*, 1984, 45: 7–9.

Pope, H.G. "Antidepressant treatment of bulimia: Preliminary experience and practical recommendation." *Journal of Clinical Psychopharmacology*, 1983, 3(5): 274–81.

Antidiabetic Drugs

CHLORPROPAMIDE

Brand Names
U.S.A.: Diabenese (Pfizer).
Canada: Apo-Chlorpropamide (Apotex), Diabenese (Pfizer), Norpropamide (Novopharm).
Great Britain: Diabenese (Pfizer), Glymese (DDSA), Melitase (Berk).

What This Drug Does
Antidiabetic.

How This Drug Affects Body Weight
By decreasing sugar excretion in the urine, chlorpropamide could cause a net retention of calories, resulting in increased formation of fat. Chlorpropamide also exhibits some antidiuretic activity. This may cause the body to decrease urine production and retain water.

Government-Approved Uses for This Drug
To lower blood sugar.

Unofficial Uses
To treat certain cases of diabetes insipidus (a rare disorder marked by extreme thirst and excessive urination).

When Not to Use This Drug
In certain diabetic ketoacidosis (excessive acid and ketones in the blood); if pregnant; in nursing mothers; if allergic to this drug or to any related drug.

Side Effects From Use of This Drug

Nausea; heartburn; vomiting; diarrhea; facial flushing; various skin reactions; various blood abnormalities.

Effects on Appetite and Body Weight as Disclosed by the Drug's Manufacturer

Loss of appetite; hunger.

Detailed Effects on Appetite and Body Weight

Weight gain: In a study of 77 obese diabetic adults, most showed weight gain during 1 year of chlorpropamide use. The average increase in body weight was 11.6 pounds, with gains continuing throughout the trial period. Some subjects put on as much as 26–29 pounds.

Water retention: A theory long held by some researchers and finally confirmed by experiment holds that chlorpropamide, when given to normal (nondiabetic) individuals, could impair water excretion. This raised concern over the possibility that those being treated with chlorpropamide for diabetes mellitus would exhibit this side effect. Two case reports presented here confirm this phenomenon.

In the first, a 76-year-old male diabetic hospitalized for urological evaluation was given chlorpropamide. Right from the outset, water elimination lagged behind fluid intake by 2–3 liters daily over a 3-day period. One day after chlorpropamide was discontinued, diuresis (increased urination) ensued, with a 5-pound weight loss (as water weight) recorded over the following 4 days.

The second case report details a 71-year-old female diabetic who had been taking chlorpropamide for 30 months. She was hospitalized with acute pulmonary edema, at which time chlorpropamide was discontinued. Rapid diuresis followed and upon rechallenge with chlorpropamide, inhibited water elimination again occurred.

In 5 of 7 normal, nondiseased subjects given intravenous chlorpropamide, a decrease in urine volume of 50% or more took place. While the clinical aim of this and similar studies has been to test chlorpropamide's value in the treatment of diabetes insipidus, the water-retaining properties of this drug might be a contributing factor toward weight gain in those being treated for diabetes mellitus.

Six patients with diabetes mellitus were given single water loads (that is, required to drink a large volume of water all at once) both with and without concurrent administration of chlorpropamide. Chlorpropamide caused impaired water excretion in all 6, inducing water retention within 3 days.

Dosage Levels at Which Effects Occur
Weight gain: Reported as low as 375mg. daily.
Water retention: Reported as low as 250mg. daily by mouth and at 500mg. daily by intravenous administration.

Remedies
Weight gain: Substitution of low-calorie foods, beverages, and snacks for normal dietary intake may aid in reversing some drug-induced weight gain.
Water retention: A decrease in daily dosage could help alleviate chlorpropamide's effects on appetite and body weight. But this must be carefully balanced against maintaining adequate therapeutic blood levels.

A switch to a different agent in the same therapeutic category could accomplish similar benefits while minimizing undesirable dietary influences. Consult your physician.

How Long It Takes Till Reversal of Drug Effects
Half the dose of chlorpropamide is cleared from the blood in 36 hours, while the drug's duration of action may persist up to 60 hours.
Water retention: In a study cited above, normal water elimination was reestablished within 3–5 days after dicontinuation of chlorpropamide.

Sources
Clarke, B.F., Duncan, L.J.P. "Comparison of chlorpropamide and metformin treatment on weight and blood glucose response of uncontrolled obsese diabetes." *Lancet*, 1968, 1: 123.

Garcia, M., et al. "Clorpropamide-induced water retention in patients with diabetes mellitus." *Annals of Internal Medicine*, 1971, 75: 549–55.

Reforzo–Membrives, J., et al. "Antidiuretic effect of 1-propyl-3-p-chlorobenzene-sulfonylurea (chlorpropamide)." *Journal of Clinical Endocrinology*, 1968, 28: 332–36.

INSULIN

Brand Names
U.S.A.: †Humuilin [various] (Lilly), †Iletin [various] (Lilly), †Insulatard NPH (Nordisk-USA), †Mixtard (Nordisk-USA), †Novolin [various] (Squibb-Novo), †Velosulin (Nordisk-USA).
Canada: Actrapid MC Pork (Connaught Novo), Humulin (Lilly), Iletin [various] (Lilly), Insulatard NPH (Nordisk), Insulin-Toronto (Connaught Novo), Intard (Nordisk), Mixtard (Nordisk), Monotard MC Pork (Connaught Novo), Novolin-Toronto (Connaught Novo), Protophane MC Pork (Connaught Novo), Velosulin Cartridge (Nordisk).
Great Britain: Actrapid (Novo; Farillon), Human Monotard (Novo; Farillon), Hypurin (Weddel), Initard 50/50 (Nordisk; Leo), Insulatard (Nordisk; Leo), Lentard MC (Novo; Farillon), Mixtard 30/70 (Nordisk; Leo), Monotard MC (Novo; Farillon), Neulente (Wellcome), Neuphane (Wellcome), Neusulin (Wellcome), Nuso Neutral Insulin (Boots; Evans Medical; Wellcome), Rapitard MC (Novo; Farillon), Semitard MC (Novo; Farillon), Ultratard MC (Novo; Farillon), Velosulin (Nordisk; Leo).

What This Drug Does
Antidiabetic.

How This Drug Affects Body Weight
Insulin promotes the conversion of food to fat. Fasting insulin levels may be 2–3 times higher than normal in obese people. This high natural insulin level may be a major cause of obesity since, in addition to promoting fat storage, it prevents its breakdown and use as a body fuel. Excessive exogenous (external) insulin administration promotes salt and water retention. Glucose deprivation after insulin use may produce low blood sugar and consequent appetite stimulation.

Government-Approved Uses for This Drug
To treat certain types of diabetes; to treat certain conditions of high blood potassium; to treat severe ketoacidosis and diabetic coma.

†Denotes over-the-counter availability in the U.S.A.

Unofficial Uses
None.

When Not to Use This Drug
If allergic to this drug or to any related drug.

Side Effects From Use of This Drug
High or low blood sugar (this is a function of proper dosing); skin rash; itching; various reactions at the site of injection; severe allergic response.

Effects on Appetite and Body Weight as Disclosed by the Drug's Manufacturer
None.

Detailed Effects on Appetite and Body Weight
Water retention; weight gain: A case report of a 16-year-old diabetic male describes treatment with increasing daily insulin doses in an effort to control diabetic complications. As a result, swelling and weight gain occurred. Facial swelling and retention of fluid in the ankles and lower legs became apparent within 4 days of the increased dosage. A total weight gain of 13.2 pounds resulted.

In one paper, a researcher presents 6 case reports of malnourished, nondiabetic children given insulin injections. A 2.5-year-old girl given insulin gained 3 pounds in 5 weeks; a 7-year-old boy gained 6 pounds in 7 weeks; a 7-year-old girl gained 16 pounds in 3 months; a 6-week-old female gained 2 pounds 13 ounces in 5 weeks; a 2-year-old boy gained a little over 3 pounds in about 1 month; a 9-year-old girl gained 12 pounds in 7 weeks. Out of a total of 40 cases of malnourished children treated with insulin by these researchers, 38 are claimed to have shown improvement.

Three cases of fluid retention and weight gain were reported by one doctor, with two of these cases presented here. A 24-year-old male was admitted to the hospital with diabetic ketoacidosis (a life-threatening complication of diabetes). Eight days after admission, he complained of swelling of the face, feet, and abdomen. By day 11, this had progressed to more generalized swelling with accompanying weight gain of 26.4 pounds over admission weight. A reduced insulin dosage resolved all complications.

The second case describes a 42-year-old insulin-dependent female diabetic who was complaining of recurrent, generalized swelling. After decreasing her insulin dosage, fluid retention decreased. Three months later, however, she returned with the same complications after increasing her daily insulin injections. With a reduction in dosage, she lost 5.5 pounds within 24 hours, with further gradual weight loss occurring.

In a study of 33 cases of malnourished psychotic adults treated with insulin, improvement was seen in about 20% of cases; 16 males in the study had an average weight gain of 3 pounds per week over a 4-week period (for a total of 12 pounds). Of the females, 13 gained 2.4 pounds on average per week over a 3-week period.

Increased appetite: A study of 30 adults (15 males and 15 females) was undertaken to determine the effects on hunger of intravenous (as opposed to the intramuscular route by which most insulin is taken) insulin injections. Within a half-hour after receiving the drug, effects on hunger were minimal. But as blood-sugar levels began to rebound upward, so did hunger. Appetite intensity continued increasing in a direct proportion to blood-sugar levels for at least 1 hour.

Treatment of anorexia nervosa: A group of 20 hospitalized patients with anorexia nervosa were treated with a combination of insulin and chlorpromazine, an antipsychotic medication. For purposes of the study, these patients were compared with 24 others treated by other means. The average weight gain of 4.4 pounds per week for the insulin-chlorpromazine group compared favorably with only a 1.25-pound increase for the control group. Unfortunately, follow-up studies conducted from 3 months to 3 years later showed only about half the patients making a lasting recovery.

Dosage Levels at Which Effects Occur
Water retention; weight gain: This occurred in children in doses as low as 9 units of insulin daily. In adults, this effect was reported as low as 10 units daily, with the most common range between 55–70 units.

Increased appetite: Reported to occur at 0.15 units per kilogram in 1 intravenous dose.

Treatment of anorexia nervosa: Reported at 40–80 units daily (combined with 1,000mg. of chlorpromazine daily).

Remedies
Water retention; weight gain: A decrease in daily insulin dosage

usually restores normal water balance and body weight. Consult your physician.

How Long It Takes Till Reversal of Drug Effects

Water retention; weight gain: In one case cited above, normal water balance and body weight were restored 3 weeks after dosage was decreased. In another instance, the condition spontaneously resolved over a 3-week period without any adjustment in dosage.

Sources

Appel, K.E., et al. "Insulin therapy in undernourished psychotic patients: Preliminary report." *Journal of the American Medical Association*, 1928, 22: 1788–89.

Barbour, O. "The use of insulin in undernourished non-diabetic children." *Archives of Pediatrics*, 1924, 41: 707–11.

Dally, P., Sargant, W. "A new treatment of anorexia nervosa." *British Medical Journal*, 1960, 1: 1770–73.

Ghadimi, H. "Amino acids and obesity." *Pediatric Annals*, 1984, 13(7): 557–63.

Sharon, M., et al. "Edema associated with improved glycemic control in an adolescent with type I diabetes." *Journal of Pediatrics*, 1987, 111(3): 403–4.

Silverstone, J.T., Besser, G.M. "Insulin, blood sugar and hunger." *Postgraduate Medical Journal*, 1971, 47(June suppl.): 427–29.

Wheatly, T., Edwards, O.M. "Insulin oedema and its clinical significance: Metabolic studies in three cases." *Diabetic Medicine*, 1985, 2(5): 400–404.

PHENFORMIN

Brand Names

U.S.A.: DBI (Geigy), Meltrol (USV).

Note: Phenformin was removed from the U.S. market in 1977 and is now available for physician use only through an Investigational New Drug (IND) Application filed with the U.S. Food and Drug Administration.

Canada: None.

Great Britain: Dibotin (Winthrop).

What This Drug Does

Antidiabetic.

How This Drug Affects Body Weight
Phenformin may decrease the absorption of some nutrients (mainly glucose) from the gastrointestinal tract. This may inhibit glucose metabolism, decreasing its use by fat tissue and limiting fat accumulation.

Government-Approved Uses for This Drug
To treat certain adult diabetes, but available to physicians only upon application to the Food and Drug Administration.

Unofficial Uses
None.

When Not to Use This Drug
In insulin-dependent diabetics; in diabetes mellitus which can be controlled by diet alone; in kidney disease or impaired kidney function; in severe liver disease; if there is a history of lactic acidosis (a condition of altered blood pH); in alcoholism; in various heart problems; in pregnancy; if allergic to this drug or to any related drug.

Side Effects From Use of This Drug
Nausea; vomiting; diarrhea.

Effects on Appetite and Body Weight as Disclosed by the Drug's Manufacturer
Unpleasant metallic taste; anorexia.

Detailed Effects on Appetite and Body Weight
Weight loss: In a long-term study of 1,027 diabetic patients who were divided into five groups, each receiving a different treatment, data after 1 year showed those given phenformin losing more weight than the other groups. Although all subjects initially lost weight, those taking phenformin continued this trend. Weight loss appeared greatest for those entering the study more than 30% overweight.

A group of 30 obese females with normal glucose tolerance (that is, nondiabetic) were given phenformin for 16 weeks. Average weight loss was 6.9 pounds compared with a control group given a placebo which gained an average 2.6 pounds.

One report details 5 obese women, 2 of whom were mildly diabetic (3 were normal), who were offered unlimited food while receiving phenformin. The study, which lasted 32 days, showed a lowered caloric intake when under the influence of phenformin, but also showed a weight loss greater than that anticipated on the basis of calorie deficit alone. The average weight loss was about 15.5 pounds.

Among 23 adult diabetics (12 females and 11 males) treated with phenformin for 6–18 months, significant weight loss occurred. Nine males lost an average of 4 pounds and 11 females lost an average of 12 pounds.

Forty-two diabetics were treated with phenformin over a 10-month period. Average weight loss reached a maximum of 5 pounds after 7 months.

A Finnish study of 19 male and 17 female diabetics treated with phenformin to lower cholesterol showed weight loss occurring in both sexes. After 3 months, males lost an average 6.4 pounds, while females lost an average 8.6 pounds.

A group of 27 nondiabetic, obese individuals enrolled in a weight-loss clinic were studied while being given various treatments, one of which was phenformin. Taken as a whole, the phenformin group showed no greater weight loss than those who were treated by diet alone. But when subjects with a family history of diabetes were grouped together, significant weight loss occurred compared to others in the study. After 15 weeks, these individuals lost an average of 26.5 pounds as compared to 16.8 pounds for all subjects.

Dosage Levels at Which Effects Occur
Weight loss: Reported as low as 50mg. daily.

Remedies
Weight loss: A decrease in daily dosage could help alleviate phenformin's effects on body weight. But this must be carefully balanced against maintaining adequate therapeutic blood levels.

A switch to a different agent in the same therapeutic category could accomplish similar benefits while minimizing undesirable dietary influences. Consult your physician.

How Long It Takes Till Reversal of Drug Effects
Weight loss: In one study cited above, researchers found that after 4 years of phenformin use, body weight tended to return to baseline values.

Sources

Alterman, S.L. "Phenformin effect on body weight, lipids and glucose regulation." *Polskie Archiwum Medycyny Wewnetrznej*, 1969, 42(3): 291–97.

Burstein, J., et al. "The effect of phenformin hydrochloride on serum cholesterol, triglycerides and body weight of nondiabetic hypercholeserolemic subjects." *Annales Medicinae Internae Fenniae*, 1968, 57(1): 15–21.

Duncan, L.J. "The effect of biguanide treatment of body-weight in diabetics and non-diabetics." *Postgraduate Medical Journal*, 1969, 45(suppl.): 13–19.

Gershberg, H., et al. "Influence of hypoglycemic agents on blood lipids and body weight in ketoacidosis-resistant diabetics." *Annals of the New York Academy of Sciences*, 1968, 148: 914.

Meinert, C.L., Schwartz, T.B. "The relationship of treatment to weight in a randomized study of maturity-onset diabetes." *Annals of the New York Academy of Sciences*, 1968, 148(3): 875–83.

Patel, D.P., Stowers, J.M. "Phenformin in weight reduction of obese diabetics." *Lancet*, 1964, 2: 282.

The Physicians' Desk Reference, 29Th ed. Oradell, New Jersey: Medical Economics Company, 1975.

Roginsky, M., Barnett, J. "Double-blind study of phenethyldiguanide in weight control of obese nondiabetic subjects." *Journal of Clinical Nutrition*, 1966, 19: 223–26.

Weller, C. "Phenformin in weight reduction of obese diabetics." *Lancet*, 1965, 1: 53.

TOLBUTAMIDE

Brand Names
U.S.A.: Oramide (Major), Orinase (Upjohn).
Canada: Apo-Tolbutamide (Apotex), Mobenol (Horner), Novobutamide (Novopharm), Orinase (Hoechst).
Great Britain: Pramidex (Berk), Rastinun (Hoechst).

What This Drug Does
Antidiabetic.

How This Drug Affects Body Weight
By stimulating the release of insulin from the pancreas, tolbutamide reduces levels of blood sugar, promoting its storage as fat. It also facilitates the conversion of amino acids into protein in muscle cells.

Government-Approved Uses for This Drug
To treat certain types of diabetes.

Unofficial Uses
None.

When Not to Use This Drug
In certain types of diabetes; if pregnant; in nursing mothers; if allergic to this drug or to any related drug.

Side Effects From Use of This Drug
Nausea; heartburn; feeling of fullness; various skin reactions including sensitivity to sunlight; various blood abnormalities; liver dysfunction; headache; low blood sugar.

Effects on Appetite and Body Weight as Disclosed by the Drug's Manufacturer
Taste alterations.

Detailed Effects on Appetite and Body Weight
Weight gain: Twenty-six diabetic patients were treated with tolbutamide for up to 10 months. Most gained weight, with an average maximum increase after 5 months of 5 pounds.

Dosage Levels at Which Effects Occur
Weight gain: Reported as low as 500mg. daily, but may occur within the usual dosage range of 250–3,000 mg.

Remedies
Weight gain: Substitution of low-calorie foods, beverages, and snacks for normal dietary intake may aid in reversing some tolbutamide-induced weight gain.

How Long It Takes Till Reversal of Drug Effects
Tolbutamide's duration of action is 6–12 hours, with half the dose cleared from the blood in 4–5 hours.

Source
Gershberg, H., et al. "Influence of hypoglycemic agents on blood lipids and body weight in ketoacidosis-resistant diabetics." *Annals of the New York Academy of Sciences*, 1968, 148: 914.

Antiepileptic Drugs

CARBAMAZEPINE

Brand Names
U.S.A.: Epitol (Lemmon), Tegretol (Geigy).
Canada: Apo-Carbamazepine (Apotex), Mazepine (ICN), Tegretol (Geigy).
Great Britain: Tegretol (Geigy).

What This Drug Does
   Anticonvulsant.

How This Drug Affects Body Weight
   May affect the limbic area of the brain, which is thought to influence bulimic behavior (overeating followed by forced vomiting and/or laxative abuse). May also cause water retention by stimulating the release of antidiuretic hormone (ADH), a substance that decreases urine production.

Government-Approved Uses for This Drug
   To control various types of epileptic seizures; to treat pain of trigeminal neuralgia (facial pain due to inflammation of the trigeminal nerve).

Unofficial Uses
   To treat neurogenic diabetes insipidus (a metabolic disease marked by thirst and excessive urination); to treat certain psychiatric disorders; to manage alcohol withdrawal; to treat cluster headaches.

When Not to Use This Drug

If there is history of bone-marrow depression; if using a monoamine oxidase inhibitor drug; if allergic to this drug or any related drug or to tricyclic antidepressant drugs.

Side Effects From Use of This Drug

Various blood abnormalities; dizziness; vertigo; drowsiness; loss of coordination; various heart problems; high or low blood pressure (reported with equal frequency); dry mouth and throat; blurred vision; various eye problems; nausea; vomiting; abdominal pain; diarrhea; dry mouth; inflammation of the mouth and tongue; difficulty in urinating; liver dysfunction; skin rash, itching, and various other dermal reactions; sweating; fever; chills; lung sensitivity; impotence.

Effects on Appetite and Body Weight as Disclosed by the Drug's Manufacturer

Loss of appetite.

Detailed Effects on Appetite and Body Weight

Treatment of bulimia: In a study of 6 patients between 20 and 34 years of age (5 females and 1 male) suffering from bulimia, a 20-week trial using carbamazepine and placebo showed 1 female responding dramatically to carbamazepine. While taking a placebo she averaged 3 binge episodes per week as compared to no bingeing during periods of active drug use.

Altered taste: In a bizarre case report, an adult male alcoholic visiting home during a break from a hospital alcohol-abuse treatment program took his brother's carbamazepine tablets in an effort to get high on "anything." He did feel high after taking large doses of the drug, but after 2 weeks of carbamazepine abuse, the drinking of alcohol imparted a very unpleasant taste, preventing its consumption. After returning to the hospital program and abstaining from both alcohol and carbamazepine use for 2 months, he again tried to take a drink. He still experienced a bad taste and only after many months of avoiding carbamazepine did normal taste sensation return.

Weight gain: Twenty-four psychiatric patients were treated with carbamazepine during a 4-week study. Those suffering from depression showed significant increases in body weight, while those who were manic did not. Those depressed patients who responded most favorably to carbamazepine treatment gained the most weight.

Appetite loss: A case report describes a 27-year-old retarded epileptic female who, when given increasing doses of carbamazepine, started losing her appetite. This progressed to the point where nasogastric tube feeding became necessary. A decrease in daily dosage resulted in improved appetite.

Water retention: In a study of 80 adult epileptics treated with carbamazepine, either alone or in combination with other antiepileptic drugs, over 13% were found to have a disturbance in the ability to excrete water from the body. In those treated with carbamazepine alone, this incidence rose to 23%.

In a study of 16 patients receiving carbamazepine for an average of almost 2 years, 5 (31%) exhibited increased levels of ADH (antidiuretic hormone) and consequent water retention.

Dosage Levels at Which Effects Occur
Treatment of bulimia: Reported at blood serum levels of 6–10mcg. per milliliter.
Altered taste: Reported as low as 800mg. daily.
Weight gain: Reported as low as 600mg. daily.
Appetite loss: Reported at 1,400mg. daily.
Water retention: Reported as low as 200mg. daily.

Remedies
Altered taste: Carbamazepine-induced taste disturbance may be countered in several ways. Taking the drug with an adequate fluid intake, chewing sugarless gum or using a mouthwash of water and lemon juice, and practicing good oral hygiene may help restore normal taste sensation.
Weight gain: Substitution of low-calorie foods, beverages, and snacks for normal dietary intake may aid in reversing some drug-induced weight gain.
Appetite loss: In the case reported above, a decrease in daily dosage to 800mg. restored normal appetite.
Water retention: In the study of 80 patients cited above, furosemide (a diuretic) was found to correct any electrolyte disturbance, restoring normal elimination of body water.

A switch to a different antiepileptic medication may also minimize any water-retaining side effects. Consult your physician.

How Long It Takes Till Reversal of Drug Effects

It takes from 12–65 hours for half the dose of carbamazepine to be cleared from the blood, depending on how long the drug has been taken. The longer the time, the quicker its elimination.
Appetite loss: In the case report cited above, appetite loss was reversed 1 week after dosage was decreased.
Altered taste: In the case cited above, normal taste returned 5 months after discontinuation of carbamazepine.

Sources

Clark, B.G., et al. "Insidious anorexia and anticonvulsant therapy." *Clinical Pharmacy*, 1986, 5(4): 287.
Halbreich, U. "Tegretol dependency and diversion of the sense of taste." *Israel Annals of Psychiatry*, 1974, 12: 328–32.
Henry, D.A., et al. "Hyponatraemia during carbamazepine treatment." *British Medical Journal*, 1977, 1: 83–84.
Joffe, R.T. "Effect of carbamazepine on body weight in affectively ill patients." *Journal of Clinical Psychiatry*, 1986, 47(6): 313–14.
Kaplan, A.S., et al. "Carbamazepine in the treatment of bulimia." *American Journal of Psychiatry*, 1983, 140(9): 1225–26.
Perucca, E., et al. "Water intoxication in epileptic patients receiving carbamazepine." *Journal of Neurology and Neurosurgery*, 1978, 41: 713–18.
Rado, J.P. "Water intoxication during carbamazepine treatment." *British Medical Journal*, 1973, 3: 479.

PHENYTOIN

Brand Names

U.S.A.: Dilantin (Parke-Davis), *Dilantin with Phenobarbital (Parke-Davis), Diphenylan (Lannett), Phenytex (Bolar).
Canada: Dilantin (Parke-Davis), Novophenytoin (Novopharm).
Great Britain: Epanutin (Parke-Davis), *Epanutin with Phenobarbitone (Parke-Davis", *Garoin (May & Baker).

What This Drug Does

Anticonvulsant.

---

*Combination drug.

How This Drug Affects Body Weight

There may be a connection between neurological abnormalities and compulsive eating disorders. Phenytoin may inhibit the appetite center of the brain by preventing nervous system stimulation in the hypothalamus. By decreasing the excitability of the nervous system, phenytoin may limit general impulsive-compulsive behavior.

Phenytoin may also inhibit antidiuretic hormone (ADH), a substance in the body that regulates water excretion. This may result in excessive water loss.

Government-Approved Uses for This Drug

To control various types of epileptic seizures.

Unofficial Uses

To treat heart-rhythm irregularities when given intravenously; to treat trigeminal neuralgia (facial pain due to inflammation of the trigeminal nerve); to treat certain skin disorders; to treat migraine headache.

When Not to Use This Drug

If a nursing mother; if allergic to this drug or to any related drug.

Side Effects From Use of This Drug

Rapid movements of the eyeball, usually from side to side; loss of coordination; slurred speech; mental confusion; dizziness; insomnia; headache; nervousness (usually temporary); nausea; vomiting; constipation; various skin reactions; various blood abnormalities; lymphatic system dysfunction; enlargement of the lips and other coarsening of facial features; overgrowth of the gums; liver dysfunction (hepatitis) and damage; bone-marrow depression; hirsutism (male-type hair growth in females); Peyronie's disease (a fibrous growth on the penis causing deflection and possible pain when erect).

Effects on Appetite and Body Weight as Disclosed by the Drug's Manufacturer

Weight gain; water retention.

Detailed Effects on Appetite and Body Weight

Treatment of compulsive eating disorder: A 79-pound, 25-year-old woman is described who, starting at the age of 15.5 years would consume enormous volumes of food, force herself to vomit, and then go to sleep. Obsessed by thoughts of food and showing an abnormal electroencephalogram (EEG) reading, she was placed on phenytoin. In 2 weeks she reported a "miracle," with no more compulsive eating episodes. Six months later, she was still symptom-free and approaching normal weight.

A group of 10 patients with compulsive eating disorder were treated with phenytoin. Four were underweight, 2 were of normal weight, and 4 were overweight. Nine of the 10 were treated successfully with phenytoin, reporting cessation of their eating compulsion.

A 23-year-old male weighing 307 pounds reported an uncontrollable urge to eat. He would consume a large meal at one restaurant and then proceed to another to repeat the process. He continued to restaurant-hop until the compulsion ended or his money ran out. His electroencephalogram (EEG) reading was abnormal and phenytoin was begun. After 8 weeks, he had lost 22 pounds without any conscious attempt to diet.

In a trial of 19 bulimics (bulimia is also a compulsive eating disorder) treated with phenytoin over a 12-week period, 6 showed a 75% reduction in binge-eating frequency. In a follow-up 18 months later, 2 of the 6 remained symptom-free.

Water loss: Eight normal subjects were given phenytoin by intravenous injection after a period of 16–20 hours of dehydration. Researchers found an increase in urine volume of 11–230%. This would seem to validate the hypothesis that phenytoin decreases the body's water volume.

Dosage Levels at Which Effects Occur
Treatment of compulsive eating disorder: Reported effective as low as 300mg. daily.
Water loss: Reported to occur at an intravenous dose of 500mg. daily.

Remedies
Treatment of compulsive eating disorder: Not applicable.
Water loss: None.

How Long It Takes Till Reversal of Drug Effects
It takes from 7–42 hours, depending on dosage and duration of therapy, for half the drug to be cleared from the blood.

Sources

Fichman, M.P., et al. "Inhibition of antidiuretic hormone secretion in diphenylhydantoin." *Archives of Neurology* (Chicago), 1970, 22: 45–53.

Green, R.S., Rau, J.H. "Treatment of compulsive eating disturbances with anticonvulsant medication." *American Journal of Psychiatry*, 1974, 131: 428–32.

Green, R.S., Rau, J.H. "The use of diphenylhydantoin in compulsive eating disorder: Further studies." In R.A. Vigersky, ed., *Anorexia Nervosa*. New York: Raven Press, 1977.

Rau, J.H., Green, R.S. "Compulsive eating: A neuropsychologic approach to certain eating disorders." *Comprehensive Psychiatry*, 1975, 16: 223–31.

Wermuth, B.M., et al. "Phenytoin treatment of the binge-eating syndrome." *American Journal of Psychiatry*, 1977, 134: 1249–53.

VALPROIC ACID

Brand Names
U.S.A.: Depakene (Abbott), Depakote (Abbott).
Canada: Depakene (Abbott).
Great Britain: Epilim (Labaz Sanofi).

What This Drug Does
Anticonvulsant.

How This Drug Affects Body Weight
May affect the hypothalamus portion of the brain which controls appetite. May also exert some effect on the storage of fat.

Government-Approved Uses for This Drug
To treat various types of epileptic seizures either alone or in combination with other drugs.

Unofficial Uses
To treat a variety of seizures including certain childhood seizure disorders.

When Not to Use This Drug
In liver disease or dysfunction; if allergic to this drug or to any related drug.

Side Effects From Use of This Drug
Various blood abnormalities; sedation; psychological changes; muscle weakness; tremors; inflammation of the mouth; nausea;

vomiting; upset stomach; abdominal cramps; constipation; inflammation of the pancreas; liver dysfunction; hair loss; irregular menses; secondary amenorrhea (cessation of menstruation); breast enlargement; galactorrhea (breast-milk flow unrelated to childbirth or nursing).

Effects on Appetite and Body Weight as Disclosed by the Drug's Manufacturer
Increased appetite; weight gain; loss of appetite.

Detailed Effects on Appetite and Body Weight
Weight gain: In a study of 63 patients taking valproic acid to control epilepsy, a 57% incidence of significant weight gain took place. Median weight increase was 16.5 pounds, with a range of 8.8–37.4 pounds. Attempts to effect weight loss by dietary restriction was difficult to accomplish while patients were still taking valproic acid.

In a group of 100 epileptic children, treatment with valproic acid caused increased appetite and excessive weight gain in 23 boys and 21 girls (44% total incidence). Although children would be expected to gain weight during the growing years, the gains shown to occur in this study exceeded those norms.

Treatment of bulimia: An 18-year-old female bulimic was given valproic acid. Within days of reaching therapeutic drug blood levels, her bulimic symptoms declined markedly. During 2 months of continued drug therapy, her binging ceased. When valproic acid was withdrawn, all bulimic symptoms reappeared within 3–4 weeks. At various intervals, when the drug was stopped, binging activity would reemerge within several days, only to remit with reintroduction of valproic acid.

Three patients suffering from bulimia, in conjunction with manic-depressive illness, were given valproic acid for 4–28 weeks. In two cases this was the only medication given and in the other instance, lithium was part of the therapy. In all three cases, marked decrease in bulimic symptoms occurred.

Dosage Levels at Which Effects Occur
Weight gain: May occur within the usual daily dosage range of 15–60mg. per kilogram of body weight (for a 150-pound man, this would be about 1,000–4,000mg. daily).

Treatment of bulimia: Reported effective at a daily dosage of 1,000–1,250mg.

Remedies
Weight gain: Substitution of low-calorie foods, beverages, and snacks for normal dietary intake may aid in reversing some valproic acid–induced weight gain.

Treatment of bulimia: Not applicable.

How Long It Takes Till Reversal Of Drug Effects
Half the dose of valproic acid is cleared from the blood within 6–16 hours. However, simultaneous use of other antiepileptic medication may decrease this to an average of 9 hours.

Sources
Dineen, H., et al. "Weight gain during treatment with valproate." *Acta Neurologica Scandinavica*, 1984, 70(2): 65–69.

Egger, J., Brett, E.M. "Effects of sodium valproate in 100 children with special reference to weight." *British Medical Journal*, 1981, 283: 577–81.

Herridge, P.L., Pope, H.G., Jr. "Treatment of bulimia and rapid-cycling bipolar disorder with sodium valproate." *Journal of Clinical Psychopharmacology*, 1985, 5: 229–30.

McElroy, S.L., et al. "Sodium valproate: Its use in primary psychiatric disorders." *Journal of Clinical Psychopharmacology*, 1987, 7: 16–24.

Antihistamines

ASTEMIZOLE

Brand Names
U.S.A.: Hismanal (Janssen).
Canada: Hismanal (Janssen).
Great Britain: Hismanal (Janssen).

What This Drug Does
  Antihistamine.

How This Drug Affects Body Weight
  A nonsedating antihistamine, astemizole partially binds serotonergic receptors in the body, functionally decreasing serotonin's effect. Since serotonin is thought to be an inhibitor of appetite,
this drug may increase the desire to eat.

Government-Approved Uses for This Drug
  To relieve symptoms of seasonal allergies; to treat symptoms
of various allergic responses.

Unofficial Uses
  None.

When Not to Use This Drug
  In newborn or premature infants; if taking a monoamine oxidase inhibitor drug; in nursing mothers; if pregnant; if allergic
to this drug or to any related drug.

Side Effects From Use of This Drug

Drowsiness; dizziness; loss of coordination; dry mouth; headache; nausea; diarrhea; abdominal pain; gas; skin rash; eczema; cough; joint pain.

Effects on Appetite and Body Weight as Disclosed by the Drug's Manufacturer

Increased appetite; increased weight.

Detailed Effects on Appetite and Body Weight

Increased appetite; increased body weight: In a study conducted in India, astemizole induced some appetite increases among 30 allergy sufferers. Two subjects reported weight increases as well.

In a double-blind study of 46 patients treated with astemizole, increased appetite was the single most common side effect reported in all phases of the trial. It affected 17% of subjects in one group and 19% in another. After 8 weeks of astemizole use, average weight gain was 2.64 pounds, with a maximum reported increase of 12.76 pounds.

In a 10–14 week study of astemizole in 55 patients, 20% reported increased appetite, averaging a weight gain of 2 pounds. When external variables were adjusted for in comparing astemizole to a placebo, 18 of 28 patients gained weight during the first month of active drug use. In those who agreed to a 1-year extended trial of astemizole, no further weight gain was noted. It is interesting to note that the main objection given by subjects to participating in long-term studies of astemizole use was the drug's effects on body weight.

Taste disturbance: In an 8-week study of 42 patients treated with astemizole, 7% complained of altered taste sensations (bitter, metallic, or other peculiar taste).

Dosage Levels at Which Effects Occur

Increased appetite; increased body weight: Reported as low as 10mg. daily.
Taste disturbance: Reported as low as 10mg. daily.

Remedies

A decrease in daily dosage could help alleviate astemizole's effects on appetite and body weight. But this must be carefully balanced against maintaining adequate therapeutic blood levels.

A switch to a different agent in the same therapeutic category could accomplish similar benefits while minimizing undesirable dietary influences. Consult your physician.

Increased appetite; increased body weight: Substitution of low-calorie foods, beverages, and snacks for normal dietary intake may aid in reversing some drug-induced weight gain.

Taste disturbance: Astemizole-induced taste disturbance may be countered in several ways. Taking the drug with an adequate fluid intake, chewing sugarless gum or using a mouthwash of water and lemon juice, and practicing good oral hygiene may help restore normal taste sensation.

How Long It Takes Till Reversal of Drug Effects

It takes about 4.3 days for half the dose of astemizole to be eliminated from the body. Since its active metabolite, desmethylastemizole, has a half-life of about 12 days, the drug's effects may linger considerably longer.

Sources

Kailasam, V., Mathews, P. "Controlled clinical assessment of astemizole in the treatment of chronic idiopathic urticaria and angioedema." *Journal of the American Academy of Dermatology*, 1987, 16(4): 797–804.

Sooknundun, M., et al. "Treatment of allergic rhinitis with a new long-acting H1 receptor antagonist: astemizole." *Annals of Allergy*, 1987, 58: 78–81.

Wihl, J.A., et al. "Effect of the nonsedative H-receptor antagonist astemizole in perennial allergic and nonallergic rhinitis." *Journal of Allergy and Clinical Immunology*, 1985, 75(6): 720–27.

CYPROHEPTADINE

Brand Names
U.S.A.: Periactin (MSD).
Canada: Periactin (MSD), Vimicon (Frosst).
Great Britain: Periactin (MSD).

What This Drug Does
Antihistamine.

How This Drug Affects Body Weight
Cyproheptadine, an inhibitor of serotonin, has been known to stimulate appetite. It has been speculated that serotonin, a chem-

ical messenger naturally occurring in the brain and intestines, may influence the subjective appreciation of hunger by inhibiting appetite. Cyproheptadine's tendency to cause drowsiness and physical inactivity has also been linked to weight gain by lowering caloric output.

Government-Approved Uses for This Drug

To relieve symptoms of seasonal hay fever and other allergic responses; to relieve itching and rash due to cold temperatures.

Unofficial Uses

As an appetite stimulant; to treat migraine cluster headaches.

When Not to Use This Drug

In glaucoma; in urinary retention; in peptic ulcer; in certain bladder and intestinal obstructions; in elderly or debilitated patients; in bronchial asthma; in newborn or premature infants; if a nursing mother; if taking a monoamine oxidase inhibitor drug; in enlarged prostate; if allergic to this drug or to any related drug.

Side Effects From Use of This Drug

Drowsiness; dizziness; loss of coordination; mental confusion; insomnia; restlessness; burning sensations of the skin; various skin reactions including sensitivity to sunlight; inner ear disturbance; visual disturbance; low blood pressure; heartbeat irregularities; blood abnormalities; fatigue; stomach upset; vomiting; diarrhea or constipation (reported with equal frequency); difficult or frequent urination; dry mouth, nose, and throat; thickened bronchial mucus; headache; chills; nasal congestion; early menses.

Effects on Appetite and Body Weight as Disclosed by the Drug's Manufacturer

Anorexia; weight gain; increased appetite; water retention.

Detailed Effects on Appetite and Body Weight

Weight gain: Cyproheptadine originally was found to stimulate the appetite and induce weight gains during studies on its use in treating childhood asthma. (It is sad to note the drug's promotion in India as a tonic and general appetite stimulant in light of that nation's real problem of food shortages.) In general, weight is gained most rapidly during the first few weeks of cyproheptadine use and is lost after its withdrawal.

Sixteen university students (13 males and 3 females), 15 of whom were below their ideal body weight, were given cyproheptadine for 4 weeks. Of the 9 who completed the trial, all gained appreciably more weight than a control group administered a placebo (an inert substance). Average weight gain for those given the active drug was 4.4 pounds versus 0.5 pound for the placebo group. All but 1 student given cyproheptadine reported greater hunger ratings than those in the control group.

In a study of 97 adults suffering from irritable-colon syndrome and who were chronically underweight, cyproheptadine had a positive effect on both appetite and body weight. After 12 weeks of treatment, the average total weight gain was about 12 pounds. Of those given the drug, 27.3% were considered successfully treated. Appetite was stimulated most in the group that initially reported a small appetite (as opposed to no appetite or moderate appetite).

In a 6-week study of 12 adults, administration of cyproheptadine to half the group over a 2-week period induced weight gains of from about 3 to almost 7 pounds, with an average of 4.84 pounds. Four of the 6 subjects receiving cyproheptadine reported increased appetite.

Treatment of anorexia nervosa: A 12-year-old female experienced 3 months of marked weight loss following dental anesthesia. After receiving a variety of antipsychotic medications and vitamin therapy, the patient went from 57 pounds to 71 pounds. At this point, cyproheptadine was initiated. Average weight gains over the next 6 months were 1.25 pounds per week. Dosage was gradually decreased after 8 months, and with withdrawal of the medication body weight stabilized at about 102 pounds. At a follow-up exam 6 months later, the patient still weighed 102 pounds.

Sixty underweight adults suffering from anorexia nervosa were enrolled in a 3-month study comparing the effectiveness of cyproheptadine to placebo. At the end of the trial, average weight gain was 6.5 pounds, most of this occurring in the first month of therapy. Those taking placebo had an average gain of 2.8 pounds. Those given the active medication reported almost twice the appetite increase claimed by those in the placebo group.

In a 12-week study of 81 anorectic patients of both sexes and of various ages, subjects were divided into five groups, each receiving different dosages of cyproheptadine ranging from none (a placebo) to 8mg. daily. At the end of 3 months, weight gains, presented as percentage increases over starting weight, ranged from 1.2% for the placebo group to 11.2% for those at the maximum daily dosage of cyproheptadine.

Dosage Levels at Which Effects Occur
Weight gain: Reported as low as 6mg. daily.
Treatment of anorexia nervosa: Reported as low as 2mg. daily. One regimen calls for a starting dose of 12mg. daily with an increase of 4mg. every 5 days if less than 1.1 pounds is gained over the previous 5 days. A maximum dose of 32mg. daily is suggested.

Remedies
Weight gain: Although commonly used to increase body weight, substitution of low-calorie foods, beverages, and snacks for normal dietary intake may aid in reversing some cyproheptadine-induced weight gain.
Treatment of anorexia nervosa: Not applicable.

How Long It Takes Till Reversal of Drug Effects
Cyproheptadine's duration of action is about 8 hours.

Sources
Benady, D.R. "Cyproheptadine hydrochloride (Periactin) and anorexia nervosa: A case report." *British Journal of Psychiatry*, 1970, 117: 681–82.

"Cyproheptadine." *Lancet*, 1978, 1: 367.

Goldberg, S.G., et al. "Cyproheptadine in anorexia nervosa." *British Journal of Psychiatry*, 1979, 134: 67–70.

Lavenstein, A.F., et al. "Effect of cyproheptadine on asthmatic children." *Journal of the American Medical Association*, 1962, 180: 912–16.

Mainguet, P. "Effect of cyproheptadine on anorexia and loss of weight in adults." *Practitioner*, 1972, 208(1248): 797–800.

Noble, R.E. "Effect of cyproheptadine on appetite and weight gain." *Journal of the American Medical Association*, 1969, 209(13): 2054–55.

Pawlowski, G.J. "Cyproheptadine: Weight-gain and appetite stimulation in essential anorexic adults." *Current Therapeutic Research, Clinical and Experimental*, 1975, 18(5): 673–78.

Silbert, M.V. "The weight gain effect of Periactin in anorexic patients." *South African Medical Journal*, 1971, 45: 374–77.

Silverstone, T., Schuyler, D. "The effect of cyproheptadine on hunger, calorie intake, and body weight in man." *Psychopharmacologia*, 1975, 40: 335–40.

Steil, J.N., et al. "Studies on the mechanism of cyproheptadine-induced weight gain in human subjects." *Metabolism*, 1970, 19(3): 192–200.

TERFENADINE

Brand Names
U.S.A.: Seldane (Merrell Dow).
Canada: None.
Great Britain: Triludan (Merrell).

What This Drug Does
Antihistamine.

How This Drug Affects Body Weight
A nonsedating antihistamine, terfenadine partially binds serotonergic receptors in the body, functionally decreasing serotonin's effect. Since serotonin is thought to be an inhibitor of
appetite, this drug may increase the desire to eat.

Government-Approved Uses for This Drug
To treat symptoms associated with various allergic responses.

Unofficial Uses
To treat certain lower respiratory bronchoconstriction and
bronchospasm.

When Not to Use This Drug
In children under 12 years; if taking a monoamine oxidase
inhibitor drug; in nursing mothers; if pregnant; if allergic to this
drug or to any related drug.

Side Effects From Use of This Drug
Drowsiness; headache; fatigue; dizziness; nervousness; weakness; abdominal distress; nausea; vomiting; changes in bowel
habits; dry mouth, nose, and throat; cough; sore throat; nosebleed; skin itching or eruption; hair loss; depression; insomnia;
nightmares; palpitation; sweating; fast heartbeat; difficulty in
urinating; visual disturbances; galactorrhea (breast-milk flow);
menstrual disorders.

Effects on Appetite and Body Weight as Disclosed by the Drug's Manufacturer
Increased appetite; weight gain.

Detailed Effects on Appetite and Body Weight
Detailed manufacturer's disclosure: Although terfenadine's official literature lists increased appetite and weight gain as potential side effects, more detailed information from independent sources is unavailable.

Appetite increase is known to occur in under 1% of those taking this medication.

Dosage Levels at Which Effects Occur
May occur at the usual daily dose of 120mg.

Remedies
Increased appetite; weight gain: Substitution of low-calorie foods, beverages, and snacks for normal dietary intake may aid in reversing some terfenadine-induced weight gain.

How Long It Takes Till Reversal of Drug Effects
Terfenadine's duration of action may persist for up to 12 hours.

Sources
Olin, B.R. (ed.). *Facts and Comparisons*. St. Louis: Facts and Comparisons, 1988.
Physicians' Desk Reference. Oradell, NJ: Medical Economics, 1988.
USP DI. Rockville, MD: The United States Pharmacopeial Convention, Inc., 1989.

Antimigraine Drugs

METHYSERGIDE

Brand Names
U.S.A.: Sansert (Sandoz).
Canada: Sansert (Sandoz).
Great Britain: Deseril (Wander).

What This Drug Does
Antimigraine.

How This Drug Affects Body Weight
Methysergide blocks or inhibits serotonin. It has been speculated that serotonin, a chemical messenger occurring naturally in the brain and intestines, may influence the subjective appreciation of hunger by inhibiting appetite.

Government-Approved Uses for This Drug
To treat migraine headache.

Unofficial Uses
None.

When Not to Use This Drug
In the presence of various diseases of the heart and circulatory system; in lung disease; in connective-tissue disorders; if there is impaired liver or kidney function; in serious infection; in debilitated states; if pregnant; if a nursing mother; in children; if allergic to this drug or to any related drug.

Side Effects From Use of This Drug

Nausea; vomiting; constipation or diarrhea (more common); stomach upset; insomnia; drowsiness; euphoria; light-headedness; weakness; hallucinations; various heart problems; constriction of the blood vessels (causing chest or abdominal pain and insufficient circulation to the lower limbs); coldness, numbness, or pain in the extremities; fast heartbeat; nasal congestion; various blood abnormalities; hair loss; facial flushing; sweating; various skin reactions; tissue damage in an area surrounding the large blood vessels of the lower back space (may cause fatigue, weight gain, backache, weakness, various urinary problems); tissue damage to the lungs.

Effects on Appetite and Body Weight as Disclosed by the Drug's Manufacturer

Water retention; weight gain.

Detailed Effects on Appetite and Body Weight

Increased appetite; weight gain: Methysergide appears to cause increased appetite and subsequent weight gain. This was first thought to be a by-product of headache relief, the drug's intended purpose, but methysergide was later found to cause this effect whether or not the drug provided pain relief.

Water retention: Water retention, primarily in the legs, is frequently encountered with methysergide use. It may be linked to lymphatic obstruction or to a disturbance of the venous and lymphatic channels, a particular hazard of this medication.

Dosage Levels at Which Effects Occur

Increased appetite; weight gain; water retention: May occur within the usual daily dosage range of 4–8mg.

Remedies

Increased appetite; weight gain: Substitution of low-calorie foods, beverages, and snacks for normal dietary intake may aid in reversing some drug-induced weight gain.

Water retention: Mild water retention may be controlled by dietary salt restriction, diuretics, or a lowering of daily dosages. If edema is severe or does not respond to these measures, physical obstruction may be at fault.

How Long It Takes Till Reversal of Drug Effects
Methysergide's duration of action is 3–4 hours.

Source
Graham, J.R. "Current therapeutics—methysergide." *Practitioner*, 1967, 198: 302–11.

Antiobesity Drugs

AMPHETAMINE

Brand Names
U.S.A.: Biphetamine (Pennwalt), Delcobese (Lemmon), Desoxyn (Abbott), Dexampex (Lemmon), Dexedrine (SKF), Ferndex (Ferndale), Methampex (Lemmon), Obetrol (Obetrol), Oxydess II (Vortech), Spancap No.1 (Vortech).
Canada: Benzedrine (SKF), Dexedrine (SKF).
Great Britain: Dexedrine (SKF), Durophet (Riker).

What This Drug Does
Appetite suppressant.

How This Drug Affects Body Weight
Believed to cause general brain stimulation. May effect a release of norepinephrine (a neurotransmitter) and, at higher doses, dopamine (a precursor of norepinephrine). This may lead to increased availability of these substances to stimulate nerve receptors. The reasons for this drug causing appetite suppression have not been definitely determined but are thought to result from direct stimulation on the satiety center in the hypothalamic and limbic areas of the brain.

Government-Approved Uses for This Drug
To treat narcolepsy (a disease marked by sudden sleep attacks); to treat hyperactivity and attention-span disorders in children; as a short-term aid to weight loss.

Unofficial Uses
None.

When Not to Use This Drug
With certain heart and circulatory disorders; if you have high blood pressure; in the presence of overactive thyroid; in glaucoma; if there is a history of drug abuse; within 14 days following the use of a monoamine oxidase inhibitor drug; if suffering from anxiety or nervous tension; if allergic to this or any related drug.

Side Effects From Use of This Drug
Rapid or irregular heartbeat; increased blood pressure; restlessness; dizziness; difficulty in sleeping; headache; euphoria; dry mouth; tremor; hives; possible psychotic experiences; diarrhea or constipation (reported with equal frequency); impotence; changes in libido.

Warning: Amphetamines have a very high addiction potential. When used in high doses over prolonged periods of time, amphetamine psychosis (a condition resembling paranoid schizophrenia) may occur. Blood pressure is elevated by amphetamines and may cause heart attacks, strokes, and various other medical crises.

Effects on Appetite and Body Weight as Disclosed by the Drug's Manufacturer
Unpleasant taste; anorexia; weight loss.

Detailed Effects on Appetite and Body Weight
Weight loss: In a study of 55 obese diabetic adults, amphetamine was added to a regimen of dietary restriction in an effort to effect weight loss in these patients. The end result was to allow them better diabetic control. Although amphetamine and related drugs should not ordinarily be administered to diabetics in view of their potential to raise blood-sugar levels and increase blood pressure, it was felt that an aggressive weight-loss program was an acceptable trade-off in these patients. Over a 1-year period 65% of subjects lost 11–77 pounds. Of 31% of these subjects taking insulin, 84% were able to decrease or discontinue its use due to better diabetic control.

In an investigation of 90 overweight subjects given amphetamine for 2.7–11.8 months following a period of diet alone, a range of weight loss of 1.1–18 pounds per month was recorded.

Initial losses were usually greater than those over longer periods of time. Most weight loss was seen in the first 1–2 months of treatment, with long-term weight loss comparable to that by diet alone.

In a 12-week trial of dextroamphetamine given to a group of obese females, the average weight loss was 6.26 pounds. The drug seemed to produce best results within the first 6 weeks, losing effectiveness after 6–8 weeks of use. Additional weight loss was minimal during the last 4 weeks of the study.

A pioneering experiment conducted in the 1930's involved 13 patients taking amphetamine. They lost an average of 16 pounds over about a 20-week period. This compared favorably with the same group averaging only a 1.67-pound loss over about a 15-week period without amphetamine. The authors of the study state that amphetamine-induced weight loss occurred at a 7 times faster rate than with diet alone. Using 14 subjects from the same population, the researchers showed the amphetamine group losing an average of 6.2 pounds in 4 weeks versus 2.7 pounds in the unmedicated group.

Treatment of bulimia: In a small-scale study of 8 bulimic patients (7 females and 1 male) given methylamphetamine by intravenous injection, the drug was found to decrease self-ratings of hunger, decrease the quantity of food consumed by all patients, and suppress bulimic symptoms. Although bulimic overeating has been considered unrelated to feelings of hunger, amphetamine may aid this condition by countering the mood that triggers bulimia.

Dosage Levels at Which Effects Occur
Weight loss: Reported as low as 10mg. daily.
Treatment of bulimia: Effective at 15mg. per 165 pounds of body weight per dose.

Remedies
Not applicable.

How Long It Takes Till Reversal of Drug Effects
Weight loss: In one study where 65% of subjects lost 11–77 pounds over 1 year of amphetamine use, 19% showed further but minor weight loss 1 year after withdrawal of the drug; 41% regained less than 10 pounds, while 40% regained 11–26 pounds.

The time it takes for half this drug's dose to be cleared from the blood varies from 7–33 hours, depending on the pH (a measure of acidity or basicity) of the urine. Acid urine will decrease this time while a basic medium will extend the duration of action. Accordingly, reversal of side effects may vary considerably after discontinuation of this drug. There is also a strong psychological component to the perception of amphetamine's effects.

Sources

Adlersberg, D., Mayer, M.E. "Results of prolonged medical treatment of obesity with diet alone, diet and thyroid preparations, and diet and amphetamine." *Journal of Clinical Endocrinology*, 1949, 9: 275.

Ong, Y.L., et al. "Suppression of bulimic symptoms with methylamphetamine." *British Journal of Psychiatry*, 1983, 143: 288–93.

Osserman, K.E., Dolger, H. "Obesity in diabetes: A study of therapy with anorexigenic drugs." *Annals of Internal Medicine*, 1951, 34: 72.

Rosenthal, G., Solomon, H.A. "Benzedrine sulfate in obesity." *Endocrinology*, 1940, 26: 807–12.

Seaton, D.A., et al. "A comparison of the appetite suppressing properties of dexamphetamine and phentermine." *Scottish Medical Journal*, 1964, 9: 482–85.

BENZOCAINE

Brand Names
U.S.A.: †Ayds Appetite Suppressant (Jeffrey Martin),†Slim-Line (Thompson).
Canada: Teething Syrup (Sabex).
Great Britain: AAA Mouth and Throat Spray (Armour), Medilave Gel (Martindale).

What This Drug Does
Anesthetic.

How This Drug Affects Body Weight
Benzocaine's anesthetic properties decrease the ability to detect sweet-tasting substances. Deadening of taste sensations may counteract a prime motivating factor in eating behavior.

---

†Denotes over-the-counter availability in the U.S.A.

Government-Approved Uses for This Drug
As an aid to weight reduction.

Unofficial Uses
None.

When Not to Use This Drug
If allergic to this drug or to any related drug.

Side Effects From Use of This Drug
Various allergic skin reactions; possible intolerance to this drug.

Effects on Appetite and Body Weight as Disclosed by the Drug's Manufacturer
None.

Detailed Effects on Appetite and Body Weight
Weight loss: In a 6-week study of 52 subjects, 34 were given benzocaine lozenges to aid in weight loss. Those remaining were given a placebo. By the sixth week, 46% of those using benzocaine lozenges lost at least 8 pounds, while similar results were reported by only 4% of the placebo group. Of those using active medication and completing the full 6-week program, 92% reported at least mild appetite suppression.

The results of treatment with benzocaine lozenges on a series of 100 overweight patients were reported by one physician. Subjects were instructed to dissolve one lozenge on the tongue 15–20 minutes before eating or whenever they felt hungry. Appetite was seen to decrease markedly after 5–7 days. Continuous use was necessary in order to maintain the drug's effect. Average weight loss was 2 pounds per week for the first 11 weeks, but after several months, one-third of the patients began to regain lost weight.

A group of 50 adults who were 12–102 pounds overweight took part in a 10-week trial using benzocaine-methylcellulose gum. One or two pieces were chewed for 5–10 minutes followed by drinking a glass of water just before meals. The gum could be chewed every few hours if patients felt hungry. Forty-five (90%) of the subjects lost weight, with an average loss of 2.3 pounds per week for the first third of the trial period and 1.8 pounds on average thereafter.

Dosage Levels at Which Effects Occur
Weight loss: When used as a lozenge, weight loss occurred at 3.25–5mg. of benzocaine per lozenge, with an average consumption quoted in one study of 17.4 lozenges daily.

Weight loss occurred when used as a candy-coated chewing gum containing methylcellulose and 4.3mg of benzocaine per piece.

Remedies
Not applicable.

How Long It Takes Till Reversal of Drug Effects
Benzocaine reaches its peak effect in about 1 minute, with a duration of action of 30–60 minutes.

Sources
Collipp, P.J. "The treatment of exogenous obesity by medical benzocaine candy: A double-blind placebo study." *Obesity and Bariatric Medicine*, 1981, 10(5): 123–25.

Gould, W.L. "Obesity and hypertension: The importance of a safe compound to control appetite." *North Carolina Medical Journal*, 1950, 11: 327.

Lindner, P.G., et al. "The future of obesity treatment (Part 1)." *Obesity and Bariatric Medicine*, 1982, 11(3): 83–88.

McClure, C.W., Brusch, C.A. "Treatment of oral syndrome obesity with non-traditional appetite control plan." *Journal of the Women's Medical Association*, 1973, 28: 239.

Plotz, M. "Obesity." *Medical Times*, 1958, 86: 860–63.

CHLORPHENTERMINE

Brand Names
U.S.A.: Chlorphen (Robinson).
Canada: Pre-Sate (Parke-Davis).
Great Britain: None.

What This Drug Does
Appetite suppressant.

How This Drug Affects Body Weight
Related to amphetamines, chlorphentermine is believed to cause general brain stimulation. It may induce release of dopamine and norepinephrine (chemical messengers) while also blocking their

removal. This can lead to increased availability of these neurotransmitters to stimulate nerve receptors. The reasons for this drug causing appetite suppression have not been definitely determined but are thought to result from direct stimulation on the satiety center in the hypothalamic and limbic areas of the brain.

Government-Approved Uses for This Drug
To aid in weight loss (short-term).

Unofficial Uses
None.

When Not to Use This Drug
In advanced arteriosclerosis; in certain cardiovascular disease; in high blood pressure; in glaucoma; in agitated states; if there is a history of drug abuse; if taking or have taken within the last 14 days any monoamine oxidase inhibitor drug; in children under 12 years of age; if allergic to this drug or to any related drug.

Side Effects From Use of This Drug
Nervousness; dizziness; insomnia; palpitations; fast heartbeat; elevation of blood pressure; dry mouth; nausea; constipation or diarrhea (reported with equal frequency); skin eruption; impotence; changes in libido.

Effects on Appetite and Body Weight as Disclosed by the Drug's Manufacturer
Unpleasant taste.

Detailed Effects on Appetite and Body Weight
Weight loss: In a 12-week study of 29 obese males taking chlorphentermine, average weight loss was 0.5 pounds per week during the course of the trial; 21 (72%) subjects lost 1–30 pounds, while 8 (28%) patients actually gained from 0.5–7.5 pounds.

In an 8-week trial where 25 obese subjects were given both chlorphentermine and placebo, average weight loss was consistently greater during active drug periods. Weight loss while on chlorphentermine ranged from 4.89–9.63 pounds, while placebo use resulted in a loss of 2.13–3.54 pounds.

In a 2-month trial of chlorphentermine, 18 patients more than 15% overweight completed the study. All were given the active drug for 4 weeks and a placebo for the same period of time.

Average weight loss during chlorphentermine use was 4.8 pounds as compared with only 0.08 pounds for the inactive preparation.

In a 12-week study of the effects of chlorphentermine, the first 6 weeks produced an average weight loss of 4.7 pounds in a group of 14 patients. Of those who lost weight, the range was 2.25–13.5 pounds. During the second 6 weeks, a group of 15 subjects given dextroamphetamine during the first period averaged only 1.8 pounds per patient of additional weight loss when taking chlorphentermine. Weight loss was more significant when chlorphentermine was the first drug used.

Dosage Levels at Which Effects Occur
Weight loss: Reported at either 25mg. taken 3 times daily (75mg. total daily dosage) or as a longer-acting dosage form of 65mg. taken once in the morning.

Remedies
Not applicable.

How Long It Takes Till Reversal of Drug Effects
Half the dose of chlorphentermine is cleared from the blood in 40 hours.

Sources
Fineberg, S.K. "Evaluation of anorexigenic agents, studies with chlorphentermine." *American Journal of Clinical Nutrition*, 1962, 11: 509–16.

Hadler, A.T. "Weight reduction with phenmetrazine and chlorphentermine, a double-blind study." *Current Therapeutic Research, Clinical and Experimental*, 1967, 9: 563–69.

Lacey, C., Hadden, D.R. "Chlorphentermine—a new 'appetite suppressant.' A crossover double-blind trial." *Ulster Medical Journal*, 1962, 31: 181–85.

Levin, J., et al. "Chlorphentermine in the management of obesity." *Practitioner*, 1963, 191: 65–70.

CHOLECYSTOKININ

Brand Names
U.S.A.: CCK (Pharmacia; was produced under this brand name but has been off the market since 1986).
Canada: Cholecystokinin [CCK] (Pharmacia).

Great Britain: Cholecystokinin (Kabi Diagnostica); Pancreo-zymin (Boots).

What This Drug Does
Diagnostic aid.

How This Drug Affects Body Weight
Cholecystokinin, a hormone manufactured in the small intes-tine, is released in response to ingested food. It may be part of a negative feedback system whereby its release signals the brain that enough food has been eaten. Based on this theory, it has been used therapeutically as a natural appetite suppressant to produce a feeling of satiety. It may also prolong gastric emptying by activating vagal nerve fibers. These act to inhibit gastric smooth muscle (one of which is the stomach).

Government-Approved Uses for This Drug
Before being removed from the U.S. market, cholecystokinin was used as a diagnostic aid for gallbladder disease, studies of the small bowel, and pancreatic insufficiency.

Unofficial Uses
None.

When Not to Use This Drug
If allergic to this drug or to any related drug.

Side Effects From Use of This Drug
Stomach ache; epigastric discomfort; flushing (if drug is given too rapidly).

Effects on Appetite and Body Weight as Disclosed by the Drug's Manufacturer
None.

Detailed Effects on Appetite and Body Weight
Decreased appetite: Many studies have confirmed cholecysto-kinin's promise as a natural appetite suppressant. These conclu-sions, however, must be tempered with its limitation of not being orally active. Intravenous infusion is the only route of adminis-tration. As an additional caveat, the drug's long-term effects have not yet been determined.

A 12-subject study was conducted to determine if cholecystokinin would have the same appetite-inhibiting effect in humans as it has in animals. All subjects were lean, healthy males who received the drug by intravenous infusion. In a 6-day protocol, the entire group showed a marked decrease in food intake.

In a group of 12 nonobese males given cholecystokinin before meals, food intake was decreased significantly as compared with the results seen with infusion of an inactive saline solution. Average decrease in food consumption was 122 grams (about 0.25 pound), with eating time shortened by about 16%.

An experiment involving 8 obese males given cholecystokinin by intravenous infusion yielded significantly inhibited food intake in 6. The average decrease in food intake over placebo (normal saline infusion) was about 13%. The duration of eating time was reduced by about 22% when subjects were given the active drug.

In a survey of the literature presented by one author, cholecystokinin use has decreased food intake by anywhere from 12–50%.

Dosage Levels at Which Effects Occur
Decreased appetite: Reported effective at the following dosages: (1) from 4–9.2 nanograms per kilogram per minute during meal; (2) at an average of 31 nanograms per kilogram per minute during meal; (3) from 1.5–3.0 Ivy Dog Units per kilogram per 15 minutes.

Remedies
Not applicable.

How Long It Takes Till Reversal of Drug Effects
Decreased appetite: Cholecystokinin has a very short duration of action and must be administered near the time of each meal.

Sources
Kissileff, H.R., et al. "Cholecystokinin-octapeptide (CCK-8) decreases food intake in man." *Clinical Research*, 1979, 27: 552A.

Kissileff, H.R., et al. "C-terminal octapeptide of cholecystokinin decreases food intake in man." *American Journal of Clinical Nutrition*, 1981, 34: 154–60.

Pi-Sunyer, X., et al. "C-terminal octapeptide of cholecystokinin decreases food intake in obese men." *Physiology and Behavior*, 1982, 29: 627–30.

Smith, G.P. "The therapeutic potential of cholecystokinin." *International Journal of Obesity*, 1984, 8(supp. 1): 35–38.

Smith G.P., et al. "The satiety effect of cholecystokinin: A progress report." *Peptides*, 1981, 2(supp. 2): 57–59.

Stacher, G.H., et al. "Cholecystokinin octapeptide decreases intake of solid food in man." *Peptides*, 1982, 3: 133–36.

DIETHYLPROPION

Brand Names
U.S.A.: Depletite-25 (Reid-Provident), Tenuate (Merrell Dow), Tenuate Dospan (Merrell Dow), Tepanil (Riker), Tepanil Ten-Tab (Riker).
Canada: Dietic (Pharbec), Nobesine (Nadeau), Propion (Pro Doc), Regibon (Medic), Tenuate (Merrell).
Great Britain: Apisate (Wyeth), Tenuate Dospan (Merrell).

What This Drug Does
Appetite suppressant.

How This Drug Affects Body Weight
Believed to cause general brain stimulation. May induce release of dopamine and norepinephrine (chemical messengers) while also blocking their removal. This can lead to increased availability of these neurotransmitters to stimulate nerve receptors. The reasons for this drug causing appetite suppression have not been definitely established but are thought to result from direct stimulation on the satiety center in the hypothalamic and limbic areas of the brain.

Government-Approved Uses for This Drug
To aid in weight loss (short-term).

Unofficial Uses
None.

When Not to Use This Drug
In advanced arteriosclerosis; in certain cardiovascular disease; in high blood pressure; in glaucoma; in agitated states; if there is a history of drug abuse; if taking or have taken within the last 14 days any monoamine oxidase inhibitor drug; in children under 12 years of age; if allergic to this drug or to any related drug.

Side Effects From Use of This Drug
Nervousness; dizziness; insomnia; palpitations; fast heartbeat; elevation of blood pressure; dry mouth; nausea; constipation or

diarrhea (reported with equal frequency); skin eruption; impotence; changes in libido; gynecomastia (enlargement of the male breasts); menstrual upset.

Effects on Appetite and Body Weight as Disclosed by the Drug's Manufacturer
Unpleasant taste.

Detailed Effects on Appetite and Body Weight
Weight loss: In a 12-week study of a patient population treated with diethylpropion and broken up into three study groups, average cumulative weight loss ranged from 9.7–14.9 pounds. In those taking the drug continuously, the figure was 14.9 pounds. Among those given diethylpropion for 4 weeks on and 4 weeks off, average weight loss was 9.7 pounds.

In a 24-week study of diethylpropion in a long-acting dosage form, administration of 1 tablet daily at 2 P.M. was compared in two groups. One group received the drug continuously and the other was given it in alternating months. The continuously dosed group realized an average total weight loss of about 21 pounds, while an average of only 15 pounds was recorded for the other group.

In a broad-based study of 121 obese patients seen in a general medical practice, diethylpropion's weight-reducing effect was studied and compared over differing lengths of time. In those taking it 2 months or less, average weight loss was 14.5 pounds. Those taking the drug for 2.1–4 months saw an average loss of 25.3 pounds; from 4.1–6 months, 26.4 pounds; from 6.1–8 months, 30 pounds; from 8.1–10 months, 46 pounds; from 10.1–12 months, 50 pounds; from 12.1–14 months, 55.2 pounds; from 14.1–16 months, 33 pounds. According to this study, diethylpropion's effects are maximized at 14 months, after which weight tends to be regained despite continued use of the drug.

In a 10-week study of 44 patients who were an average 56 pounds overweight, subjects were split into two groups. One received diethylpropion and the other a placebo. Average total weight loss for those taking the active drug was 14.8 pounds, while those on placebo lost an average of only 9 pounds.

In a Danish study of 43 subjects who were 20–80% overweight and who completed 12 weeks of diethylpropion use, the median weight loss was 18.5 pounds, with 72% losing 11 pounds or more.

Dosage Levels at Which Effects Occur
Weight loss: The usual daily dose of diethylpropion is 75mg., taken either all at once in a long-acting dosage form, or 3 times daily as a 25mg. tablet.

Remedies
Not applicable.

How Long It Takes Till Reversal of Drug Effects
It takes about 3 hours for diethylpropion to be eliminated from the body, depending on the pH (a measure of acidity or basicity) of the urine. Acid urine will decrease this time, while a basic medium will extend the duration of action. There is also a strong psychological component to the perception of diethylpropion's effects.

Sources
Bolding. O.T. "Diethylpropion hydrochloride: An effective appetite suppressant." *Current Therapeutic Research*, 1974, 16: 40–48.

LeRiche, W.H., Csima, A. "A long-acting appetite suppressant." *Canadian Medical Association Journal*, 1967, 97: 1016.

Malchow-Møller, A., et al. "Ephedrine as an anorectic: The story of the 'Elsinore Pill.'" *International Journal of Obesity*, 1981, 5: 183–87.

Matthews, P.A. "Diethylpropion in the treatment of obese patients seen in general practice." *Current Therapeutic Research*, 1975, 17: 340–46.

Nolan, G.R. "Use of an anorexic drug in a total weight reduction program in private practice." *Current Therapeutic Research, Clinical and Experimental*, 1975, 18(2): 332–37.

EPHEDRINE

Brand Names
U.S.A.: †*Amesec (Glaxo) †Efed II (Alto), †Ephedrine Sulfate (various manufacturers), †Efedron Nasal (Hyrex), †Vatronol Nose Drops (Vicks Health Care).

† Denotes over-the-counter availability in the U.S.A.
*Combination drug.

Canada: Manufactured under generic name "ephedrine" by A&H, Abbott, S&N.

Great Britain
*Amesec (Lilly), *Asmapax (Nicholas), *Asthma Dellipsoids D17 (Pilsworth), *Bronchial Dellipsoids D15 (Pilsworth), *Bronchotone (Rorer), *CAM (Rybar), *Expansyl Spansule (SKF), *Franol (Winthrop), *Iodo-Ephedrine (Philip Harris), *Phyldrox (Carlton), *Tedral (General Diagnostics).

What This Drug Does
Stimulates the sympathetic (involuntary) nervous system.

How This Drug Affects Body Weight
Ephedrine is believed to cause general brain stimulation. It has not been definitely determined why this drug causes appetite suppression but the phenomenon is thought to result from direct stimulation on the satiety center in the hypothalamic and limbic areas of the brain. Ephedrine may also increase energy expenditure and, to a lesser degree, decrease the appetite. It may increase the body's metabolic rate without increasing food intake.

Government-Approved Uses for This Drug
To treat various allergic disorders such as bronchial asthma; to treat nasal congestion; to treat low blood pressure; to treat sudden fainting caused by complete heart block (Stokes-Adams syndrome); to treat narcolepsy (sudden sleep attacks).

Unofficial Uses
As an appetite suppressant.

When Not to Use This Drug
In certain glaucoma; if receiving certain anesthetics; with certain thyroid abnormalities; in diabetes; with high blood pressure; with certain heart problems; if allergic to this drug or to any related drug.

Side Effects From Use of This Drug
Insomnia; nervousness; dizziness; headache; mental confusion; muscle weakness; euphoria; excessive sweating; fast heart-

*Combination drug.

beat; palpitations; high blood pressure; dry nose and throat; nausea; vomiting; difficulty in urinating; difficult breathing.

Effects on Appetite and Body Weight as Disclosed by the Drug's Manufacturer
Loss of appetite.

Detailed Effects on Appetite and Body Weight
Weight loss: An Italian study of 10 obese females given ephedrine for 2 months showed an average weight loss of about 5.3 pounds when combined with a low-calorie diet. A placebo group (given an inert substitute capsule) plus the same low-calorie diet averaged only about a 1.4-pound loss.

A Danish report detailing the effects of ephedrine on 5 females over a 3-month period revealed an energy expenditure about 10% greater than that of nonmedicated subjects. This translates into a loss of 184 calories per 24 hours in ephedrine-treated subjects due to an increased metabolic rate.

In a study of 41 patients who were 20–80% overweight and received a combination of ephedrine and caffeine for 12 weeks, a median weight loss of 17.82 pounds was reported; 74% of subjects lost 11 pounds or more.

Dosage Levels at Which Effects Occur
Weight loss: Reported within a range of 60–150mg. daily.

Remedies
Weight loss: Not applicable.

How Long It Takes Till Reversal of Drug Effects
Ephedrine's duration of action when taken by mouth is 3–5 hours, except for long-acting dosage forms, whose effects may persist for up to 12 hours.

Sources
Astrup, A., et al. "The effect of chronic ephedrine treatment on substrate utilization, the sympathoadrenal activity, and energy expenditure during glucose-induced thermogenesis in man." *Metabolism*, 1986, 35: 260–65.
Malchow-Møller, A., et al. "Ephedrine as an anorectic: The story of the 'Elsinore Pill.' " *International Journal of Obesity*, 1981, 5: 183–87.
Pasquali, R., et al. "Does ephedrine promote weight loss in low-energy-adapted obese women?" *International Journal of Obesity*, 1987, 11(2): 163–68.

FENFLURAMINE

Brand Names
U.S.A.: Pondimin (Robins).
Canada: Ponderal (Servier), Pondimin (Robins).
Great Britain: Ponderax (Servier).

What This Drug Does
Appetite suppressant.

How This Drug Affects Body Weight
Fenfluramine has been claimed to induce weight loss without central nervous system stimulation. Serotonin, a chemical involved in nerve-impulse transmission in the brain, may influence craving for carbohydrate food. Fenfluramine increases brain concentrations of serotonin by stimulating its release, as well as by blocking its neuronal uptake. This causes a decrease in carbohydrate intake. The drug may stimulate the satiety center of the hypothalamus as well as increase glucose utilization in the body.

Government-Approved Uses for This Drug
As an aid to short-term weight loss.

Unofficial Uses
To treat autistic children with elevated serotonin levels.

When Not to Use This Drug
If taking or have taken within the last 14 days any monoamine oxidase inhibitor drug; in alcoholics; in glaucoma; in advanced arteriosclerosis; in high blood pressure; in agitated states; if allergic to this drug or to any related drug.

Side Effects From Use of This Drug
Dizziness; loss of coordination; headache; mood changes; anxiety; insomnia; weakness; fatigue; palpitations; high or low blood pressure (reported with equal frequency); chest pain; blurred vision; eye irritation; diarrhea or constipation (reported with equal frequency); dry mouth; nausea; vomiting; abdominal pain; painful urination; frequent urination; skin rash, itching or burning sensation; sweating; chills; fever; changes in libido.

Effects on Appetite and Body Weight as Disclosed by the Drug's Manufacturer
Unpleasant taste.

Detailed Effects on Appetite and Body Weight
Weight loss: In one fenfluramine study, obese subjects who were prone to consuming most of their excess calories as snack foods were divided into two groups—those who craved mostly carbohydrates and those who craved noncarbohydrates. Both groups were given fenfluramine for 3 months. Thirteen of the 24 carbohydrate cravers lost 2% or more of their body weight by the end of the first month. They maintained or bettered this loss throughout the balance of the study. Among noncarbohydrate cravers, most showed no weight change.

In a study of long-term fenfluramine users, 42 obese females who lost at least 13.2 pounds during 26 weeks of drug use were split into two equal groups, one of which was given the active drug and the other a placebo. At the end of 1 year, among those receiving fenfluramine as a sustained-release dosage form, 8 maintained their weight loss, 7 regained the lost weight, and 6 failed to complete the study.

In a 20-week study of fenfluramine's effects on 41 obese women, average weight loss ranged from 4.62–19.36 pounds, depending on the dosage taken. Greater weight loss was in direct correlation to increased blood drug levels.

Thirty-one women, all clinically obese (at least 20% overweight), were given fenfluramine for 9 months. At the end of the study, average weight loss was 26.1 pounds, with most of the loss occurring in the first half of the study.

Fifty obese women who were unsuccessful in losing weight by any other means participated in a 12-week trial to test the effectiveness of fenfluramine. Divided evenly into two groups, one of which took the active drug and the other a placebo, the fenfluramine group lost an average of 9.3 pounds, while the others gained 0.4 pounds.

Decreased appetite: In a 5-day trial of 11 volunteers, fenfluramine administration decreased carbohydrate food consumption by 50% or more in 3 (27%) and by 10–50% in 4 others (36%).

Dosage Levels at Which Effects Occur
Weight loss: Reported as low as 30mg. daily.

Decreased appetite: Reported to occur at a dose of 20mg. given 1 hour before snacking.

Remedies
Not applicable.

How Long It Takes Till Reversal of Drug Effects
Half the dose of fenfluramine is cleared from the blood within 20 hours. This time may be decreased to about 11 hours if the urine is kept acidic and passed rapidly.

Sources
Douglas, J.G., et al. "Longer term efficacy of fenfluramine in obesity." *Lancet*, 1983, 1: 384.

Hudson, K.D. "The anorectic and hypotensive effect of fenfluramine in obesity." *Journal of the Royal College of General Practitioners*, 1977, 27: 497.

Innes, J.A., et al. "Plasma fenfluramine levels, weight loss and side effects." *British Medical Journal*, 1977, 2: 1322–25.

Munro, J.F. "The management of obesity" in Symposium: Anorexia Nervosa and Obesity. *Journal of the Royal College of Physicians of Edinburgh*, 1973, 42: 100.

Munro, J.F., et al. "Treatment of refractory obesity with fenfluramine." *British Medical Journal*, 1966, 2: 624–25.

Steel, J.M., et al. "A comparative trial of different regimens of fenfluramine and phentermine in obesity." *Practitioner*, 1973, 211: 232–36.

Steel, J.M., Briggs, W. "Withdrawal depression in obese patients after fenfluramine treatment." *British Medical Journal*, 1972, 3: 26.

Wurtman, J., et al. "Fenfluramine suppresses snack intake among carbohydrate cravers but not among noncarbohydrate cravers." *International Journal of Eating Disorders*, 1987, 6(6): 687–99.

GLUCOMANNAN

Brand Names
U.S.A.: Marketed as "glucomannan" by various manufacturers.
Canada: None.
Great Britain: None.

What This Drug Does
Alleged to promote weight loss.

How This Drug Affects Body Weight
The bulk-forming properties of glucomannan are claimed to be responsible for its effect on weight loss: 3 grams of gluco-

mannan will absorb about 300ml. of water (10 ounces). When taken before meals, the added bulk produced in the stomach is said to cause subjects to eat less.

Glucomannan is also alleged to facilitate faster transport of food particles through the gastrointestinal tract. This is supposed to allow less time for absorption of calories, promoting elimination of undigested food. Glucomannan has also been described as forming a gel around food particles, reducing caloric gain from eating.

Government-Approved Uses for This Drug
None.

Unofficial Uses
To promote weight loss (evidence of its effectiveness has still not been submitted to the FDA).

When Not to Use This Drug
If allergic to this drug or to any related drug.

Side Effects From Use of This Drug
None.

Effects on Appetite and Body Weight as Disclosed by the Drug's Manufacturer
Alleged to promote weight loss.

Detailed Effects on Appetite and Body Weight
Weight loss: A plant fiber indigenous to the Orient and processed from the konjac root, glucomannan has been touted as the "weight loss secret that's been in the Orient for over 500 years." To date, no manufacturer of this product has been able to supply the Food and Drug Administration with evidence of its effectiveness in weight loss.

An 8-week trial involving 20 obese females (20% or more over ideal body weight) was designed to test the effectiveness of glucomannan in weight loss and as a cholesterol-lowering agent. The subjects were assigned to two equal groups, with one receiving the active product and the other a placebo. After 4 weeks, the glucomannan group lost an average of 4.9 pounds; after 8 weeks the loss totaled 5.5 pounds. The placebo group actually gained an average of 1.5 pounds after 8 weeks.

Dosage Levels at Which Effects Occur
Weight Loss: Reported to occur at a daily dose of 3 grams (1 gram taken 1 hour before each of 3 daily meals with 8 ounces of water).

Remedies
Not applicable.

How Long It Takes Till Reversal of Drug Effects
Unknown.

Sources
Covington, T.R. "Vitamins: Part 1—Common myths." *Facts and Comparisons Drug Newsletter*, 1987, 6(7): 54–55.

Walsh, D.E., et al. "Effect of glucomannan on obese patients: A clinical study." *International Journal of Obesity*, 1981, 8(1): 289–93.

Willis, J. "About body wraps, pills and other magic wands for losing weight." *FDA Consumer*, 1982, 16: 18–20.

GUARANA

Brand Names
U.S.A.: Guarana (marketed by various manufacturers).
Canada: Guarana (marketed by various manufacturers).
Great Britain: Guarana (marketed by various manufacturers).

What This Drug Does:
Claimed to suppress appetite and aid in weight loss.

How This Drug Affects Body Weight
Since its active ingredient is caffeine, guarana affects the body in the same way as this substance. It stimulates all levels of the central nervous system, including parts of the brain and the spinal cord. This may cause suppression of appetite and subsequent weight loss.

Government-Approved Uses for This Drug
Among caffeine's approved uses is as an aid to restoring mental alertness and in staying awake.

Unofficial Uses
As an aid to appetite suppression and weight loss.

When Not to Use This Drug
If allergic to this drug or to any related drug.

Side Effects From Use of This Drug
[As listed for caffeine.] Insomnia; nervousness; ringing in the ears; muscle tremor; visual disturbance; headache; light-headedness; nausea; vomiting; diarrhea; stomach pain; fast heart-beat and other heart-rhythm irregularities.

Effects on Appetite and Body Weight as Disclosed by the Drug's Manufacturer
[As listed for caffeine.] Increased urination.

Detailed Effects on Appetite and Body Weight
Appetite suppression; weight loss: Once an official entry in the United States Pharmacopeia (1882–1926) and the National Formulary (1926–1947), guarana has been touted as possessing cocaine-like energizing properties. It has been claimed to impart a sense of euphoria, making it "a diet that's fun . . . [and allows you to] pep up as you slim down."

Although guarana's action originally was thought to be derived from "guaranine," an alkaloid present in the product, it was later determined that the real active ingredient was caffeine. Pure guarana contains 4% caffeine. Those diet products claiming to produce a "natural high" deliver about 80mg. of caffeine per tablet, or an amount equal to slightly less than that available in one cup of coffee.

Dosage Levels at Which Effects Occur
Appetite suppression; weight loss: Each tablet of guarana contains about 80mg. of caffeine.

Remedies
Not applicable.

How Long It Takes Till Reversal of Drug Effects
It takes 3–7.5 hours (average 3.5 hours) for half the dose of caffeine to be cleared from the blood.

Source
Uretsky, S.D. "A pharmacists' guide to quack weight products." *American Pharmacy*, 1985, NS25 (2): 24–29.

GUAR GUM

Brand Names
U.S.A.: *†D-S-S Compound (Wolins), *†Gentlax B (Blair), *†Guarsol (Western Research).
Canada: None.
Great Britain: Decorpa (Norgine; no longer marketed).

What This Drug Does
Appetite suppressant and weight-loss aid.

How This Drug Affects Body Weight
Guar gum, a dietary gelling fiber obtained from the cluster bean, is composed of the sugars galactose and mannose. It is claimed to slow the rate of gastric emptying, increasing feelings of fullness after meals.

Government-Approved Uses for This Drug
None.

Unofficial Uses
As an appetite suppressant and weight-loss aid; used to treat duodenal ulcers.

When Not to Use This Drug
If allergic to this drug or to any related drug.

Side Effects From Use of This Drug
Gas; loose stools.

Effects on Appetite and Body Weight as Disclosed by the Drug's Manufacturer
None.

Detailed Effects on Appetite and Body Weight
Decreased appetite; weight loss: In a series of experiments involving obese patients, subjects were given guar gum twice daily for 10 weeks. The objective was to study several of guar

*Combination drug.
†Denotes over-the-counter availability in the U.S.A.

gum's effects, one of which was its influence on body weight. The substance was given as a granulated powder stirred into water and taken just before lunch and dinner. Subjects were asked not to consciously alter their normal eating habits. After 8 weeks, an average of 9.5 pounds was lost, and after 10 weeks another group's loss averaged 15.6 pounds.

In a study of the appetite-inhibiting effects of guar gum in 11 healthy volunteers (4 males and 7 females), subjects were first standardized for 1 week to determine their normal food intake. After 1 week of guar-gum use, taken a half-hour before each of the two largest daily meals, about a 10% decrease in food consumption was recorded. Weight loss was slightly over 1 pound in normal subjects and over 3 pounds in the obese.

Twenty-one obese patients were alternately given wheat bran or guar gum twice daily, 1 week on each, by the same protocol as described above. Over a period of about 6.6 weeks (3.3 weeks on each substance), it was not surprising to find that guar gum produced decreased feelings of hunger, especially during lunch and dinner.

In a 4-month study of 33 females with high cholesterol, subjects were divided into three groups. One was given guar gum, one a placebo, and the last no treatment at all. Of the 10 women given guar gum and completing the trial, average weight loss was 5.5 pounds. Guar gum was found to cause decreased intestinal absorption of one or more dietary components.

Dosage Levels at Which Effects Occur
Decreased appetite; weight loss: Reported effective at 16 grams daily (8 grams taken a half-hour before the day's two largest meals with a glass of water).

Guar gum has been effectively used as a component in bread; 7.5 grams of the substance per roll, eaten 4 times a day provides the necessary daily requirement.

Remedies
Not applicable.

How Long It Takes Till Reversal of Drug Effects
Although not specifically stated in the experiments cited above, it can be inferred that guar gum's optimum effects were obtained shortly after each dose, given just before meals. This

would seem to indicate that its effects did not last more than a few hours.

Sources

Evans, E., Miller, D.S. "Bulking agents in the treatment of obesity." *Nutrition and Metabolism*, 1975, 18: 199–203.

Harju, E.J., Larmi, T.K. "Effect of guar gum added to the diet of patients with duodenal ulcer." *Journal of Parenteral and Enteral Nutrition*, 1985, 9(4): 496–500.

Hill, M.A., et al. "The preparation and use of guar gum bread in diet therapy." *Human Nutrition, Applied Nutrition*, 1981, 38(3): 227–28.

Krotkiewski, M. "Effect of guar gum on body-weight, hunger ratings and metabolism in obese subjects." *British Journal of Nutrition*, 1984, 52(1): 97–105.

Tuomilehto, J., et al. "Effect of guar gum on body weight and serum lipids in hypercholesterolemic females." *Acta Medica Scandinavica*, 1980, 208: 45–48.

MAZINDOL

Brand Names
U.S.A.: Mazanor (Wyeth), Sanorex (Sandoz).
Canada: Sanorex (Sandoz), Teronac (Anca).
Great Britain: Teronac (Wander).

What This Drug Does
Appetite suppressant.

How This Drug Affects Body Weight
Related to amphetamines, mazindol is believed to cause general brain stimulation. It may induce the release of dopamine and norepinephrine (chemical messengers) while also blocking their removal. This can lead to increased availability of these neuro-transmitters to stimulate nerve receptors. Mazindol is thought to exert most of its effects on the limbic system (an area of the brain associated with emotions and feelings). The reasons for this drug causing appetite suppression have not been definitely determined.

Government-Approved Uses for This Drug
As a short-term aid in weight loss.

Unofficial Uses
None.

When Not to Use This Drug
In glaucoma; in agitated states; in patients with history of drug abuse; if taking or have taken within the last 14 days any mono-amine oxidase inhibitor drug; in children under 12 years of age; if allergic to this drug or to any related drug.

Side Effects From Use of This Drug
Nervousness; restlessness; dizziness; insomnia; headache; depression; drowsiness; weakness; muscle tremors; fast heart-beat; palpitations; dry mouth; diarrhea or constipation (reported with equal frequency); nausea; difficulty in urinating; skin rash; sweating; impotence; changes in libido.

Effects on Appetite and Body Weight as Disclosed by the Drug's Manufacturer
Unpleasant taste.

Detailed Effects on Appetite and Body Weight
Weight loss: In a three-study series measuring weight loss in patients treated with mazindol, different dosages and protocols were compared. The first trial involved 7 weeks of continuous use and yielded an average total weight loss of 7.64 pounds. The second of the series lasted 9 weeks and compared the same total daily dose given once daily and 3 times a day. Both methods gave similar results, with an average total loss of about 11 pounds. The third trial compared continuous and intermittent mazindol use over 18 weeks. Those on continuous medication lost an average of 12.9 pounds versus 11 pounds for those taking it 4 weeks on alternating with 2 weeks off.

Of 19 patients who were more than 20% over their ideal body weight and who completed a 12-week study of the effects of mazindol, average weight loss was about 3 pounds. The range of weight change was from a 5.94-pound weight gain to an 18.92-pound weight loss. Maximum loss occurred at 6 weeks, with only 5 patients (those recording the greatest total weight loss) losing any weight during the last half of the trial.

In a 12-week study involving 20 patients taking mazindol and 20 taking a placebo, average weight loss for those taking the active drug was about 15 pounds while the others averaged only about 3.5 pounds. Of the mazindol group, 65% lost at least 1.1 pounds per week during the course of the trial while only 1 placebo subject equaled this.

Forty obese individuals participated in a 12-week study to test the effectiveness of mazindol. At the end of the 3 months, average weight loss was 18.5 pounds as compared with a 2.4-pound loss in a second control group given a placebo.

Of 50 obese male volunteers, half of whom received mazindol for 4 weeks and half of whom were given a placebo, those on active medication showed an average weight loss of 0.9 pounds per week. This was 3–4 times greater than the placebo group.

A group of 158 obese adults was divided into three groups, each of which was placed on a five-phase weight-loss plan. The groups alternated among periods of diet, placebo, and mazindol use in sequences that totaled 15 weeks. Diet alone was found to be more effective in early phases of weight-loss programs, but as time progressed, mazindol use became more effective. This was borne out by results showing greatest weight loss to occur in those groups given mazindol in later phases of the trial. Average weight loss for the three groups ranged from about 16–22 pounds.

Dosage Levels at Which Effects Occur
Weight loss: Reported as low as 1mg. daily. The average therapeutic range for mazindol is 3–6 mg. daily.

Remedies
Weight loss: Not applicable.

How Long It Takes Till Reversal of Drug Effects
Weight loss: In one study cited above, 68% of those monitored 2 weeks after withdrawal of mazindol had gained back 2.2 pounds of the average 3 pounds lost during the drug trial. The authors of the study claim this figure might have been higher if all 19 patients had been available for follow-up.

Mazindol's therapeutic effects are evident up to 15 hours after the last dose.

Sources
Conte, A. "Evaluation of Sanorex—a new appetite suppressant." *Obesity and Bariatric Medicine*, 1973, 2: 104.
DeFelice, E.A., et al. "Double-blind comparison of placebo and 42-548, a new

appetite suppressant, in obese volunteers." *Current Therapeutic Research, Clinical and Experimental*, 1969, 11: 256–62.

Enzi, G., et al. "Short-term and long-term clinical evaluation of a non-amphetamine anorexiant (mazindol) in the treatment of obesity." *Journal of International Medical Research*, 1976, 4: 305–18.

Heber, K.R. "Double-blind trial of mazindol in overweight patients." *Medical Journal of Australia*, 1975, 2: 566–67.

Schwartz, L.N. "A non-amphetamine anorectic agent: Preclinical background and a double-blind clinical trial." *Journal of International Medical Research*, 1975, 3: 328–32.

Smith, R.G., et al. "Double-blind evaluation of mazindol in refractory obesity." *British Medical Journal*, 1975, 3: 284.

METHYLCELLULOSE

Brand Names
U.S.A.: Citrucel (Lakeside), Cologel (Lilly).
Canada: MC (E-Z-EM).
Great Britain: None.

What This Drug Does
Laxative.

How This Drug Affects Body Weight
Methylcellulose swells when mixed with water, forming bulk in the stomach and creating feelings of fullness.

Government-Approved Uses for This Drug
Short-term treatment of constipation.

Unofficial Uses
As a diet aid.

When Not to Use This Drug
In the presence of vomiting or other signs of appendicitis; in acute surgical abdomen; in fecal impaction; in intestinal obstruction; in presence of undiagnosed abdominal pain; if allergic to this drug or to any related drug.

Side Effects From Use of This Drug
Abdominal cramping; diarrhea; nausea; vomiting; perianal irritation; weakness; dizziness; gas; obstruction of the esophagus,

stomach, small intestine, or rectum due to accumulation of bulking agent.

Effects on Appetite and Body Weight as Disclosed by the Drug's Manufacturer
None.

Detailed Effects on Appetite and Body Weight
Decreased appetite; weight loss: In a study of the appetite-inhibiting effects of methylcellulose in 11 healthy volunteers (4 males and 7 females), subjects were first standardized for 1 week to determine their normal food intake. After 1 week of methylcellulose use, taken a half-hour before each of the two largest daily meals, about a 10% decrease in food consumption was recorded. Weight loss was about 1.3 pounds in normal subjects and almost 4 pounds in the obese.

The researchers caution, however, that large doses of methylcellulose, such as those given in this study, may cause intestinal obstruction. They rated the granule form of methylcellulose better than tablets since the latter often do not disintegrate quickly enough in the stomach to swell in the presence of water.

Dosage Levels at Which Effects Occur
Decreased appetite; weight loss: Reported effective at a daily dose of 15.5 grams (4.5–6 grams a half-hour before each meal taken with water).

Remedies
Not applicable.

How Long It Takes Till Reversal of Drug Effects
Decreased appetite; weight loss: Although the authors of the above study claim weight loss was permanent, this seems unlikely. Since methylcellulose is not absorbed into the body, its effects probably last only as long as its transit time through the gastrointestinal system.

Source
Evans, E., Miller, D.S. "Bulking agents in the treatment of obesity." *Nutrition and Metabolism*, 1975, 18: 199–203.

PHENDIMETRAZINE

Brand Names
U.S.A.: Adipost (Ascher), Adphen (Ferndale), Alphazine (Vitarine), Anorex (Dunhall), Bacarate (Reid-Provident), Bontril PDM (Carnrick), Bontril Slow-Release (Carnrick), Cam-Metrazine (Camall), Di-Ap-Trol (Foy), Di-Metrex (Private Formulations), Dyrexan-OD (Trimen), Hyrex 105 (Hyrex), Melfiat (Reid-Provident), Melfiat-105 Unicelles (Reid-Provident), Metra (Forest), Obalan (Lannett), Obeval (Vale), Obezine (Pharm. Basics), Phenazine (MM Mast), Phenzine (Mallard), Plegine (Ayerst), Prelu-2 (Boehringer Ingelheim), Slyn-LL (Edwards), Sprx (Reid-Provident), Statobex (Lemmon), Statobex-G (Lemmon), Trimstat (Laser), Trimtabs (Mayrand), Weh-less (Hauck), Weightrol (Vortech), X-Trozine (Rexar).
Canada: None.
Great Britain: None.

What This Drug Does
Appetite suppressant.

How This Drug Affects Body Weight
Related to amphetamines, phendimetrazine is believed to cause general brain stimulation. It may induce release of dopamine and norepinephrine (chemical messengers) while also blocking their removal. This can lead to increased availability of these neurotransmitters to stimulate nerve receptors. The reasons that this drug causes appetite suppression have not been definitely determined but are thought to result from direct stimulation on the satiety center in the hypothalamic and limbic areas of the brain.

Government-Approved Uses for This Drug
To aid in weight loss (short-term).

Unofficial Uses
None.

When Not to Use This Drug

In advanced arteriosclerosis; in certain cardiovascular disease; in high blood pressure; in glaucoma; in agitated states; if there is a history of drug abuse; if taking or have taken within the last 14 days any monoamine oxidase inhibitor drug; in children under 12 years of age; if allergic to this drug or to any related drug.

Side Effects From Use of This Drug

Nervousness; dizziness; insomnia; palpitations; fast heartbeat; elevation of blood pressure; dry mouth; nausea; constipation; diarrhea; skin eruption; impotence; changes in libido.

Effects on Appetite and Body Weight as Disclosed by the Drug's Manufacturer

Unpleasant taste.

Detailed Effects on Appetite and Body Weight

Weight loss: In a 12-week study, 90 adults (65 males and 25 females), all of whom were at least 10% overweight, were divided into two equal groups. One group received a placebo and the other active medication; 36 completed the entire course of phendimetrazine therapy and 35 finished the placebo regimen. Phendimetrazine use induced an average weight loss of 0.62 pounds per week, while the placebo resulted in a weekly reduction of only 0.09 pounds.

Of 20 obese patients completing a 6-month study of the effectiveness of phendimetrazine versus a placebo, average weight loss for the active drug over 3 months was 6.96 pounds. This compared favorably to a loss of only 0.33 pounds for the placebo. This works out to a 20 times greater weight loss with phendimetrazine.

Dosage Levels at Which Effects Occur

Weight loss: Reported to occur at a daily dose of 105mg. This may be given either as a sustained-action tablet taken once a day, or as a 35mg. tablet taken 3 times daily.

Remedies

Weight loss: Not applicable.

How Long It Takes Till Reversal of Drug Effects

Weight loss: It takes about 3 hours for phendimetrazine to be eliminated from the body, depending on the pH (a measure of acidity or basicity) of the urine. Acid urine will decrease this time, while a basic medium will extend the duration of action.

Sources

Hadler, A.J. "Sustained-acting phendimetrazine in obesity." *Journal of Clinical Pharmacology*, 1968, 8: 113–17.
Ressler, C., Schneider, S.H. "Clinical evaluation of phendimetrazine bitartrate." *Clinical Pharmacology and Therapeutics*, 1961, 2: 727.

PHENMETRAZINE

Brand Names
U.S.A.: Preludin (Boehringer Ingelheim).
Canada: None.
Great Britain: Preludin (Boehringer Ingelheim; no longer marketed).

What This Drug Does
Appetite suppressant.

How This Drug Affects Body Weight
Related to amphetamines, phenmetrazine is believed to cause general brain stimulation. It may induce the release of dopamine and norepinephrine (chemical messengers) while also blocking their removal. This can lead to increased availability of these neurotransmitters to stimulate nerve receptors. The reasons that this drug causes appetite suppression have not been definitely determined but are thought to result from direct stimulation on the satiety center in the hypothalamic and limbic areas of the brain.

Government-Approved Uses for This Drug
To aid in weight loss (short-term).

Unofficial Uses
None.

When Not to Use This Drug
In advanced arteriosclerosis; in certain cardiovascular disease; in high blood pressure; in glaucoma; in agitated states; if there

is a history of drug abuse; if taking or have taken within the last 14 days any monoamine oxidase inhibitor drug; in children under 12 years of age; in nursing mothers; if allergic to this drug or to any related drug.

Side Effects From Use of This Drug

Nervousness; dizziness; insomnia; palpitations; fast heartbeat; elevation of blood pressure; dry mouth; nausea; constipation or diarrhea (reported with equal frequency); skin eruption; impotence; changes in libido.

Effects on Appetite and Body Weight as Disclosed by the Drug's Manufacturer

Unpleasant taste.

Detailed Effects on Appetite and Body Weight

Weight loss: In a 12-week study of 24 obese patients given phenmetrazine, 18 lost from 2–23.5 pounds, with an average weekly weight loss of 0.52 pounds. Five subjects actually gained weight (from 0.5–12 pounds).

In a trial of phenmetrazine where the drug was given to 60 obese patients over a period of 2–14 weeks (average 9.6 weeks), all but 1 subject lost weight. Maximum reported loss was 35 pounds, with an average total loss of 18.8 pounds for all subjects.

In a 10-week German study of 50 overweight patients given phenmetrazine, subjects lost an average of 1.9 pounds weekly during the course of the trial.

In a 3-month study of 30 overweight patients, about half received phenmetrazine and half a placebo. All those taking the active medication lost an average of 1.34 pounds per week; total weight loss averaged 15.25 pounds. Those on placebo lost an average 0.24 pounds weekly with a total average loss of only 3.02 pounds.

In a group of 84 overweight patients seen in private office practice and treated with phenmetrazine for an average of about 5 weeks, mean weight loss was 7.7 pounds. Average weekly loss was 1.55 pounds.

Some members of a group of 45 obese individuals attending an obesity clinic were given phenmetrazine for an average of about 7 weeks. Mean weight loss per week was 1.5 pounds.

In a study of 55 overweight patients who were given both

phenmetrazine and a placebo, average weight loss while taking phenmetrazine was 1.25 pounds per week over an average of 9.07 weeks. Those taking a placebo averaged a loss of only 0.19 pounds weekly.

Dosage Levels at Which Effects Occur
Weight loss: Reported to occur within a range of 25–75mg. daily.

Remedies
Weight loss: Not applicable.

How Long It Takes Till Reversal of Drug Effects
It takes about 3 hours for phenmetrazine to be eliminated from the body, depending on the pH (a measure of acidity or basicity) of the urine. Acid urine will decrease this time, while a basic medium will extend the duration of action.

Sources
Berneike, K.H. "Beitrag zur medikamentösen fettsuchbehandlung." *Medizinische Klinik*, 1954, 49: 478–81.

Fazekas, J.K., et al. "A study of the effectiveness of certain anorexigenic agents." *American Journal of the Medical Sciences*, 1958, 236: 692–99.

Gelvin, E.P., et al. "Phenmetrazine in management of obesity." *American Journal of Digestive Disorders*, 1956, 1: 155–59.

Hadler, A.T. "Weight reduction with phenmetrazine and chlorphentermine, a double-blind study." *Current Therapeutic Research, Clinical and Experimental*, 1967, 9: 563–69.

Howard, L.A., et al. "Complicated obesity: Clinical evaluation of a timed-release anorectic agent." *Current Therapeutic Research, Clinical and Experimental*, 1964, 6: 659–64.

Natenshon, A.L. "Clinical evaluation of a new anorexic agent, phenmetrazine hydrochloride (Preludin)." *American Practitioner*, 1956, 7: 1456–59.

Ressler, C. "Treatment of obesity with phenmetrazine hydrochloride, a new anorexiant." *Journal of the American Medical Association*, 1957, 165: 135–38.

PHENTERMINE

Brand Names
U.S.A.: Adipex-P (Lemmon), Dapex-37.5 (Ferndale), Fastin (Beecham), Ionamin (Penwalt), Obe-Nix (Holloway), Obephen (Mallard), Obermine (Forest), Obestin-30 (Ferndale), Oby-Trim

(Rexar), Ona-Mast (MM Mast), Parmine (Parmed), Phentamine (Major), Phentrol (Vortech), Tora (Reid-Provident), Unifast Unicelles (Reid-Provident), Wilpowr (Foy).
Canada: Fastin (Beecham), Ionamin (Penwalt).
Great Britain: Duromine (Carnegie), Ionamin (Lipha).

What This Drug Does
Appetite suppressant.

How This Drug Affects Body Weight
Related to amphetamines, phentermine is believed to cause general brain stimulation. It may induce release of dopamine and norepinephrine (chemical messengers) while also blocking their removal. This can lead to increased availability of these neurotransmitters to stimulate nerve receptors. The reasons that this drug causes appetite suppression have not been definitely determined but are thought to result from direct stimulation on the satiety center in the hypothalamic and limbic areas of the brain.

Government-Approved Uses for This Drug
To aid in weight loss (short-term).

Unofficial Uses
None.

When Not to Use This Drug
In advanced arteriosclerosis; in certain cardiovascular disease; in high blood pressure; in glaucoma; in agitated states; if there is a history of drug abuse; if taking or have taken within the last 14 days any monoamine oxidase inhibitor drug; in children under 12 years of age; if allergic to this drug or to any related drug.

Side Effects From Use of This Drug
Nervousness; dizziness; insomnia; palpitations; fast heartbeat; elevation of blood pressure; dry mouth; nausea; constipation or diarrhea (reported with equal frequency); skin eruption; impotence; changes in libido.

Effects on Appetite and Body Weight as Disclosed by the Drug's Manufacturer
Unpleasant taste.

Detailed Effects on Appetite and Body Weight

Weight loss: In a 36-week study comparing the effectiveness of phentermine to diet alone and to intermittent versus continuous phentermine use, the drug proved superior to dieting alone. While dieters lost an average of 10.5 pounds, those on continuous phentermine lost an average of 27 pounds. Those alternating 4 weeks on and 4 weeks off the medication lost an average of 28.7 pounds.

Of 30 obese patients who completed an 18-week evaluation of phentermine use, weight loss averaged 16.1 pounds during 14 weeks of active medication, as compared with a 3.9-pound average loss for those given a placebo.

In a series of 86 overweight individuals given phentermine for an average of 1 month, mean daily weight loss was about 0.25 pound. Weight loss was found to be about the same whether high- or low-dose phentermine was given.

In a 12-week trial of phentermine given to a group of obese women, average weight loss was 5.87 pounds. The drug seemed to produce most weight loss during the first 6 weeks of use. It started losing its effectiveness after 6–8 weeks and showed minimal benefits during the last 4 weeks of the trial.

In a 20-week study of 34 obese females receiving phentermine, average weight loss was about 14 pounds, with 9 women losing 22 pounds or more. Most loss was attributed to phentermine-induced sustained appetite suppression.

Decreased appetite: Six moderately overweight adult females were studied for the effects of phentermine on hunger. This single-dose drug trial showed caloric intake to be decreased by 25–33% in direct proportion to the dose of phentermine given.

Dosage Levels at Which Effects Occur

Weight loss: Reported as low as 15mg. daily.
Decreased appetite: Reported as low as 15mg. daily.

Remedies

Weight loss: Not applicable.
Decreased appetite: Not applicable.

How Long It Takes Till Reversal of Drug Effects

It takes about 3 hours for phentermine to be eliminated from the body, depending on the pH (a measure of acidity or basicity) of the urine. Acid urine will decrease this time, while a basic medium will extend the duration of action.

Sources

Douglas, A., et al. "Plasma phentermine levels, weight loss and side effects." *International Journal of Obesity*, 1983, 7: 591.

Freed, S.C., Hays, E.E. "A new nonamphetamine anorectic agent." *American Journal of the Medical Sciences*, 1959, 238: 55–59.

Langlois, K.J., et al. "A double-blind clinical evaluation of the safety and efficacy of phentermine hydrochloride (Fastin) in the treatment of exogenous obesity." *Current Therapeutic Research, Clinical and Experimental*, 1974, 16: 289–96.

Munro, J.J., et al. "Comparison of continuous and intermittent anorectic therapy in obesity." *British Medical Journal*, 1968, 1: 352.

Seaton, D.A., et al. "A comparison of the appetite suppressing properties of dexamphetamine and phentermine." *Scottish Medical Journal*, 1964, 9: 482–85.

Silverstone, T. "The anorectic effect of a long-acting preparation of phentermine (duromine)." *Psychopharmacologia*, 1972, 25: 315–20.

PHENYLPROPANOLAMINE

Brand Names

U.S.A.: †Accutrim Maximum Strength (Ciba), *†Appedrine (Thompson), †Control (Thompson), †Dex-A-Diet (O'Connor), *†Dex-A-Diet Plus Vitamin C (O'Connor), *†Dex-A-Diet Plus Vitamins (O'Connor), † Dexatrim-15 (Thompson), *†Dexatrim-15 w/Vitamin C (O'Connor), *†Dexatrim Plus Vitamins (O'-Connor), †Diadax (O'Connor), *†Extra Strength Grapefruit Diet Plan w/Diadax (O'Connor), *†Grapefruit Diet Plan w/Diadax (O'Connor), *†Grapefruit Diet Plan w/Diadax, Vitamin Fortified (O'Connor), †Prolamine (Thompson), †Propagest (Carnrick), †Resolution I Maximum Strength (Lee), †Resolution II Half-Strength (Lee), ‡Rhindecon (McGregor), †Sucrets Cold Decongestant Formula (Beecham), †Unitrol (Republic).
Canada: Coldecon (Parke-Davis).
Great Britain: *Totolin (Galen).

*Combination drug.
†Denotes over-the-counter availability in the U.S.A.
‡Denotes prescription-only status in the U.S.A.

What This Drug Does
Decongestant; appetite suppressant.

How This Drug Affects Body Weight
Phenylpropanolamine is believed to cause general brain stimulation. It may induce release of dopamine and norepinephrine (chemical messengers) while also blocking their removal. This can lead to increased availability of these neurotransmitters to stimulate nerve receptors. The reasons that this drug causes appetite suppression have not been definitely determined but are thought to result from direct stimulation on the satiety center in the hypothalamic and limbic areas of the brain.

Government-Approved Uses for This Drug
As a nasal, sinus, and eustachean tube decongestant; as a short-term aid to weight reduction.

Unofficial Uses
None.

When Not to Use This Drug
If taking or have taken within 14 days any monoamine oxidase inhibitor drug; in severe high blood pressure; in coronary artery disease; in nursing mothers; if allergic to this drug or to any related drug.

Side Effects From Use of This Drug
Anxiety; restlessness; headache; light-headedness; dizziness; tremor; insomnia; hallucinations; convulsions; heart-rhythm irregularities; blood pressure changes; palpitations; various heart problems; blurred vision and other eye problems; nausea; vomiting; painful urination; breathing difficulties; sweating.

Effects on Appetite and Body Weight as Disclosed by the Drug's Manufacturer
None.

Detailed Effects on Appetite and Body Weight
Decreased appetite: Sixteen adult subjects underwent a 10-day study to evaluate the appetite-suppressant effects of phenylpropanolamine. Each subject was given the active drug or a placebo (5 days of each) 30 minutes before eating. At the end of the

study, phenylpropanolamine had reduced meal intake by an average of 27% over placebo.

In a second experiment by the same researchers, identical in all ways to the above except for using twice as many subjects, only a 5% reduction in meal consumption over placebo was seen with phenylpropanolamine use. The authors do not adequately explain this disparity in the results of the two studies.

Weight loss: Although phenylpropanolamine is recognized as an effective method of short-term weight loss, much of its advertising is misleading or overstated. One promoter says it will ". . . turn ugly fat into harmless water and flow out of your system by the gallon," while another ad promises to turn your body into a "fat blowtorch."

In a large-scale 4-week study of 77 obese adults, about half were given a phenylpropanolamine/caffeine/multivitamin preparation and the other half a placebo. In the active drug group, males lost a median (half above and half below) of 8 pounds and females 4 pounds. The placebo group showed a median loss of 4.5 pounds in males and 2 pounds in females. Of all patients taking the phenylpropanolamine preparation, 27% lost 10 pounds or more while only 12% did so in the other group.

Seventy adults took part in a 4-week study to determine phenylpropanolamine's ability to effect weight loss over a 2-week period. Subjects were given either the active drug or a placebo for 2 weeks, 30 minutes before each of 3 daily meals. The groups then switched drugs for an additional 2 weeks. Those taking phenylpropanolamine in the first 2 weeks lost an average of just over 2 pounds, while the placebo group averaged a 1.23-pound loss. In the second 2 weeks, those on active medication lost an average 1.4 pounds compared with the placebo group's gain of 0.16 pounds. Taking all subjects as a whole without regard for the sequencing of medication, an average weight loss of 1.7 pounds was recorded for phenylpropanolamine versus 0.54 pounds lost with placebo.

Dosage Levels at Which Effects Occur

Decreased appetite: Reported to occur at 25mg. daily before a meal in a single-dose study. To benefit from this effect on a full-day basis, this dose should be repeated before each meal.

Weight loss: Reported to occur at a daily dose of 75mg. (25mg. given 3 times daily).

Remedies
Not applicable.

How Long It Takes Till Reversal of Drug Effects
Half the dose of phenylpropanolamine is cleared from the blood in 3–4 hours.

Sources
Covington, T.R. "Obesity: Health implications and approaches to management." *Facts and Comparisons Drug Newsletter*, 1987, 6(9): 65–67.

Griboff, S.I., et al. "A double-blind clinical evaluation of a phenylpropanolamine-caffeine-vitamin combination and a placebo in the treatment of exogenous obesity." *Current Therapeutic Research, Clinical and Experimental*, 1975, 17: 535–43.

Hoebel, B.G., et al. "Appetite suppression by phenylpropanolamine in humans." *Obesity and Bariatric Medicine*, 1975, 4(5): 192–97.

Hoebel, B.G., et al. "Body weight decreased in humans by phenylpropanolamine taken before meals." *Obesity and Bariatric Medicine*, 1975, 4(5): 200–206.

Silverman, H.I. "Phenylpropanolamine—Misused? Or simply abused?" *American Journal of Pharmacy*, 1963, 135: 45–54.

SPIRULINA

Brand Names
U.S.A.: Marketed as "spirulina" by various manufacturers.
Canada: None.
Great Britain: None.

What This Drug Does
Food supplement.

How This Drug Affects Body Weight
Claimed to contain the amino acid phenylalanine, spirulina may act on the brain's appetite center to "switch off" hunger pangs.

Government-Approved Uses for This Drug
As a food supplement.

Unofficial Uses
To promote weight loss.

When Not to Use This Drug
If allergic to this substance or to any related product.

Side Effects From Use of This Drug
None.

Effects on Appetite and Body Weight as Disclosed by the Drug's Manufacturer
None.

Detailed Effects on Appetite and Body Weight
Weight loss: Based on its phenylalanine content, spirulina is claimed to suppress the appetite. But a 1979 FDA advisory panel found no evidence to support this claim. Although various marketers of spirulina have claimed it promotes major weight loss, this dark green powder or pill, available in health food stores, has yet to be proven effective for this use.

Spirulina is derived from a species of blue-green alga (*Spirulina maxima*) that grows in brackish ponds and lakes located in mild and hot climates. Although it contains many vitamins and minerals, these amounts are negligible when taken according to label directions.

In animal studies, substitution of one-third of the daily dietary protein quota with spirulina had no measurable effect on reducing food consumption. Although the experiment did find value in the product as a nutrient, it was deemed worthless as a diet aid in both animals and humans.

Some researchers caution that consuming large quantities of spirulina may be harmful. Because algae, which are high in nucleic acid content, are the source of spirulina, spirulina's conversion to uric acid in the body may induce kidney stones or gout.

Dosage Levels at which Effects Occur
Weight loss: Unknown.

Remedies
Weight loss: Not applicable.

How Long It Takes Till Reversal of Drug Effects
Unknown.

Sources

Maranesi, M., et al. "Nutritional studies on spirulina maxima." *Acta Vitaminologica et Enzymologica*, 1984, 6(4): 295–394.

Willis, J. "About body wraps, pills and other magic wands for losing weight." *FDA Consumer*, 1982, 16: 18–20.

STARCH BLOCKER

Brand Names
U.S.A.: The FDA removed starch blocker from the U.S. market pending scientific testing for its safety and effectiveness.
Canada: None.
Great Britain: None.

What This Drug Does
Diet aid (unproven).
Note: Because starch blocker was so popular during the time it was available to the public, and due to the radical nature of its approach to dieting, it is included here for informational purposes only.

How This Drug Affects Body Weight
Starch blocker is alleged to block or impede the breakdown of starch in the body by inhibiting amylase, an enzyme responsible for the digestion of carbohydrates.

Government-Approved Uses for This Drug
None. The FDA reclassified this product from a food substance to a drug, effectively removing it from the U.S. market.

Unofficial Uses
As an aid to weight reduction.

When Not to Use This Drug
If allergic to this drug or to any related drug.

Side Effects From Use of This Drug
Nausea; vomiting; diarrhea; stomach pains; worsening of diabetes.

Effects on Appetite and Body Weight as Disclosed by the Drug's Manufacturer
None.

Detailed Effects on Appetite and Body Weight
Weight loss: Starch blocker, originally a food substance but now considered a drug by the FDA, was claimed to allow one to eat up to 600 calories daily of starchy foods like bread, potatoes, and pasta without those calories being absorbed. It was removed from the market pending scientific testing for safety and effectiveness. Those using the product prior to this time had developed nausea, diarrhea, vomiting, and stomach pains. It posed a potential danger to diabetics because they might mistakenly rely on starch blocker's effects to calculate their daily caloric intake.

Although the FDA reclassified this substance as a drug, effecting its removal from the U.S. marketplace, the early 1980's saw more than 200 different starch blocker products available in health food stores. Although its effectiveness has so far not been proven, it represents an ingenious approach to achieving diet goals and may one day again be available.

Dosage Levels at Which Effects Occur
Weight loss: Unknown.

Remedies
Weight loss: Not applicable.

How Long It Takes Till Reversal of Drug Effects
Unknown.

Sources
Willis, J. "About body wraps, pills and other magic wands for losing weight." *FDA Consumer*, 1982, 16: 18–20.

Parker, W.A., et al. "Obesity: Health aspects—drug treatment." *U.S. Pharmacist*, 1984, 9(7): 35–51.

Anti-Parkinson Drugs

LEVODOPA

Brand Names
U.S.A.: Bendopa (ICN), Dopar (Norwich Eaton), Laradopa (Roche), *Sinemet (MSD).
Canada: Laradopa (Roche), *Prolopa (Roche), Sinemet (MSD).
Great Britain: Berkdopa (Berk), Brocadopa (Brocades), Laradopa (Roche), *Madopar (Roche), *Sinemet (MSD), *Sinemet Plus (MSD).

What This Drug Does
Anti-Parkinson agent.

How This Drug Affects Body Weight
The weakness and inactivity often seen in those with anorexia nervosa have been thought to resemble some symptoms of Parkinson's disease. Since evidence of brain dopamine deficiency has been linked to anorexia nervosa, levodopa has been suggested as a possible treatment. Weight loss attributed to levodopa use may be due to increased fat breakdown caused by the effects of a drug-induced increased in circulating insulin levels.

Government-Approved Uses for This Drug
To treat Parkinson's disease (a nervous disorder involving fixed mask-like facial expressions; trembling hands, legs, and arms; stiff arm and leg movements).

*Combination drug.

Unofficial Uses
To relieve herpes zoster (shingles) pain.

When Not to Use This Drug
If taking or have taken within 14 days any monoamine oxidase inhibitor drug; in narrow-angle glaucoma; if you have undiagnosed skin lesions or history of melanoma; in nursing mothers; if allergic to this drug or to any related drug.

Side Effects From Use of This Drug
Various involuntary muscle movements; psychiatric disturbance; memory loss; nervousness; anxiety; euphoria; dream disturbance; fatigue; severe depression; suicidal thoughts; hallucinations; various blood disturbances; dizziness upon standing; heart irregularities; flushing; high blood pressure; various visual disturbances; nasal discharge; nausea; vomiting; constipation or diarrhea (reported with equal frequency); gas; epigastric (stomach and intestinal) pain; hiccups; excessive salivation; dry mouth; urinary disturbance; liver toxicity; dark perspiration; rapid, shallow breathing; priapism (prolonged, often painful erection unrelated to sexual desire).

Effects on Appetite and Body Weight as Disclosed by the Drug's Manufacturer
Loss of appetite; weight gain or loss; bitter taste; altered taste; water retention.

Detailed Effects on Appetite and Body Weight
Weight loss: A group of 7 elderly Parkinson sufferers treated with levodopa for 1–3 years showed an average weight loss of almost 14 pounds. This was compared with a normal control group that lost an average of only 1 pound during the same time period.

In a study of 100 patients with Parkinson's disease, treatment with levodopa for 2 months resulted in 5 subjects complaining of loss of appetite and subsequent weight loss.

Altered taste: Of 100 patients treated with levodopa for Parkinson's disease, 22 reported changes in taste sensation. This phenomenon has been described as a strange metallic or garlic-like taste in the mouth. It persisted for up to 2 months after beginning levodopa use.

In a study of 514 patients treated with Sinemet (a combination product containing levodopa and carbidopa), 4.5% reported altered taste sensation ranging from a mild to a total taste loss. The most common complaints were a metallic or plastic taste, with meat being the most frequently affected food. Drinks sometimes were characterized as having a benzene taste. Taste changes were first reported 3–32 weeks after beginning drug treatment (average 12 weeks), with a duration of from 2–40 weeks. The authors note that the lower incidence of taste-change their group experienced (4.5%) versus the 22% incidence described in the first study stems from the lower dose of levodopa required in the combination product Sinemet. The addition of the second ingredient, carbidopa, allows the effective dose of levodopa to be lowered by 75–80%.

Treatment of anorexia nervosa: In a report describing 9 patients (aged 13–22) suffering from anorexia nervosa and treated with levodopa, use of the drug for 16–27 days resulted in 5 of the 9 (56%) gaining from 6.6–12.1 pounds.

Six female sufferers of anorexia nervosa were treated with levodopa for 2–4 weeks. Four of the 6 responded with weight gains ranging from 7–12 pounds.

Dosage Levels at Which Effects Occur

Weight loss: Reported as low as 2,000mg. daily.

Altered taste: Reported as low as 375mg. daily.

Treatment of anorexia nervosa: Reported as low as 200mg. daily but final daily dosages ranged as high as 3,000mg.

Remedies

Weight loss: A decrease in daily dosage could help alleviate levodopa's effects on appetite and body weight. But this must be carefully balanced against maintaining adequate therapeutic blood levels. Consult your physician.

Altered taste: Levodopa-induced taste disturbance may be countered in several ways. Taking the drug with an adequate fluid intake, chewing sugarless gum or using a mouthwash of water and lemon juice, and practicing good oral hygiene may help restore normal taste sensation.

How Long It Takes Till Reversal of Drug Effects

Weight loss: Half the dose of levodopa is cleared from the blood within 1–3 hours.

Altered taste: In one case cited above, discontinuation of levodopa did not improve taste loss even after 1 month. At 2 months, the patient noted some improvement.

Sources

Barbeau, A. "L-Dopa therapy past, present and future." *Arizona Medicine*, 1970, 27 (7): 1–4.

Johanson, A.J., Knorr, N.J. "L-Dopa as treatment for anorexia nervosa." In R.A. Vigersky, ed., *Anorexia Nervosa*. New York: Raven Press, 1977.

Johanson, A.J., Knorr, N.J. "Treatment of anorexia nervosa by levodopa." *Lancet*, 1974, 2: 591.

Siegfried, J., Zumstein, H. "Changes in taste under L-Dopa therapy." *Zeitschrift fur Neurologie*, 1971, 200: 345–48.

Vardi, J., et al. "Weight loss in patients treated long-term with levodopa." *Journal of the Neurological Sciences*, 1976, 30: 33–40.

Willoughby, J.M.T. "Drug-induced abnormalities of taste sensation." *Adverse Drug Reaction Bulletin*, 1983, 100: 368–71.

Antipsychotic Drugs

CHLORPROMAZINE

Brand Names
U.S.A.: Clorazine (Pasadena), Ormazine (Hauck), Promapar (Parke-Davis), Promaz (Keene), Sonazine (Cord), Thorazine (SKF), Thor-Prom (Major).
Canada: Apo-chlorpromazine (Apotex), Chlor-Promanyl (Technilab), Largactil (Rhône-Poulenc), Novochlorpromazine (Novopharm).
Great Britain: Chloractil (DDSA), Dozine (R.P. Drugs), Largactil (May & Baker).

What This Drug Does
Antipsychotic.

How This Drug Affects Body Weight
Chlorpromazine may influence glucose metabolism, causing elevation of sugar levels in the body. It may also cause direct appetite stimulation through its action on the hypothalamus (feeding center in the brain). Weight gain may be caused by chlorpromazine-induced lifting of depression and subsequent appetite improvement.

Government-Approved Uses for This Drug
As an antipsychotic; to control the manic phase of manic-depressive illness; to relieve anxiety prior to surgery; to treat hyperactivity in children; to control nausea and vomiting; to treat hiccups.

Unofficial Uses
None.

When Not to Use This Drug
In coma; in bone-marrow depression; if using large amounts of narcotics, barbiturates, alcohol; in certain blood abnormalities; in the presence of Parkinson's disease; in certain brain damage; in circulatory collapse; in heart disease; in severe low or high blood pressure; if allergic to this drug or to any related drug.

Side Effects From Use of This Drug
Drowsiness; liver dysfunction (jaundice); various blood abnormalities; heart irregularities; Parkinson-like reactions (fixed mask-like facial expression; trembling hands, legs, and arms; stiff arm and leg movements); epileptic seizures; various skin reactions including sensitivity to sunlight; high or low blood sugar; dry mouth; nasal congestion; constipation; difficulty in urinating; visual disturbances; changes in body temperature; bone-marrow depression; breast-milk flow; moderate female breast engorgement; cessation of menstruation; enlargement of the male breasts; priapism (prolonged, often painful erection unrelated to sexual desire); false positive pregnancy test.

Effects on Appetite and Body Weight as Disclosed by the Drug's Manufacturer
Increased appetite; overeating; weight gain; anorexia.

Detailed Effects on Appetite and Body Weight
Weight gain: In a 12-week study of 77 schizophrenics treated with chlorpromazine, the average weight gain after 4 weeks was 5.5 pounds. After 12 weeks, an average increase of 8.2 pounds was reported.

One researcher has suggested that, in his experience, chlorpromazine causes a steady weight gain of about 1.65 pounds per week. This levels off after a total of 15.4–22 pounds has been added to a subjects's initial body weight.

In a short-term trial of 18 psychotics given chlorpromazine, the average weight increase for the 6-day course of drug treatment was 1.8 pounds. Weight returned to normal rather abruptly after discontinuation of chlorpromazine. This rapid change in body weight so closely parallelled starting and stopping of the drug that the authors of the report felt it to be conclusive proof of chlorpromazine's implication in this phenomenon.

In a study of 179 patients treated with chlorpromazine, weight gain was shown to occur in all subjects. An average of 15.9% (range 11.7%–20.2%) over maximum ideal weight was recorded over a 1–2 year period. After this time, weight gains tended to stabilize.

In a report describing 20 female schizophrenics treated with chlorpromazine for over 1 year, 11 (55%) had weight gains of more than 20%. All were of normal weight prior to chlorpromazine treatment.

Fluid retention: A 45-year-old female schizophrenic taking chlorpromazine for 2 years complained of severe fluid retention during this time. Examination revealed swelling of the face, breasts, abdomen, and ankles. Several diuretic drugs were administered with no success. When chlorpromazine was discontinued, a weight loss of 26.4 pounds occurred and all swelling ceased. After 6 months, chlorpromazine was restarted. This resulted in a 33-pound weight gain and renewed swelling. Withdrawal of chlorpromazine again resulted in rapid weight loss and reduced swelling.

Treatment for anorexia nervosa: A group of 20 hospitalized patients with anorexia nervosa were treated with chlorpromazine and insulin (40–80 units daily). For evaluation purposes, these subjects were compared with 24 other patients treated with other regimens. The chlorpromazine-insulin group gained an average of 4.4 pounds per week, as opposed to only about 1.25 pounds per week in the control group. Unfortunately, in follow-up studies of from 3 months to 3 years, only about half the subjects made a lasting recovery.

In a series of 21 hospitalized patients with anorexia nervosa, all were treated with chlorpromazine for a minimum of 8 weeks. When checked 18 months later, 71% had maintained normal body weight, although only about 50% exhibited normal eating behavior.

Dosage Levels at Which Effects Occur
Weight gain: Reported as low as 20mg. daily.
Fluid retention: Reported at 400mg. daily.
Treatment for anorexia nervosa: Reported as low as 150mg. daily.

Remedies

A decrease in daily dosage could help alleviate chlorpromazine's effects on appetite and body weight. But this must be carefully balanced against maintaining adequate therapeutic blood levels.

A switch to a different agent in the same therapeutic category could accomplish similar benefits while minimizing undesirable dietary influences. Consult your physician.

Weight gain: Substitution of low-calorie foods, beverages, and snacks for normal dietary intake may aid in reversing some drug-induced weight gain.

How Long It Takes Till Reversal of Drug Effects

Half this drug is cleared from the body within 10 to 20 hours.

Weight gain: In one case, weight gain was reversed within 3 days after discontinuation of chlorpromazine.

Sources

Amdisen, A. "Drug-produced obesity: Experience with chlorpromazine, perphenazine, and clopenthixol." *Danish Medical Bulletin*, 1964, 11: 182–89.

Brown, J.D. "Drugs causing weight gain." *British Medical Journal*, 1974, 1: 168.

Caffey, E.M. "Experiences with large-scale interhospital cooperative research in chemotherapy." *American Journal of Psychiatry*, 1961, 117: 713–19.

Crisp, A.H. "Some aspects of the evaluation, presentation and follow-up of anorexia nervosa." *Proceedings of the Royal Society of Medicine*, 1965, 58: 814–20.

Dally, P.J., Sargant, W.A. "A new treatment of anorexia nervosa." *British Medical Journal*, 1960, 1: 1770–73.

Johnson, C., et al. "Psychopharmacological treatment of anorexia nervosa and bulimia. Review and synthesis." *Journal of Nervous and Mental Diseases*, 1983, 171(9): 524–34.

Osterman, E., Lassenius, B. "Complications following treatment with chlorpromazine." *Nordisk Medicin*, 1956, 55: 798–801.

Sletten, I.W., Gershon, S. "The effect of chlorpromazine on water and electrolyte balance." *Journal of Nervous and Mental Diseases*, 1966, 142(1): 25–31.

Witz, L., et al. "Chlorpromazine-induced fluid retention masquerading as idiopathic oedema." *British Medical Journal*, 1987, 294 (6575): 807–8.

HALOPERIDOL

Brand Names
U.S.A.: Haldol (McNeil).
Canada: Apo-Haloperidol (Apotex), Haldol (McNeil), Peridol (Technilab).
Great Britain: Haldol (Janssen), Serenace (Searle).

What This Drug Does
Antipsychotic.

How This Drug Affects Body Weight
Unknown. Haloperidol inhibits the action of dopamine (a chemical messenger) in the brain. Although dopamine is thought to act as an appetite depressant, and haloperidol theoretically should cause weight gain, the drug has been shown to cause the opposite, weight loss.

Government-Approved Uses for This Drug
As an antipsychotic; to treat Tourette's disorder (a condition characterized by facial twitches, uncontrolled arm and shoulder motions, and spontaneous and often obscene vocalizations); to control various behavioral problems in children (such as excitability, attention-span difficulties, and excessive aggression).

Unofficial Uses
To control vomiting; to control acute psychotic episodes.

When Not to Use This Drug
In coma or certain central nervous system depression; in Parkinson's disease; if allergic to this drug or to any related drug.

Side Effects From Use of This Drug
Blurred vision; dry mouth; nausea; vomiting; diarrhea or constipation (reported with equal frequency); excessive salivation; various blood abnormalities; sedation; Parkinson-like symptoms (fixed mask-like facial expression; trembling hands, legs, and arms; stiff arm and leg movements); fast heartbeat; blood pressure changes; changes in electrocardiogram; breathing difficulties; liver abnormalities; difficult urination; skin rash; hair loss;

lactation (breast-milk flow); breast engorgement; mastalgia (breast pain); menstrual irregularities; gynecomastia (enlargement of the male breasts; impotence; increased libido.

Effects on Appetite and Body Weight as Disclosed by the Drug's Manufacturer
Loss of appetite.

Detailed Effects on Appetite and Body Weight
Weight loss: In a study of 14 schizophrenics treated with haloperidol for 12 weeks, 6 subjects (43%) showed a weight loss of 10 pounds.

Dosage Levels at Which Effects Occur
Weight loss: Reported at an average daily dosage of 12.3mg. over a 12-week period.

Remedies
A decrease in daily dosage could help alleviate haloperidol's effects on appetite and body weight. But this must be carefully balanced against maintaining adequate therapeutic blood levels.

A switch to a different agent in the same therapeutic category could accomplish similar benefits while minimizing undesirable dietary influences. Consult your physician.

How Long It Takes Till Reversal of Drug Effects
It may take as long as 38 hours for half the dose of haloperidol to clear from the blood.

Source
Serafetinides, E.A., et al. "Haloperidol, clopenthixol, and chlorpromazine in chronic schizophrenia." *Journal of Nervous and Mental Diseases*, 1972, 154(1): 31–42.

LITHIUM

Brand Names
U.S.A.: Cibalith-S (Ciba), Eskalith (SKF), Eskalith CR (SKF), Lithane (Miles), Lithobid (Ciba), Lithonate (Reid-Rowell), Lithotabs (Reid-Rowell).

Canada: Carbolith (ICN), Lithane (Pfizer), Lithizine (Technilab).
Great Britain: Camcolit (Norgine), Liskonum (SKF), Litarex (Weddel), Phasal (Pharmex), Priadel (Delandale).

What This Drug Does
Antimanic.

How This Drug Affects Body Weight
Lithium may increase blood glucose (sugar) levels, effecting enhanced sensitivity to insulin. This could result in more glucose being taken into body tissues. Lithium may stimulate glycogen synthesis, a process by which glucose is stored in the liver and muscles.

Weight gains reported from lithium use may be secondary to increased thirst, promoting high intake of sugar-containing beverages. Lithium may alter taste sensations by accumulating in the olfactory bulb (responsible for smell), as well as in the caudate and pituitary areas of the brain.

Government-Approved Uses for This Drug
To treat the manic phase of manic-depressive illness.

Unofficial Uses
To raise the density of neutrophils (white blood cells) in patients whose count is affected by cancer chemotherapy and in children with chronic neutropenia (decreased white blood cell count); to prevent cluster and certain migraine headaches.

When Not to Use This Drug
In certain kidney disease; in certain heart disease; in severe dehydration or sodium depletion; if pregnant; in nursing mothers; in children under 12 years old; if allergic to this drug or to any related drug.

Side Effects From Use of This Drug
Reversible increase in white blood cell (leukocytes) count; muscle tremors; drowsiness; headache; confusion; restlessness; dizziness; coma; blackouts; seizures; various brain dysfunction; impaired speech; loss of coordination; various heart and circulatory disorders; ringing in the ears; visual impairment; nausea; vomiting; diarrhea; dry mouth; urinary abnormalities and difficulties; high blood sugar (temporary); goiter; thyroid abnor-

malities; itching and rash; drying and thinning of the hair; impotence/sexual dysfunction.

Effects on Appetite and Body Weight as Disclosed by The Drug's Manufacturer

Loss of appetite; weight loss; metallic taste.

Detailed Effects on Appetite and Body Weight

Weight gain: One group of researchers describe about one-third of patients taking lithium and attending a clinic to have experienced weight gains of from 11–33 pounds.

In a 30-month trial of lithium on 44 patients, an average weight gain of 8.9 pounds was seen, with one woman gaining 46 pounds. Gains were seen as a function of time and were progressive in some subjects.

Of 70 patients taking lithium and evaluated over a 2- to 10-year period, 45 (two-thirds) reported average weight gains of 22 pounds. Of those who had a weight problem before taking lithium, 88% had weight gains while taking the drug; 57% of those without previous weight problems also gained weight on lithium. Increased appetite was reported by one-third of subjects and nearly all complained of increased thirst. There was a significant correlation found between increased fluid intake and weight gains.

In a long-term study of 8 patients maintained on lithium, all showed large initial weight gains. Although no further gains were noted, the patients maintained this increased level of body weight. The study, which varied in length from 1–6 years, showed higher body weight remaining constant. One male who discontinued lithium use showed immediate weight loss, but it was quickly regained when he was restarted on the drug.

Body weight was monitored over a 12-month period in a group of 74 patients taking lithium. Weight changes correlated to individual response to lithium therapy, with greatest gains seen in those responding most favorably to treatment. The group as a whole averaged more than a 10-pound weight gain over the 1-year period. Those whose condition was not improved by lithium gained no weight on average, while those helped somewhat had intermediate weight gains. Those who were obese prior to lithium treatment or had a family history of obesity were more prone to gain weight while taking lithium.

Manic depressives have been shown to exhibit large weight changes in response to mood swings. In a British study of 8 such patients placed on long-term lithium therapy, all showed an often large initial weight gain which then stabilized. After this time, only small weight changes were noted over several years of taking the drug. Most of the weight gained is described as an increase in fat and "solid" tissue, a view supported by evidence that total body water remained constant in part of the group.

Water retention: Due to lithium's potential toxicity when dietary salt intake is restricted, patients using the drug are cautioned to maintain adequate salt levels in their diet. Although high blood sodium levels undoubtedly influence water retention in the body, lithium has been shown to increase urinary excretion of aldosterone (a hormone that causes sodium retention) during initial use of the drug. A group of 9 manic depressives treated with lithium were studied for water retention. Ankle swelling was noted in all 9, but only when diet included high sodium levels. Water-weight gain was 2–3 pounds.

Taste change: A 50-year-old man reported a strange and unpleasant taste associated with butter and celery, starting a few days after beginning lithium therapy. This new flavor seemed superimposed on the original taste and cooked celery also assumed an unpleasant smell. The patient was switched from butter to margarine, but after about 2 weeks margarine also developed an unpleasant taste, as did cream and mild cheese. Additionally, some vegetables such as onions imparted a slightly disagreeable taste. Discontinuation of lithium saw a return to normal taste sensation.

A case report describes a 35-year-old psychotic female patient who, after severe manic-depressive illness, was placed on lithium. She reported a complete loss of the ability to taste salt. To compensate, she was adding up to half a shaker of salt to her soup and a quarter-inch on her steak. Successful lithium therapy depends on adequate dietary salt intake; too little causes lithium toxicity, while too much depresses lithium blood levels. In this case, doctors were unable to determine the cause of lowered drug blood levels until they discovered the patient's extreme response to her taste changes.

In a study group of more than 450 patients treated with lithium, about 1 in 20 complained of butter and similar dairy products tasting spoiled. An even greater percentage noted that celery had a different taste.

Treatment of anorexia nervosa: One researcher described two case reports of adult female sufferers of long-term anorexia nervosa who were being treated with lithium. One gained over 13 pounds in 2 weeks, and after another 12 weeks had gained a total of 26 pounds. She maintained this weight for 1 year while under continuous lithium treatment. The other case involved a female who, when treated with the drug, gained almost 20 pounds in 6 weeks.

Dosage Levels at Which Effects Occur
Weight gain: Reported as low as 900mg. daily.
Water retention: Reported as low as 900mg. daily.
Taste change: Reported as low as 750mg. daily.
Treatment of anorexia nervosa: Reported as low as 1,000mg. daily.

Remedies
Weight gain: Substitution of low-calorie foods, beverages, and snacks for normal dietary intake may aid in reversing some drug-induced weight gain.

A decrease in daily dosage could help alleviate lithium's effects on appetite and body weight. But this must be carefully balanced against maintaining adequate therapeutic blood levels.

Water retention: In one case described above, administration of spirinolactone (a diuretic and aldosterone inhibitor), 100mg. daily for 2 days, reversed water retention.

Taste change: Lithium-induced taste disturbance may be countered in several ways. Taking the drug with an adequate fluid intake, chewing sugarless gum or using a mouthwash of water and lemon juice, and practicing good oral hygiene may help restore normal taste sensation.

How Long It Takes Till Reversal of Drug Effects
Weight gain: Some researchers report that patients often continue to gain weight, even after discontinuation of lithium. Among those whose weight does decrease, it may never reach predrug levels.

Water retention: It may take as long as 24 hours for half the dose of lithium to be cleared from the blood.

Taste change: In one case report cited above, taste returned to normal 2 days after discontinuation of lithium. In another instance, this took 3 days.

Sources

Barcai, A. "Lithium in adult anorexia nervosa. A pilot study." *Acta Psychiatrica Scandinavica*, 1977, 55: 97–102.

Bressler, B. "An unusual side-effect of lithium." *Psychosomatics*, 1980, 21: 688–89.

Demers, R., Heninger, G. "Pretibial edema and sodium retention during lithium carbonate treatment." *Journal of the American Medical Association*, 1970, 214: 1845–48.

Dempsey, G.M., et al. "Treatment of excessive weight gain in patients taking lithium." *American Journal of Psychiatry*, 1976, 133: 1082–84.

Duffield, J.E. "Side effects of lithium carbonate." *British Medical Journal*, 1973, 1(5851): 491.

Grof, P., et al. "Lithium stabilization and weight gain." In T.A. Ban et al., eds., *Psychopharmacology, Sexual Disorders and Drug Abuse*. Amsterdam: Elsevier/North-Holland Biomedical Press BV, 1973, pp. 323–27.

Himmelhoch, J.M., Hanin, I. "Side effects of lithium carbonate." *British Medical Journal*, 1974, 4: 233.

Kerry, R.J., et al. "Weight changes in lithium responders." *Acta Psychiatrica Scandinavica*, 1970, 46: 238–43.

O'Connell, R.A. "Lithium's site of action: Clues from side effects." *Comprehensive Psychiatry*, 1971, 12: 224–29.

Schou, M., et al. "Pharmacological and clinical problems of lithium prophylaxis." *British Journal of Psychiatry*, 1970, 116: 615–19.

Vendsborg, P.B., et al. "Lithium treatment and weight gain." *Acta Psychiatrica Scandinavica*, 1976, 53: 139–47.

MOLINDONE

Brand Names
U.S.A.: Moban (DuPont).
Canada: None.
Great Britain: None.

What This Drug Does
Antipsychotic.

How This Drug Affects Body Weight
May exert an appetite-inhibiting effect on the central nervous system. May also increase body movement activity, resulting in the burning of more calories.

Government-Approved Uses for This Drug
To treat psychosis.

Unofficial Uses
None.

When Not to Use This Drug
In severe central nervous system depression or coma; in children under 12 years of age; if allergic to this drug or to any related drug.

Side Effects From Use of This Drug
Drowsiness; dry mouth; blurred vision; dizziness or dizziness upon standing; nasal congestion; fast heartbeat; nausea; vomiting; constipation; various skin reactions; various blood abnormalities; liver dysfunction (jaundice); Parkinson-like symptoms (fixed mask-like facial expression; trembling hands, legs, and arms; stiff arm and leg movements); amenorrhea (cessation of menstruation); resumption of menses in previously amenorrheic women; galactorrhea (breast-milk flow unrelated to childbirth or nursing); gynecomastia (enlargement of the male breasts); increased libido.

Effects on Appetite and Body Weight as Disclosed by the Drug's Manufacturer
Loss of appetite; weight loss or gain.

Detailed Effects on Appetite and Body Weight
Loss of appetite: In a group of 11 schizophrenic males given molindone for a maximum of 13 weeks, appetite decreased during the first 3 weeks, but was somewhat restored thereafter. This paralleled a slight drop in body weight which was then reversed. **Weight loss:** Nine hospitalized schizophrenic patients (4 males and 5 females) aged 26–62 were switched from their previous psychotropic medication to molindone for 3 months. All showed weight loss ranging from 1.8–37 pounds, with an average loss of 16.7 pounds. Six reported no appetite change, while 2 reported a decrease and 1 an increase.

In a study of 15 adults taking molindone (3 males and 12 females) for 12 weeks, none gained weight and 4 (27%) lost more than 10 pounds.

A 2-month study of 30 schizophrenics given molindone showed an average weight loss of 9.9 pounds.

The therapeutic effect of molindone was compared with another antipsychotic drug, trifluoperazine, in a group of 24 schizophrenics. During the 9-week trial, patients on molindone gained an average of only 0.9 pounds versus an average gain of 4.1 pounds in those taking trifluoperazine. While molindone users did show slightly increased body weight, this was considered insignificant when compared with trifluoperazine, as well as with many other psychotropic medications that tend to cause weight gain.

In a study of 23 patients treated with molindone for 6–19 months, a mean weight loss of 5.6 pounds was recorded. Five subjects lost 10 pounds or more (maximum 24 pounds, average 15.7 pounds), while 5 gained an average of 3.6 pounds.

Weight gain: In a 3-month survey of 6 schizophrenic patients taking molindone, an average weight gain of about 20 pounds was recorded. In the first month, the average increase was about 5 pounds; after 2 months the average gain was 15 pounds.

Dosage Levels at Which Effects Occur
Loss of appetite: Reported as low as 5mg. daily.
Weight loss: Reported as low as 5mg. daily.
Weight gain: Reported to occur at an average daily dosage of 143mg.

Remedies
Loss of appetite: The maintenance of adequate fluid intake and the avoidance of excessive alcohol use may aid in reversing molindone-induced appetite loss.

Weight loss: A decrease in daily dosage could help alleviate molindone's effects on appetite and body weight. But this must be carefully balanced against maintaining adequate therapeutic blood levels.

A switch to a different agent in the same therapeutic category could accomplish similar benefits while minimizing undesirable dietary influences. Consult your physician.

Weight gain: Substitution of low-calorie foods, beverages, and snacks for normal dietary intake may aid in reversing some drug-induced weight gain.

How Long It Takes Till Reversal of Drug Effects
Molindone's duration of action may persist for 24–36 hours.

Sources

Clark, M.L., et al. "Molindone in chronic schizophrenia." *Clinical Pharmacology and Therapeutics*, 1970, 11, 680–88.

Gallant, D.M., et al. "Molindone: A cross-over evaluation of capsule and tablet formulation in severely ill schizophrenic patients." *Current Therapeutic Research, Clinical and Experimental*, 1973, 15: 915–18.

Gallant, D.M., Bishop, M.P. "Molindone: A controlled evaluation in chronic schizophrenic patients." *Current Therapeutic Research, Clinical and Experimental*, 1968, 10: 441–47.

Gardos, G., Cole, J.O. "Weight reduction in schizophrenics by molindone." *American Journal of Psychiatry*, 1977, 134: 302–4.

Kellner, R., et al. "Long-term study of molindone hydrochloride in chronic schizophrenics." *Current Therapeutic Research, Clinical and Experimental*, 1976, 20: 686–93.

Parent, M.M., et al. "Effect of molindone on weight change in hospitalized schizophrenic patients." *Drug Intelligence and Clinical Pharmacy*, 1986, 20: 873–75.

Sugerman, A.A., Herrmann, J. "Molindone: An indole derivative with antipsychotic activity." *Clinical Pharmacology and Therapeutics*, 1967, 8: 261–65.

PERPHENAZINE

Brand Names
U.S.A.: *Etrafon (Schering), *Triavil (MSD), Trilafon (Schering).
Canada: Apo-Perphenazine (Apotex), *Etrafon (Schering), Phenazine (ICN), *Triavil (MSD), Trilafon (Schering).
Great Britain: Fentazin (Allen & Hanburys).

What This Drug Does
Antipsychotic.

How This Drug Affects Body Weight
Probably causes weight gain by lifting depression and improving appetite.

Government-Approved Uses for This Drug
To treat symptoms of psychotic disorders; to control nausea, vomiting, and hiccups.

---

*Combination drug.

Unofficial Uses
None.

When Not to Use This Drug
In coma; in bone-marrow depression; if using large amounts of narcotics, barbiturates, or alcohol; in certain blood abnormalities; in the presence of Parkinson's disease; in certain brain damage; in circulatory collapse; in heart disease; if there is severe low or high blood pressure; in children under 12 years of age; if allergic to this drug or to any related drug.

Side Effects From Use of This Drug
Various blood abnormalities; extrapyramidal reactions; Parkinson-like symptoms (fixed mask-like facial expression; trembling hands, legs, and arms; stiff arm and leg movements); sedation; brain-wave changes; dizziness or dizziness upon standing; fast heartbeat; blurred vision and other eye problems; dry mouth; constipation; difficult urination; dark urine color; liver dysfunction; various skin reactions including sensitivity to sunlight; lactation (breast-milk flow), galactorrhea (breast-milk flow unrelated to childbirth or nursing), and moderate breast enlargement in females; gynecomastia (enlargement of the breasts) in males (at high doses); disturbances in menstrual cycle; amenorrhea (cessation of menstruation); changes in libido; inhibition of ejaculation; false positive pregnancy test.

Effects on Appetite and Body Weight as Disclosed by the Drug's Manufacturer
Weight gain or loss; increased appetite; loss of appetite.

Detailed Effects on Appetite and Body Weight
Weight gain: In a study of 83 patients treated with perphenazine, weight gain was shown to occur in all patients. An average gain of 8% (range 6.3–9.5%) over their maximum ideal body weight was recorded over 1–2 years of perphenazine use. After this time, weight tended to stabilize at the higher level.

In a group of 77 schizophrenics treated with perphenazine for 12 weeks, average weight gain after 1 month was 3.27 pounds. After 3 months, this increased to an average gain of 7.38 pounds.

Dosage Levels at Which Effects Occur
Weight gain: Reported as low as 9mg. daily.

Remedies
Weight gain: Substitution of low-calorie foods, beverages, and snacks for normal dietary intake may aid in reversing some drug-induced weight gain.

How Long It Takes Till Reversal of Drug Effects
Weight gain: Although half the dose of perphenazine is eliminated from the body in 10–12 hours, traces of the drug may be found in the urine for up to 6 months.

Sources
Amdisen, A. "Drug-produced obesity: Experience with chlorpromazine, perphenazine, and clopenthixol." *Danish Medical Bulletin*, 1964, 11: 182–89.
Klett, C.J., Caffey, E.M.T. "Weight changes during treatment with phenothiazine derivatives." *Journal of Neuropsychiatry*, 1960, 2: 102–8.

PIMOZIDE

Brand Names
U.S.A.: Orap (McNeil).
Canada: Orap (McNeil).
Great Britain: Orap (Janssen).

What This Drug Does
Antipsychotic.

How This Drug Affects Body Weight
Anorexia nervosa may be related to hyperactivity of dopamine receptors. Dopamine is a chemical transmitter in the nervous system which may depress the appetite. Pimozide is a selective blocker of dopamine activity which may reverse some of its effects.

Government-Approved Uses for This Drug
To treat Tourette's disorder (a condition characterized by facial twitches, uncontrolled arm and shoulder motions, and spontaneous and often obscene vocalizations).

Unofficial Uses
None.

When Not to Use This Drug

In treating simple tics unassociated with Tourette's disorder; to treat drug-induced tics; in various heart-rhythm irregularities; if taking certain other drugs affecting cardiac function; in severe toxic central nervous system depression; in coma; in children under 12 years; if allergic to this drug or to any related drug.

Side Effects From Use of This Drug

Parkinson-like symptoms (fixed mask-like facial expression; trembling hands, legs, and arms; stiff arm and leg movements); various abnormalities in heart function; dry mouth; diarrhea or constipation (reported with equal frequency); thirst; increased salivation; nausea; vomiting; gastrointestinal distress; muscle tightness; stooped posture; headache; drowsiness; insomnia; speech disorder; changes in handwriting appearance; seizures; dizziness or dizziness upon standing; tremor; fainting; depression; visual problems; urinary difficulties; changes in blood pressure; fast heartbeat; skin rash or irritation; sweating; chest pain; menstrual disorders; breast secretions; impotence; loss of libido.

Effects on Appetite and Body Weight as Disclosed by the Drug's Manufacturer

Increased appetite; loss of appetite; taste change; weight gain or loss.

Detailed Effects on Appetite and Body Weight

Treatment of anorexia nervosa: A case report describes a 17-year-old male with anorexia nervosa who was treated with pimozide for 1 month. Improvement was dramatic after 3 weeks, with the patient showing a weight gain of about 20 pounds and eradication of his obsession with body weight.

Eighteen female patients aged 15–36 and suffering from anorexia nervosa participated in a trial to test the value of pimozide as a possible treatment. The study was done over a 6-week period, 3 weeks on pimozide and 3 weeks on a placebo, with the sequence of medication reversed between two subgroups. Both groups showed pimozide to induce significantly greater weight gains than placebo.

In a study of 8 women with anorexia nervosa, 5 were treated with pimozide and copper sulfate for 5 weeks. Average weight gain for this group was slightly over 1 pound per week.

Dosage Levels at Which Effects Occur
Treatment of anorexia nervosa: Found to be effective at 3–12mg. daily.

Remedies
Treatment of anorexia nervosa: Not applicable.

How Long It Takes Till Reversal of Drug Effects
Half the dose of pimozide is eliminated from the body in about 55 hours.

Sources
Hoes, M.J. "Copper sulfate and pimozide for anorexia nervosa." *Journal of Orthomolecular Psychiatry*, 1980, 9: 48–51.

Plantley, F. "Pimozide in the treatment of anorexia nervosa." *Lancet*, 1977, 1: 1105.

Vandereycken, W., Pierloot, R. "Pimozide combined with behavior therapy in the short-term treatment of anorexia nervosa." *Acta Psychiatrica Scandinavica*, 1982, 66: 445–50.

PROCHLORPERAZINE

Brand Names
U.S.A.: Chlorazine (Major), Compazine (SKF).
Canada: Stemetil (Rhône-Poulenc).
Great Britian: Stemetil (May & Baker), Vertigon (SKF).

What This Drug Does
Antipsychotic; antinausea.

How This Drug Affects Body Weight
Prochlorperazine may influence glucose metabolism, causing elevation of its levels in the body. It may also cause direct appetite stimulation through its action on the hypothalamus (the feeding center in the brain). Prochlorperazine may also cause weight gain by lifting depression and improving appetite.

Government-Approved Uses for This Drug
To treat psychosis; to treat anxiety; to control nausea and vomiting.

Unofficial Uses
None.

When Not to Use This Drug

In coma; in bone-marrow depression; with use of large amounts of narcotics, barbiturates, alcohol; in certain blood abnormalities; in the presence of Parkinson's disease; with certain brain damage; in circulatory collapse; in heart disease; in severe low or high blood pressure; in pediatric surgery; in children under 2 years of age or under 20 pounds; if allergic to this drug or to any related drug.

Side Effects From Use of This Drug

Drowsiness; liver dysfunction (jaundice); various blood abnormalities; heart irregularities; Parkinson-like reactions (fixed mask-like facial expression; trembling hands, legs, and arms; stiff arm and leg movements); epileptic seizures; various skin reactions including sensitivity to sunlight; dry mouth; nasal congestion; constipation; difficulty in urinating; visual disturbances; fever or lowered body temperature; bone-marrow depression; amenorrhea (cessation of menstruation); inhibition of ejaculation; priapism (prolonged, often painful erection unrelated to sexual desire); galactorrhea (breast-milk flow unrelated to childbirth or nursing); gynecomastia (enlargement of the male breasts); menstrual irregularities; false positive pregnancy test.

Effects on Appetite and Body Weight as Disclosed by the Drug's Manufacturer

Increased appetite; weight gain.

Detailed Effects on Appetite and Body Weight

Weight gain: In a 12-week study of 84 schizophrenics treated with prochlorperazine, weight gain after 4 weeks averaged 4.4 pounds. After 12 weeks, the average total gain increased to 7.15 pounds.

Dosage Levels at Which Effects Occur

Weight gain: Reported as low as 25mg. daily.

Remedies

Weight gain: Substitution of low-calorie foods, beverages, and snacks for normal dietary intake may aid in reversing some drug-induced weight gain.

How Long It Takes Till Reversal of Drug Effects
Duration of action may persist for up to 3–4 hours (up to 12 hours in extended-release form).

Source
Klett, C.J., Caffey, E.M.T. "Weight changes during treatment with phenothiazine derivatives." *Journal of Neuropsychiatry*, 1960, 2: 102–8.

TRIFLUOPERAZINE

Brand Names
U.S.A.: Stelazine (SKF), Suprazine (Major), TFP (Cord).
Canada: Apo-Trifluoperazine (Apotex), Novoflurazine (Novopharm), Solazine (Horner), Stelazine (SKF , Terflulzine (ICN), Triflurin (Technilab).
Great Britain: *Stelabid (SKF), Stelazine (SKF).

What This Drug Does
Antipsychotic.

How This Drug Affects Body Weight
Probably causes weight gain by lifting depression and improving appetite.

Government-Approved Uses for This Drug
To treat psychotic disorders; to control excessive anxiety, tension, and agitation associated with illness or neurosis.

Unofficial Uses
None.

When Not to Use This Drug
In coma; in severe central nervous system depression; in certain blood abnormalities; in bone-marrow depression; in certain liver problems; if allergic to this drug or to any related drug.

Side Effects From Use of This Drug
Drowsiness; dry mouth; constipation; difficult urination; dizziness; various skin reactions; insomnia; muscle spasms; Parkinson-like symptoms (fixed mask-like facial expression; trembling

*Combination drug.

hands, legs, and arms; stiff arm and leg movements); weakness; fatigue; amenorrhea (cessation of menstruation); lactation (breast-milk flow); priapism (prolonged, often painful erection unrelated to sexual desire); inhibition of ejaculation; galactorrhea (breast-milk flow unrelated to childbirth or nursing); gynecomastia (enlargement of the male breasts); menstrual irregularities; false positive pregnancy test.

Effects on Appetite and Body Weight as Disclosed by the Drug's Manufacturer
Anorexia; increased appetite; weight gain.

Detailed Effects on Appetite and Body Weight
Weight gain: In a group of 24 schizophrenic patients, 12 of whom were treated with trifluoperazine during a 9-week trial, an average weight gain of 4.1 pounds was reported.

Dosage Levels at Which Effects Occur
Weight gain: Reported as low as 10mg. daily.

Remedies
Weight gain: Substitution of low-calorie foods, beverages, and snacks for normal dietary intake may aid in reversing some trifluoperazine-induced weight gain.

How Long It Takes Till Reversal of Drug Effects
It may take up to 20 hours for half the dose of trifluoperazine to be eliminated from the body.

Source
Gallant, D.M., Bishop, M.P. "Molindone: A controlled evaluation in chronic schizophrenic patients." *Current Therapeutic Research, Clinical and Experimental*, 1968, 10: 441–47.

TRIFLUPROMAZINE

Brand Names
U.S.A.: Vesprin (Squibb).
Canada: Novoflurazine (Novopharm), Solazine (Horner), Stelazine (SKF), Terfluzine (ICN), Triflurin (Technilab).
Great Britain: Vesprin (Squibb).

What This Drug Does
Antipsychotic.

How This Drug Affects Body Weight
Triflupromazine may influence glucose metabolism, causing elevation of its levels in the body. It may also cause direct appetite stimulation through its action on the hypothalamus (feeding center in the brain). Triflupromazine may cause weight gain by lifting depression and improving appetite.

Government-Approved Uses for This Drug
To treat certain psychotic disorders; to control severe nausea and vomiting.

Unofficial Uses
None.

When Not to Use This Drug
In coma; in bone-marrow depression; if using large amounts of narcotics, barbiturates, alcohol; in certain blood abnormalities; in the presence of Parkinson's disease; in certain brain damage; in circulatory collapse; in heart disease; in severe low or high blood pressure; in children under 2.5 years; if allergic to this drug or to any related drug.

Side Effects From Use of This Drug
Drowsiness; liver dysfunction (jaundice); various blood abnormalities; heart irregularities; Parkinson-like reactions (fixed mask-like facial expression; trembling hands, legs, and arms; stiff arm and leg movements); epileptic seizures; various skin reactions including sensitivity to sunlight; changes in blood-sugar levels; dry mouth; nasal congestion; constipation; difficulty in urinating; visual disturbances; changes in body temperature; bone-marrow depression; breast-milk flow; moderate female breast engorgement; cessation of menstruation; enlargement of the male breasts; priapism (prolonged, often painful erection unrelated to sexual desire); false positive pregnancy test.

Effects on Appetite and Body Weight as Disclosed by the Drug's Manufacturer
Increased appetite; overeating; weight gain; anorexia.

Detailed Effects on Appetite and Body Weight
Weight gain: In a 12-week study of 69 schizophrenics given

triflupromazine, an average weight gain of about 1.5 pounds was seen after 4 weeks. At 12 weeks, this rose to an average gain of 4.54 pounds.

Dosage Levels at Which Effects Occur
Weight gain: Reported as low as 50mg. daily.

Remedies
Weight gain: Substitution of low-calorie foods, beverages, and snacks for normal dietary intake may aid in reversing some triflupromazine-induced weight gain.

How Long It Takes Till Reversal of Drug Effects
Half the dose of triflupromazine is eliminated from the body in 10–20 hours.

Source
Klett, C.J., Caffey, E.M.T. "Weight changes during treatment with phenothiazine derivatives." *Journal of Neuropsychiatry*, 1960, 2: 102–8.

Cholesterol-Lowering Drugs

CHOLESTYRAMINE

Brand Names
U.S.A: Questran (Mead Johnson).
Canada: Questran (Bristol).
Great Britain: Questran (Bristol-Meyers).

What This Drug Does
  Antihyperlipidemic.

How This Drug Affects Body Weight
  Cholestyramine combines with bile acid, a product of cholesterol synthesis, to form an insoluble complex which is then excreted from the body.

Government-Approved Uses for This Drug
  To reduce high blood cholesterol levels; to relieve itching associated with partial biliary obstruction.

Unofficial Uses
  To treat certain colitis; to treat certain diarrheas; to treat certain pesticide poisoning; to treat digitalis toxicity.

When Not to Use This Drug
  In pregnant women; if there is complete biliary obstruction; if allergic to this drug or to any related drug.

Side Effects From Use of This Drug
Constipation; hemorrhoids; fatty stools; gas; nausea; vomiting; skin rash or irritation; tongue or perianal irritation; vitamin A, D, and K deficiency.

Effects on Appetite and Body Weight as Disclosed by the Drug's Manufacturer
Anorexia; weight gain or loss; edema; sour taste.

Detailed Effects on Appetite and Body Weight
Detailed manufacturer's disclosure: Although cholestyramine's official literature lists loss of appetite, changes in body weight, water retention, and sour taste as potential side effects, more detailed information from independent sources is unavailable.

Dosage Levels at Which Effects Occur
May occur within the normal daily dosage range of 16–32 grams.

Remedies
Loss of appetite; weight loss: The maintenance of adequate fluid intake and the avoidance of excessive alcohol use may aid in restoring normal appetite.

Weight gain: Substitution of low-calorie foods, beverages, and snacks for normal dietary intake may aid in reversing some cholestyramine-induced weight gain.

Water retention: Possible use of a diuretic may help rid the body of excess water. This should only be attempted under the supervision of a doctor.

Taste change: Cholestyramine-induced taste disturbance may be countered in several ways. Taking the drug with an adequate fluid intake, chewing sugarless gum or using a mouthwash of water and lemon juice, and practicing good oral hygiene may help restore normal taste sensation.

How Long It Takes Till Reversal of Drug Effects
Cholestyramine is minimally absorbed from the gastrointestinal tract. Blood cholesterol levels are generally reduced within 1–2 days after beginning the drug. It takes about 2–4 weeks for cholestyramine's cholesterol-lowering effects to dissipate after its withdrawal.

Sources

Olin, B.R. (ed.). *Facts and Comparisions*. St. Louis: Facts and Comparisons, 1988.

Physicians' Desk Reference. Oradell, NJ: Medical Economics, 1988.

USP DI, Rockville, MD: The United States Pharmacopeial Convention, Inc., 1989.

CLOFIBRATE

Brand Names

U.S.A.: Atromid-S (Ayerst).

Canada: Atromid-S (Ayerst), Claripex (ICN), Novofibrate (Novopharm).

Great Britain: Atromid-S (ICI).

What This Drug Does

Antihyperlipidemic.

How This Drug Affects Body Weight

Inhibits early cholesterol formation by accelerating the breakdown of low-density and very-low-density lipoproteins (precursors to cholesterol). It also inhibits formation of very-low-density lipoprotein in the liver.

Government-Approved Uses for This Drug

To help reduce high blood-cholesterol levels under certain conditions.

Unofficial Uses

None.

When Not to Use This Drug

In pregnant women; in nursing mothers; in cases of certain liver or kidney dysfunction; if allergic to this drug or to any related drug.

Side Effects From Use of This Drug

Weakness; fatigue; nausea; vomiting; diarrhea; inflammation of the mouth; upset stomach; gas; blood abnormalities; gallstones; liver dysfunction; various skin reactions; dryness of the hair; muscle and joint pain; fever; impotence; decreased libido; gynecomastia (enlargement of the male breasts).

Effects on Appetite and Body Weight as Disclosed by the Drug's Manufacturer
Weight gain; overeating.

Detailed Effects on Appetite and Body Weight
Weight gain: In a long-term study of 9 patients treated with clofibrate to lower serum cholesterol levels, an average weight gain of 4.4 pounds was recorded the first year. Thereafter, no significant changes in body weight occurred for 7–9 years of the study.

Dosage Levels at Which Effects Occur
Weight gain: Reported at 2 grams daily.

Remedies
Weight gain: Substitution of low-calorie foods, beverages, and snacks for normal dietary intake may aid in reversing some drug-induced weight gain.

How Long It Takes Till Reversal of Drug Effects
It takes from 6–25 hours for half this drug to be cleared from the blood. In patients with compromised kidney function, this may be extended as long as 113 hours.

Source
Stuyt, P.M., et al. "Long-term treatment of type III hyperlipoprotenaemia with clofibrate." *Atherosclerosis*, 1981, 40(3–4): 329–36.

Corticosteroids

COLESTRIPOL

Brand Names
U.S.A.: Colestid (Upjohn).
Canada: Colestid (Upjohn).
Great Britain: Colestid (Upjohn).

What This Drug Does
Antihyperlipidemic.

How This Drug Affects Body Weight
Colestipol combines with bile acid, a product of cholesterol synthesis, to form an insoluble complex which is then excreted from the body.

Government-Approved Uses for This Drug
To reduce high blood cholesterol levels.

Unofficial Uses
To treat digitalis toxicity.

When Not to Use This Drug
In pregnant women; if there is complete biliary obstruction; if allergic to this drug or to any related drug.

Side Effects From Use of This Drug
Constipation; hemorrhoids; fatty stools; gas; nausea; vomiting; skin rash or irritation; tongue or perianal irritation; vitamin A, D, and K deficiency.

Effects on Appetite and Body Weight as Disclosed by the Drug's Manufacturer
Anorexia.

Detailed Effects on Appetite and Body Weight
Detailed manufacturer's disclosure: Although colestipol's official literature lists loss of appetite as a potential side effect, more detailed information from independent sources is unavailable.

Dosage Levels at Which Effects Occur
May occur within the normal daily dosage range of 15–30 grams.

Remedies
Loss of appetite: The maintenance of adequate fluid intake and the avoidance of excessive alcohol use may aid in restoring normal appetite.

How Long It Takes Till Reversal of Drug Effects
Colestipol is minimally absorbed from the gastrointestinal tract. Blood cholesterol levels are generally reduced within 1–2 days after beginning the drug. It takes about 1 month for colistipol's cholesterol-lowering effects to dissipate after its withdrawal.

Source
Olin, B.R. (ed.). *Facts and Comparisons*. St. Louis: Facts and Comparisons, 1988.

Physicians' Desk Reference. Oradell, NJ: Medical Economics, 1988.

USP DI Rockville, MD: The United States Pharmacopeial Convention, Inc., 1989.

DEXTROTHYROXINE

Brand Names
U.S.A.: Choloxin (Flint).
Canada: Choloxin (Flint).
Great Britain: Choloxin (Travenol).

What This Drug Does
Antihyperlipidemic.

How This Drug Affects Body Weight
Stimulates the liver to increase the breakdown and excretion of cholesterol, lowering its level in the body.

Government-Approved Uses for This Drug
To treat high blood cholesterol levels (in those with normal thyroid function and no heart disease).

Unofficial Uses
To treat underactive thyroid in patients with heart disease who cannot tolerate other thyroid supplements.

When Not to Use This Drug
In organic heart disease and various other cardiac problems; with most conditions of high blood pressure; in advanced liver or kidney disease; with high iodine levels; if pregnant; in nursing mothers; if allergic to this drug or to any related drug.

Side Effects From Use of This Drug
Angina pectoris and various other cardiac dysfunction; insomnia; nervousness; tremors; headache; ringing in the ears; dizziness; numbness or tingling sensations; psychic changes; nausea; vomiting; constipation; diarrhea; hair loss; skin rash and itching; visual disturbances; sweating; flushing; fever; increased urination; hoarseness; muscle pain; menstrual irregularities; changes in libido.

Effects on Appetite and Body Weight as Disclosed by the Drug's Manufacturer
Decreased appetite; weight loss; edema.

Detailed Effects on Appetite and Body Weight
Detailed manufacturer's disclosure: Although dextrothyroxine's official literature lists decreased appetite, weight loss, and water retention as potential side effects, more detailed information from independent sources is unavailable.

Dosage Levels at Which Effects Occur
May occur within the usual daily dosage range of 4–8 mg.

Remedies
Loss of appetite; weight loss: The maintenance of adequate fluid intake and the avoidance of excessive alcohol use may aid in restoring normal appetite.

Water retention: Possible use of a diuretic may help rid the body of excess water. This should only be attempted under the supervision of a doctor.

How Long It Takes Till Reversal of Drug Effects
Half the dose of dextrothyroxine is cleared from the blood in about 18 hours. Blood cholesterol levels are generally reduced within 1–2 months after beginning the drug. It takes about 6 weeks to 3 months for dextrothyroxine's cholesterol-lowering effects to dissipate after its withdrawal.

Sources
Olin, B.R. (ed.). *Facts and Comparisons.* St. Louis: Facts and Comparisons, 1988.
Physicians' Desk Reference. Oradell, NJ: Medical Economics, 1988.
USP DI Rockville, MD: The United States Pharmacopeial Convention, Inc., 1989.

GEMFIBROZIL

Brand Names
U.S.A.: Lopid (Parke-Davis).
Canada: Lopid (Parke-Davis).
Great Britain: Lopid (Parke-Davis).

What This Drug Does
Antihyperlipidemic.

How This Drug Affects Body Weight
Probably inhibits the breakdown of peripheral fat stores. Also reduces the synthesis of triglycerides in the liver.

Government-Approved Uses for This Drug
To reduce high blood triglyceride levels.

Unofficial uses
None.

When Not to Use This Drug
In severe liver or kidney dysfunction; in preexisting gallbladder disease; in children; in nursing mothers; if allergic to this drug or to any related drug.

Side Effects From Use of This Drug

Upset stomach; abdominal pain; gas; diarrhea; nausea; vomiting; constipation; fatigue; vertigo; headache; dizziness; skin rash or itching; painful extremities; elevated liver enzymes; various blood abnormalities.

Effects on Appetite and Body Weight as Disclosed by the Drug's Manufacturer

Weight loss; edema; taste perversion.

Detailed Effects on Appetite and Body Weight

Detailed manufacturer's disclosure: Although gemfibrozil's official literature lists weight loss, water retention, and taste changes as potential side effects, more detailed information from independent sources is unavailable.

Dosage Levels at Which Effects Occur

May occur within the usual daily dosage range of 900–1,500 mg.

Remedies

Weight loss: The maintenance of adequate fluid intake and the avoidance of excessive alcohol use may aid in restoring normal appetite.

Water retention: Possible use of a diuretic may help rid the body of excess water. This should only be attempted under the supervision of a doctor.

Taste change: Gemfibrozil-induced taste disturbance may be countered in several ways. Taking the drug with an adequate fluid intake, chewing sugarless gum or using a mouthwash of water and lemon juice, and practicing good oral hygiene may help restore normal taste sensation.

How Long It Takes Till Reversal of Drug Effects

Half the dose of gemfibrozil is cleared from the blood in 1.5 hours after a single dose. Blood triglyceride levels are generally reduced within 2–5 days after beginning the drug. Peak effects are usually reached in 4 weeks.

Sources

Olin, B.R. (ed.). *Facts and Comparisons*. St. Louis: Facts and Comparisons, 1988.

Physicians' Desk Reference. Oradell, NJ: Medical Economics, 1988.
USP DI Rockville, MD: The United States Pharmacopeial Convention, Inc., 1989.

PREDNISOLONE

Brand Names
U.S.A.: Articulose-50 (Seatrace), Cortalone (Halsey), Delta-Cortef (Upjohn), Fernisolone-P (Ferndale), Hydeltrasol (MSD), Hydeltra-T.B.A. (MSD), Key-Pred (Hyrex), Meticortelone (Schering), Niscort (Kay), Nor-Pred T.B.A. (Vortech), Pediapred (Fisons), Predaject-50 (Mayrand), Predalone (Forest), Predcor (Hauck), Predicort (Dunhall), Prednisol TBA (Pasadena), Prelone (Muro), Solu-Pred (Carter-Glogau), Sterane (Pfipharmecs).
Canada: Meticortelone (Schering), Nova-Pred (Nova), Novo-prednisolone (Novopharm).
Great Britain: Codelcortone (MSD), Deltacortril Enteric (Pfizer), Deltalone (DDSA), Delta Phoricol (Wallace; Farrillon), Deltastab (Boots), Marsolone (Marshall's), Precortisyl (Roussel), Ultracortenol (Ciba).

What This Drug Does
Adrenal cortical steroid.

How This Drug Affects Body Weight
Prednisolone may suppress the hypothalamic-pituitary axis, part of the body's endocrine system. It has been suggested that prednisolone's potential to cause high blood sugar may unmask latent diabetes.

Government-Approved Uses for This Drug
To treat certain endocrine disorders; to treat various arthritic conditions; to treat various collagen (connective tissue) diseases; to treat various skin disorders; to treat various allergic responses.

Unofficial Uses
None.

When Not to Use This Drug

In widespread fungal infections of the blood; during use of live virus vaccines; if already receiving large amounts of this drug or a similar drug; if allergic to this drug or to any related drug.

Side Effects From Use of This Drug

High blood pressure; potassium loss; muscle weakness; bone decomposition; loss of muscle mass; peptic ulcer with perforation or bleeding; inflammation of the pancreas; inflammation or ulceration of the esophagus; delayed wound healing; various skin reactions; increased sweating; convulsions; increased skull pressure; headache; vertigo; growth suppression in children; Cushing's syndrome (excessive function of the pituitary gland); loss of diabetic control; congestive heart failure (in certain predisposed patients); various eye disorders including glaucoma; decreased resistance to infection; various mental disturbances; menstrual irregularities; hirsutism (male-type hair growth in females); increase or decrease in motility or number of spermatozoa.

Effects on Appetite and Body Weight as Disclosed by the Drug's Manufacturer

Water retention and swelling; increased appetite; weight gain.

Detailed Effects on Appetite and Body Weight

Increased appetite: A study of 61 cancer patients complaining of poor appetite or weight loss was conducted over a 5-week period. In assessments at weeks 2 and 5 of the study, it was determined that prednisolone was more effective than placebo in improving the subjects' appetite.

Dosage Levels at Which Effects Occur

Increased appetite: Reported effective at a daily dose of 15mg.

Remedies

Increased appetite: Not applicable.

How Long It Takes Till Reversal of Drug Effects

Although half the dose of prednisolone is cleared from the blood in 2–3.5 hours, its effects may persist for up to a day and a half.

Source
Willox, J.C., et al. "Prednisolone as an appetite stimulant in patients with cancer." *British Medical Journal [Clin. Res.]*, 1984, 288(6410): 27.

PREDNISONE

Brand Names
U.S.A.: Cortan (Halsey), Delta-Dome (Miles), Deltasone (Upjohn), Fernisone (Ferndale), Liquid Pred (Muro), Meticorten (Schering), Orasone (Reid-Rowell), Panasol (Seatrace), Paracort (Parke-Davis), Prednicen-M (Central), Servisone (Lederle), SK-Prednisone (SKF), Sterapred (Mayrand), Wojtab (Roxane).
Canada: Apo-Prednisone (Apotex), Colisone (Frosst), Deltasone (Upjohn), Novoprednisone (Novopharm), Paracort (Parke-Davis), Winpred (ICN).
Great Britain: Decortisyl (Roussel), Deltacortone (MSD), Econosone (DDSA), Marsone (Marshall's).

What This Drug Does
Adrenal cortical steroid.

How This Drug Affects Body Weight
Prednisone may suppress the hypothalamic-pituitary axis, part of the body's endocrine system. It has been suggested that prednisone's potential to cause high blood sugar may unmask latent diabetes.

Government-Approved Uses for This Drug
To treat certain endocrine disorders; to treat various arthritic conditions; to treat various collagen (connective tissue) diseases; to treat various skin disorders; to treat various allergic responses.

Unofficial Uses
None.

When Not to Use This Drug
In widespread fungal infections of the blood; during use of live virus vaccines; if already receiving large amounts of this drug or a similar drug; if allergic to this drug or to any related drug.

Side Effects From Use of This Drug

High blood pressure; potassium loss; muscle weakness; bone decomposition; loss of muscle mass; peptic ulcer with perforation or bleeding; inflammation of the pancreas; inflammation or ulceration of the esophagus; delayed wound healing; various skin reactions; increased sweating; convulsions; increased skull pressure; headache; vertigo; growth suppression in children; Cushing's syndrome (excessive function of the pituitary gland); loss of diabetic control; congestive heart failure (in certain predisposed patients); various eye disorders including glaucoma; decreased resistance to infection; various mental disturbances; menstrual irregularities; hirsutism (male-type hair growth in females); increase or decrease in motility or number of spermatozoa.

Effects on Appetite and Body Weight as Disclosed by the Drug's Manufacturer

Water retention and swelling; increased appetite; weight gain.

Detailed Effects on Appetite and Body Weight

Weight gain: In a study of 36 asthmatic patients treated with a variety of cortisones, 1 subject noted weight gain while taking prednisone. The 57-year-old man gained almost 18 pounds in 28 months of prednisone therapy.

Weight loss: In the same study of 36 asthmatic patients as described above, several subjects reported weight loss while taking prednisone. A 55-year-old male exhibited a 7.7-pound weight loss over 28 months, while a 59-year-old man reported losing 18 pounds in 24 months. A 68-year-old female lost about 10 pounds in 19 months; a 76-year-old woman dropped 10.6 pounds in 2 years.

Dosage Levels at Which Effects Occur

Weight gain: Reported as low as 10mg. daily.
Weight loss: Reported as low as 10mg. daily.

Remedies

Weight gain: Substitution of low-calorie foods, beverages, and snacks for normal dietary intake may aid in reversing some prednisone-induced weight gain.
Weight loss: A decrease in daily dosage could help alleviate

prednisone's effects on body weight. But this must be carefully balanced against maintaining adequate therapeutic blood levels.

A switch to a different agent in the same therapeutic category could accomplish similar benefits while minimizing undesirable influences. Consult your physician.

How Long It Takes Till Reversal of Drug Effects
While half the dose of prednisone is cleared from the blood in about 1 hour, its duration of action may persist up to 36 hours.

Source
Lindholm, B. "Body cell mass during long-term treatment with cortisone and anabolic steroids in asthmatic subjects." *Acta Endocrinologica* (Copenhagen), 1967, 55 (2): 222–39.

PROBUCOL

Brand Names
U.S.A.: Lorelco (Merrel Dow).
Canada: Lorelco (Dow).
Great Britain: Lurselle (Merrell).

What This Drug Does
Antihyperlipidemic.

How This Drug Affects Body Weight
Probucol decreases the transport of cholesterol from the intestine. It is also thought to inhibit cholesterol production.

Government-Approved Uses for This Drug
To reduce high cholesterol levels.

Unofficial Uses
None.

When Not to Use This Drug
If pregnant; if breast-feeding; in children; in certain heart arrhythmias and other heart problems; if allergic to this drug or to any related drug.

Side Effects From Use of This Drug

Diarrhea; gas; abdominal pain; nausea; vomiting; sweating; dizziness; headache; various blood abnormalities; skin rash; insomnia; blurred vision; ringing in the ears; impotence.

Effects on Appetite and Body Weight as Disclosed by the Drug's Manufacturer

Anorexia; edema; diminished sense of taste and smell.

Detailed Effects on Appetite and Body Weight:

Detailed manufacturer's disclosure: Although probucol's official literature lists loss of appetite, water retention and diminished sense of taste and smell as potential side effects, more detailed information from independent sources is unavailable.

Dosage Levels At Which Effects Occur

May occur within the normal daily dosage range of 500–1,000 mg.

Remedies

Loss of appetite: The maintenance of adequate fluid intake and the avoidance of excessive alcohol use may aid in restoring normal appetite.

Water retention: Possible use of a diuretic may help rid the body of excess water. This should only be attempted under the supervision of a doctor.

Taste change: Probucol-induced taste disturbance may be countered in several ways. Taking the drug with an adequate fluid intake, chewing sugarless gum or using a mouthwash of water and lemon juice, and practicing good oral hygiene may help restore normal taste sensation.

How Long It Takes Till Reversal of Drug Effects

Probucol accumulates in the body's fat tissue and may remain in the fat and blood for 6 months or more after the last dose.

Sources

Olin, B.R. (ed.). *Facts and Comparisons.* St. Louis: Facts and Comparisons, 1988.

Physicians' Desk Reference. Oradell, NJ: Medical Economics, 1988.

USP DI Rockville, MD: The United States Pharmacopeial Convention, Inc., 1989.

TRIAMCINOLONE

Brand Names
U.S.A.: Acetospan (Reid-Provident), Amcort (Keene), Aristocort (Lederle), Aristospan (Lederle), Articulose L.A. (Seatrace), Atolone (Major), BayTac-40 (Bay), BayTac-D (Bay), Cenocort A-40 (Central), Cenocort Forte (Central), Cino 40 (Reid-Provident), Kenacort (Squibb), Kenaject (Mayrand), Kenalog-10 (Squibb), Kenalog-40 (Squibb), Kenalone (Kay), Tac-D (Parnell), Tracilon (Savage), Tramacort-40 (Bolan), Triacin 40 (Vortech), Triacort (Kay), Triam-A (Hyrex), Triam Forte (Hyrex), Triamolone 40 (Forest), Triamonide 40 (Forest), Tri-Kort (Keene), Trilog (Hauck), Tristoject (Mayrand).
Canada: Aristocort (Lederle), Aristospan hexacetonide (Lederle), Triamacort (ICN).
Great Britain: Adcortyl (Squibb), Ledercort (Lederle), Lederspan (Lederle).

What This Drug Does
Adrenal cortical steroid.

How This Drug Affects Body Weight
Triamcinolone may suppress the hypothalamic-pituitary axis, part of the body's endocrine system. It has been suggested that triamcinolone's potential to cause high blood sugar may unmask latent diabetes. Weight loss may occur at high doses due to a catabolic (breaking down) process which may affect protein tissue and cause dehydration. Although triamcinolone is claimed to lack the salt-retaining properties (responsible for water retention in the body) of its parent compound cortisone, studies, as well as its official literature, have shown this phenomenon to occur with its use.

Government-Approved Uses for This Drug
To treat certain endocrine disorders; to treat various arthritic conditions; to treat various collagen (connective tissue) diseases; to treat various skin disorders; to treat various allergic responses.

Unofficial Uses
None.

When Not to Use This Drug
In widespread fungal infections of the blood; during use of live virus vaccines; if already receiving large amounts of this drug or a similar drug; if allergic to this drug or to any related drug.

Side Effects From Use of This Drug
High blood pressure; potassium loss; muscle weakness; bone decomposition; peptic ulcer with perforation or bleeding; inflammation of the pancreas; inflammation or ulceration of the esophagus; delayed wound healing; various skin reactions; increased sweating; convulsions; increased skull pressure; headache; vertigo; growth suppression in children; Cushing's syndrome (excessive function of the pituitary gland); loss of diabetic control; congestive heart failure (in certain predisposed patients); various eye disorders including glaucoma; decreased resistance to infection; various mental disturbances; amenorrhea (cessation of menstruation) and other menstrual irregularities; increase or decrease in motility or number of spermatozoa.

Effects on Appetite and Body Weight as Disclosed by the Drug's Manufacturer
Water retention and swelling; loss of muscle mass; increased appetite; weight gain.

Detailed Effects on Appetite and Body Weight
Weight gain: In a study of 20 asthmatic patients on long-term corticosteroid therapy, 16 of whom were taking triamcinolone, weight gain was found to have occurred in 15% of cases.

Of 29 sufferers of systemic lupus erythematosis (SLE) treated with triamcinolone, weight gain over an average of 4 months was reported in 3 patients. One woman gained 29 pounds during the first 6 weeks of therapy.

A weight gain of almost 30 pounds was reported in a 40-year-old male asthmatic treated with triamcinolone for 22 months.

A 63-year-old asthmatic man given triamcinolone for 31 months reported a 10-pound weight gain.

Water retention: In a study of 20 asthmatic patients on long-term corticosteroid treatment, 16 of whom were taking triamcinolone, water retention was reported to have occurred in 10% of cases.

Appetite loss; weight loss: In a comprehensive study of 74 patients treated with triamcinolone for rheumatoid arthritis, loss of appetite and weight loss were reported. In those treated with the drug for less than 90 days, almost 16% complained of suppressed appetite. Weight loss ranged from 6–12 pounds. In those treated longer than 90 days, weight loss ranged from 8–30 pounds.

Of 29 patients treated with triamcinolone for systemic lupus erythematosis (SLE), 18 reported a mean weight loss of 10.7 pounds during an average 4 months of therapy. Maximum recorded weight loss was 18 pounds. Most patients noted a gradual weight reduction over the course of treatment.

Dosage Levels at Which Effects Occur
Weight gain: Reported as low as 2mg. daily.
Water retention: Reported to occur within a daily dose range of 2–8mg.
Appetite loss; weight loss: Reported as low as 4mg. daily.

Remedies
Weight gain: Substitution of low-calorie foods, beverages, and snacks for normal dietary intake may aid in reversing some triamcinolone-induced weight gain.
Water retention: A decrease in daily dosage could help alleviate triamcinolone's effect on water retention. But this must be carefully balanced against maintaining adequate therapeutic blood levels.

Dietary salt restriction may also be helpful in reversing edema. Consult your physician.

How Long It Takes Till Reversal of Drug Effects
Half the dose of triamcinolone is cleared from the blood in a minimum of 200 minutes, often longer. Its duration of effect may persist up to 3 days.

Sources
Dubois, E.L. "Triamcinolone in the treatment of systemic lupus erythematosis." *Journal of the American Medical Association*, 1958, 167: 1590.
Freyberg, R.H., et al. "Further experiences with Δ1, 9 alpha fluoro 16 alpha hydroxyhydrocortisone (triamcinolone) in treatment of patients with rheumatoid arthritis." *Arthritis and Rheumatism*, 1958, 1: 215–29.

Lindholm, B. "Body cell mass during long-term cortisone treatment in asthmatic subjects." *Acta Endocrinologica* (Copenhagen), 1967, 55(2): 202–21.

Lindholm, B. "Body cell mass during long-term treatment with cortisone and anabolic steroids in asthmatic subjects." *Acta Endocrinologica* (Copenhagen), 1967, 55(2): 222–39.

Tuft, L., et al. "Long-term corticosteroid therapy in chronic asthmatic patients." *Annals of Allergy*, 1971, 29(6): 287–93.

Diuretic Drugs

ACETAZOLAMIDE

Brand Names
U.S.A.: Ak-Zol (Akorn), Dazamide (Major), Diamox (Lederle).
Canada: Acetazolam (ICN), Diamox (Lederle).
Great Britain: Diamox (Lederle).

What This Drug Does
Diuretic.

How This Drug Affects Body Weight
By blocking the enzyme carbonic anhydrase, acetazolamide enhances the kidneys' excretion of sodium, potassium, bicarbonate, and water.

Government-Approved Uses for This Drug
To treat glaucoma; as a diuretic; to treat epilepsy; to treat acute mountain sickness experienced at high altitudes.

Unofficial Uses
To treat periodic paralysis (a rare inherited disorder).

When Not to Use This Drug
In the presence of low sodium and/or potassium blood levels; in certain kidney and liver diseases; in certain glaucomas; in adrenal gland failure; in certain blood imbalances; if allergic to this drug, to any related drug, or to sulfa drugs.

Side Effects From Use of This Drug
Infrequent but may include drowsiness; burning, itching, or tingling of the skin; stomach upset; nausea; blood abnormalities; liver problems.

Effects on Appetite and Body Weight as Disclosed by the Drug's Manufacturer
Loss of appetite.

Detailed Effects on Appetite and Body Weight
Loss of appetite; weight loss: In a study encompassing 92 patients with chronic glaucoma who were treated with carbonic anhydrase inhibitor drugs (either acetazolamide or acetohexamide), about 48% complained of a complex of symptoms including appetite loss and weight loss.

In another study of 70 patients receiving acetazolamide, only about 6% reported loss of appetite.

Dosage Levels at Which Effects Occur
Loss of appetite; weight loss: Reported as low as 500mg. daily.

Remedies
Loss of appetite; weight loss: A decrease in daily dosage could help alleviate acetazolamide's effects on appetite and body weight. But this must be carefully balanced against maintaining adequate therapeutic blood levels.

The maintenance of adequate fluid intake and the avoidance of excessive alcohol use may aid in reversing appetite loss.

The addition of sodium bicarbonate, 56–70 milliequivalents (mEq.) orally per day, dramatically reversed weight loss and loss of appetite in 42% of those taking carbonic anhydrase inhibitor drugs. About 21% reported partial relief of these drug side effects.

How Long It Takes Till Reversal of Drug Effects
Acetazolamide's duration of action in the body is 8–12 hours.

Sources
Becker, B. "Use of methazolamide (Neptazane) in the therapy of glaucoma." *American Journal of Ophthalmology*, 1960, 49:1307–11.
Epstein, D.L., Grant, M. "Carbonic anhydrase inhibitor side effects." *Archives of Ophthalmology*, 1977, 95: 1378–82.

BUMETANIDE

Brand Names
U.S.A.: Bumex (Roche).
Canada: None.
Great Britain: Burinex (Leo).

What This Drug Does
Diuretic.

How This Drug Affects Body Weight
It inhibits the reabsorption of sodium and chloride in the kidneys, causing increased water excretion.

Government-Approved Uses for This Drug
To rid the body of excess fluid associated with congestive heart failure and various other conditions.

Unofficial Uses
None.

When Not to Use This Drug
If there is a lack of urine output; in hepatic (liver) coma; if there is severe electrolyte depletion; in nursing mothers; if allergic to this drug or to any related drug.

Side Effects From Use of This Drug
Dizziness or dizziness upon standing; headache; dehydration; deafness (temporary); nausea; low blood potassium; high blood uric acid; low blood calcium; high blood sugar; skin rash; muscle pain and tenderness; premature ejaculation; difficulty maintaining an erection.

Effects on Appetite and Body Weight as Disclosed by the Drug's Manufacturer
Anorexia.

Detailed Effects on Appetite and Body Weight
Detailed manufacturer's disclosure: Although bumetanide's official literature lists loss of appetite as a potential side effect, more detailed information from independent sources is unavailable.

Dosage Levels at Which Effects Occur

May occur within the usual oral daily dosage range of 0.5–2mg.

Remedies

Loss of appetite: The maintenance of adequate fluid intake and the avoidance of excessive alcohol use may aid in restoring normal appetite.

How Long It Takes Till Reversal of Drug Effects

While half the dose of bumetanide is cleared from the blood within 60–90 minutes, its duration of action may persist up to 6 hours.

Sources

Olin, B.R. (ed.). *Facts and Comparisons*. St. Louis: Facts and Comparisons, 1988.
Physicians' Desk Reference. Oradell, NJ: Medical Economics, 1988.
USP DI. Rockville, MD: The United States Pharmacopeial Convention, Inc., 1989.

CHLOROTHIAZIDE

Brand Names

U.S.A.: *Aldochlor (MSD), *Chloroserpine (Schein), Diachlor (Major), *Diupres (MSD), Diuril (MSD).
Canada: Diuril (Frosst).
Great Britain: Saluric (MSD).

What This Drug Does

Diuretic.

How This Drug Affects Body Weight

By inhibiting the reabsorption of sodium in the kidneys, it causes increased excretion of water.

Government-Approved Uses for This Drug

To rid the body of excess fluid associated with congestive heart failure and various other conditions; to treat high blood pressure.

*Combination drug.

Unofficial Uses
In combination with amiloride or allopurinol to prevent calcium kidney stones; to correct various problems of calcium absorption, metabolism, and elimination; to treat diabetes insipidus (a metabolic disease marked by thirst and excessive urination).

When Not to Use This Drug
If there is a lack of urine output; if a nursing mother; if allergic to this drug or to any related drug.

Side Effects From Use of This Drug
Stomach upset; nausea; vomiting; cramps; diarrhea; constipation; liver dysfunction (jaundice); inflammation of the pancreas; dizziness or dizziness upon standing; vertigo; burning sensations of the skin; headache; various blood abnormalities; various skin reactions including sensitivity to sunlight; high blood sugar and uric acid; muscle spasm and weakness; blurred vision.

Effects on Appetite and Body Weight as Disclosed by the Drug's Manufacturer
Anorexia; bitter taste; weight loss.

Detailed Effects on Appetite and Body Weight
Detailed manufacturer's disclosure: Although chlorothiazide's official literature lists loss of appetite, bitter taste, and weight loss as potential side effects, more detailed information from independent sources is unavailable.

Dosage Levels at Which Effects Occur
May occur within the usual daily dosage range of 500–2,000mg.

Remedies
Loss of appetite; weight loss: The maintenance of adequate fluid intake and the avoidance of excessive alcohol use may aid in restoring normal appetite.
Bitter taste: Chlorothiazide-induced taste disturbance may be countered in several ways. Taking the drug with an adequate fluid intake, chewing sugarless gum or using a mouthwash of water and lemon juice, and practicing good oral hygiene may help restore normal taste sensation.

How Long It Takes Till Reversal of Drug Effects
Half the dose of chlorothiazide is cleared from the blood within 1–2 hours, with a duration of action lasting from 6–12 hours.

Sources
Olin, B.R. (ed.). *Facts and Comparisons*. St. Louis: Facts and Comparisons, 1988.
Physicians' Desk Reference. Oradell, NJ: Medical Economics, 1988.
USP DI. Rockville, MD: The United States Pharmacopeial Convention, Inc., 1989.

FUROSEMIDE

Brand Names
U.S.A.: Lasix (Hoechst-Roussel).
Canada: Apo-Furosemide (Apotex), Furoside (ICN), Lasix (Hoechst), Neo-Renal (Neolab), Novosemide (Novopharm), Uritol (Horner).
Great Britain: Diumide-K (Napp), Dryptal (Berk), Frusetic (Unimed), Frusid (DDSA), Fur-O-Ims (IMS), Lasikal (Hoechst), *Lasilactone (Hoechst), Lasix (Hoechst), Lasix+K (Hoechst), Min-I-Jet Furosemide Injection (IMS).

What This Drug Does
Diuretic.

How This Drug Affects Body Weight
Furosemide-induced loss of body water due to increased urination may cause compensatory mechanisms in the body to attempt to conserve sodium and water. These processes may overwhelm the diuretic effects of furosemide, causing a net water gain rather than a loss. Furosemide stimulates the renin-angiotensin system, a delicate balance affecting kidney function. This can cause increased levels of aldosterone (a hormone produced by the kidneys), a condition that may cause salt and fluid retention.

Government-Approved Uses for This Drug
To rid the body of excess fluid associated with congestive heart failure and various other conditions; to treat high blood pressure.

Unofficial Uses
None.

*Combination drug.

When Not to Use This Drug

In women contemplating pregnancy; if urine output is impaired; if a nursing mother; if allergic to this drug or to any related drug.

Side Effects From Use of This Drug

Mouth irritation; stomach upset; nausea; vomiting; abdominal cramps; constipation; liver dysfunction (jaundice); inflammation of the pancreas; dizziness or dizziness upon standing; burning sensations of the skin; headache; blurred vision; ringing in the ears or hearing loss; various blood abnormalities; various skin reactions including sensitivity to sunlight; high blood sugar and uric acid; muscle spasm and weakness; bladder spasm; restlessness; thrombophlebitis (swelling of a vein, often accompanied by a blood clot).

Effects on Appetite and Body Weight as Disclosed by the Drug's Manufacturer

Loss of appetite.

Detailed Effects on Appetite and Body Weight

Water retention: Use of furosemide, as well as other diuretics, to treat trivial complaints such as monthly menstrual swelling may actually increase water retention and cause patients to become dependent on continued use of these drugs.

Although furosemide is used to rid the body of excess water, it has the potential to cause the reverse. Two case reports describe women given furosemide to treat periodic menstrual fluid retention. In one instance, ankle and facial swelling became worse with furosemide use than with no drug at all. After taking furosemide for 18 months, the patient still had enough ankle and leg swelling to warrant admission into the hospital. After 11 drug-free days, sodium intake was reduced and the patient began losing water weight. One month after furosemide was withdrawn, the patient had lost a total of 13.2 pounds of water weight.

The second case describes a woman who, after 1 year of taking furosemide to treat water retention, still had intermittent swelling of the fingers, face, and ankles. Whenever she attempted to discontinue the drug, swelling increased to such an extent that furosemide use had to be resumed. Placed in the hospital and taken off the drug, she gained over 7 pounds of water weight in

4 days, with visible swelling of the face, hands, and ankles. After 3 furosemide-free weeks, swelling subsided and body weight decreased to normal.

Dosage Levels at Which Effects Occur
Water retention: Reported as low as 40mg. daily.

Remedies
Water retention: Discontinuation of furosemide is the only known remedy.

How Long It Takes Till Reversal of Drug Effects
Water retention: In the cases cited above, withdrawal of furosemide resulted in decreased swelling and a return to normal body weight within 3–4 weeks.

With half this drug cleared from the blood in slightly under 1 hour, its effects may persist from 6–8 hours.

Source
MacGregor, G.A., et al. "Diuretic-induced oedema." *Lancet*, 1975, 1: 489–92.

HYDROCHLOROTHIAZIDE

Brand Names
U.S.A: *Aldactazide (Searle),*Aldoril (MSD), *Apresazide (Ciba), *Apresodex (Rugby), *Apresoline-Esidrix (Ciba), *Aprozide (Major), Aquazide H (Western Research), *Cam-ap-es (Camall), *Capozide (Squibb), *Cherapas (Kay), Chlorzide (Foy), Diaqua (Hauck), Diu-Scrip (Scrip), *Dralserp (Vitarine), *Dyazide (SKF), Esidrix (Ciba), *Esimil (Ciba), *H-H-R (Schein), *H.R.-50 (Towne Paulsen), *Hydral (Reid-Provident), *Hydrap-Es (Vitarine), *Hydra-Zide (Par), Hydro-Chlor (Vortech), Hydro-D (Halsey), HydroDiuril (MSD), Hydromal (Mallard), *Hydro Plus (Reid-Provident), *Hydropres (MSD), *Hydro-Reserp (Camall), *Hydroserp (Reid-Provident), *Hydro-Serp (Vitarine), *Hydroserpine (Schein), *Hydrosine (Major), Hydro-T (Major), *Hydrotensin (Mayrand), Hydro-Z-50 (Mayrand), *Inderide (Ayerst), *Lo-

*Combination drug.

pressor HCT (Geigy), *Mallopress (Mallard), *Maxzide (Lederle), Mictrin (Econo Med), *Moduretic (MSD), Oretic (Abbott), *Oreticyl (Abbott), *Rezide (Edwards), *Ser-A-Gen (Goldline), *Seralazide (Lannett), *Ser-Ap-Es (Ciba), *Serpasil-Apresoline (Ciba), *Serpasil-Esidrix (Ciba), *Serpazide (Major), *Spironazide (Schein), *Spirozide (Schein), Thiuretic (Parke-Davis), *Timolide (MSD), *Tri-Hydroserpine (Rugby), *Unipres (Reid-Rowell), Zide (Reid-Provident).
Canada: *Aldactazide (Searle), *Aldoril (MSD), Apo-Hydrochlorothiazide (Apotex), Diuchlor-H (Medic), *Dyazide (SKF), Esidrix (Ciba), HydroDiuril (MSD), *Hydropres (MSD), *Inderide (Ayerst), *Ismelin-Esidrix (Ciba), *Moduret (MSD), Natrimax (Triamon), Nefrol (Riva), Neo-Codema (Neolab), Novohydrazide (Novopharm), *Ser-Ap-Es (Ciba), Urozide (ICN).
Great Britain: Direma (Dista), Esidrex (Ciba), Esidrex-K (Ciba), HydroSaluric (MSD).

What This Drug Does
Diuretic.

How This Drug Affects Body Weight
By inhibiting the reabsorption of sodium in the kidneys, it causes increased excretion of water.

Government-Approved Uses for This Drug
To rid the body of excess fluid associated with congestive heart failure and various other conditions; to treat high blood pressure.

Unofficial Uses
In combination with amiloride or allopurinol to prevent calcium kidney stones; to correct various problems of calcium absorption, metabolism, and elimination; to treat diabetes insipidus (a metabolic disease marked by thirst and excessive urination).

When Not to Use This Drug
If there is a lack of urine output; if breast-feeding; if allergic to this drug or to any related drug.

Side Effects From Use of This Drug
Stomach upset; nausea; vomiting; cramps; diarrhea; constipation; liver dysfunction (jaundice); inflammation of the pancreas; dizziness or dizziness upon standing; vertigo; burning sensations of the skin; headache; various blood abnormalities;

various skin reactions including sensitivity to sunlight; high blood sugar and uric acid; muscle spasm and weakness; blurred vision.

Effects on Appetite and Body Weight as Disclosed by the Drug's Manufacturer
Anorexia; bitter taste; weight loss.

Detailed Effects on Appetite and Body Weight
Detailed manufacturer's disclosure: Although hydrochlorothiazide's official literature lists loss of appetite, bitter taste, and weight loss as potential side effects, more detailed information from independent sources is unavailable.

Dosage Levels at Which Effects Occur
May occur within the usual daily dosage range of 50–200mg.

Remedies
Loss of appetite; weight loss: The maintenance of adequate fluid intake and the avoidance of excessive alcohol use may aid in restoring normal appetite.
Bitter taste: Hydrochlorothiazide-induced taste disturbance may be countered in several ways. Taking the drug with an adequate fluid intake, chewing sugarless gum or using a mouthwash of water and lemon juice, and practicing good oral hygiene may help restore normal taste sensation.

How Long It Takes Till Reversal of Drug Effects:
Half the dose of hydrochlorothiazide is cleared from the blood within 6–15 hours. The duration of this drug's therapeutic effects is 6–12 hours.

Sources
Olin, B.R. (ed.). *Facts and Comparisons*. St. Louis: Facts and Comparisons, 1988.
Physicians' Desk Reference. Oradell, NJ: Medical Economics, 1988.
USP DI. Rockville, MD: The United States Pharmacopeial Convention, Inc., 1989.

INDAPAMIDE

Brand Names
U.S.A.: Lozol (USV).

Canada: Lozide (Servier).
Great Britain: Natrilix (Servier).

What This Drug Does
Diuretic.

How This Drug Affects Body Weight
It inhibits sodium reabsorption in the kidneys, increasing urinary excretion of water.

Government-Approved Uses for This Drug
To treat high blood pressure; to rid the body of fluid associated with congestive heart failure.

Unofficial Uses
None.

When Not to Use This Drug
If there is a lack of urine output; if breast-feeding; if allergic to this drug or to any related drug.

Side Effects From Use of This Drug
Headache; irritability; nervousness; dehydration; nausea; dizziness upon standing; inflammation of the pancreas; low blood potassium; high blood concentration of uric acid; gout; various skin reactions including sensitivity to sunlight; muscle cramps and spasms; impotence or reduced libido.

Effects on Appetite and Body Weight as Disclosed by the Drug's Manufacturer
Anorexia; bitter taste; weight loss.

Detailed Effects on Appetite and Body Weight
Detailed manufacturer's disclosure: Although indapamide's official literature lists loss of appetite, bitter taste, and weight loss as potential side effects, more detailed information from independent sources is unavailable.

Dosage Levels at Which Effects Occur
May occur within the usual daily dosage range of 2.5–5mg.

Remedies
Loss of appetite; weight loss: The maintenance of adequate fluid intake and the avoidance of excessive alcohol use may aid in restoring normal appetite.

Bitter taste: Indapamide-induced taste disturbance may be countered in several ways. Taking the drug with an adequate fluid intake, chewing sugarless gum or using a mouthwash of water and lemon juice, and practicing good oral hygiene may help restore normal taste sensation.

How Long It Takes Till Reversal of Drug Effects
Although half this drug's dose is cleared from the blood within 14 hours, indapamide's effects may persist for up to 36 hours.

Sources
Olin, B.R. (ed.). *Facts and Comparisons*. St. Louis: Facts and Comparisons, 1988.
Physicians' Desk Reference. Oradell, NJ: Medical Economics, 1988.
USP DI. Rockville, MD: The United States Pharmacopeial Convention, Inc., 1989.

METHAZOLAMIDE

Brand Names
U.S.A.: Neptazane (Lederle).
Canada: Neptazane (Lederle).
Great Britain: None.

What This Drug Does
Diuretic.

How This Drug Affects Body Weight
By blocking the enzyme carbonic anhydrase, methazolamide enhances the kidneys' excretion of sodium, potassium, bicarbonate, and water.

Government-Approved Uses for This Drug
To treat glaucoma.

Unofficial Uses
To treat periodic paralysis (a rare inherited disorder).

When Not to Use This Drug
In the presence of low sodium and/or potassium blood levels; in certain kidney and liver diseases; in certain glaucomas; in the

presence of suprarenal gland failure; in certain blood imbalances; if allergic to this drug or to any related drug.

Side Effects From Use of This Drug

Drowsiness; burning, itching, or tingling of the skin; nausea; vomiting; stomach upset; blood abnormalities; liver problems.

Effects on Appetite and Body Weight as Disclosed by the Drug's Manufacturer

Loss of appetite.

Detailed Effects on Appetite and Body Weight

Loss of appetite; weight loss: In a study encompassing 92 patients with chronic glaucoma, about 48% complained of a symptom complex including loss of appetite and weight loss while being treated with carbonic anhydrase inhibitor drugs. Methazolamide was one of these drugs.

In another report involving 70 patients treated with methazolamide, 20% complained of loss of appetite.

Dosage Levels at Which Effects Occur

Loss of appetite; weight loss: Reported as low as 150mg. daily.

Remedies

Loss of appetite; weight loss: The maintenance of adequate fluid intake and the avoidance of excessive alcohol use may aid in reversing appetite loss.

Administration of sodium bicarbonate (56–70 mEq. by mouth daily) dramatically reversed complaints of weight and appetite loss in 42% of subjects in one study cited above. About 21% reported partial relief.

How Long It Takes Till Reversal of Drug Effects

Loss of appetite; weight loss: Methazolamide has a duration of action of from 10–18 hours.

Sources

Becker, B. "Use of methazolamide (Neptazane) in the therapy of glaucoma." *American Journal of Ophthalmology*, 1960, 49: 1307–11.

Epstein, D.L., Grant, M. "Carbonic anhydrase inhibitor side effects." *Archives of Ophthalmology*, 1977, 95: 1378–82.

Gastrointestinal Drugs

BELLADONNA

Brand Names
U.S.A.: ★Belladenal-S (Sandoz), Belladonna Extract (Lilly), Belladonna Tincture (various manufacturers), ★Bellergal-S (Sandoz).
Canada: ★Belladenal (Sandoz),★Bellandenal Spacetabs (Sandoz).
Great Britain: ★Bellergal (Sandoz), ★Bellocarb (Sinclair), ★Climacteric Dellipsoids D19 (Pilsworth).

What This Drug Does
Anticholinergic.

How This Drug Affects Body Weight
By blocking the action of acetylcholine (a chemical messenger) on the vagus nerve, belladonna decreases movement of the gastrointestinal tract and inhibits acid secretion in the stomach.

Government-Approved Uses for This Drug
To treat peptic ulcer; to treat various digestive disorders; to treat painful menstruation; to control bed-wetting; to treat Parkinsonism; to treat motion sickness.

Unofficial Uses
None.

★Combination drug.

When Not to Use This Drug

In certain glaucomas and other eye problems; in fast heartbeat and various other cardiac irregularities; in various obstructive diseases of the gastrointestinal tract; in intestinal paralysis; in ulcerative colitis; in liver disease; in urinary tract obstruction; in kidney disease; in myasthenia gravis (a chronic condition associated with muscle weakness and tiredness); if allergic to this drug or to any related drug.

Side Effects From Use of This Drug

Dry mouth; difficulty in swallowing; constipation; nausea; vomiting; headache; insomnia; drowsiness; dizziness; nervousness; weakness; mental confusion or excitement (in the elderly); fast heartbeat; palpitations; blurred vision; dilated pupils; various eye abnormalities; difficulty in urinating; impotence; various skin reactions; decreased sweating; nasal congestion.

Effects on Appetite and Body Weight as Disclosed by the Drug's Manufacturer

Loss of taste.

Detailed Effects on Appetite and Body Weight

Weight loss: In a study of 45 patients, most of whom were obese, tincture of belladonna given alone or in combination with phenobarbital or bromides (this was a 1940 study when bromides were in common use) diminished appetite in 40 subjects. Whether belladonna was given by itself or with these other drugs, similar results were obtained.

Dosage Levels at Which Effects Occur

Weight loss: Unknown.

Remedies

Not applicable.

How Long It Takes Till Reversal of Drug Effects

Atropine, the main alkaloid of belladonna, is 94% eliminated in the urine in 24 hours. Belladonna's therapeutic effects usually persist for about 4 hours.

Source

Greene, J.A. "Effect of belladonna on appetite of patients with obesity and with other disease." *Journal of Laboratory and Clinical Medicine*, 1940, 26: 477–78.

CHENODIOL

Brand Names
U.S.A.: Chenix (Reid-Rowell).
Canada: None.
Great Britain: Chendol (Weddel), Chenofalk (Armour).

What This Drug Does
Gallstone solubilizing agent.

How This Drug Affects Body Weight
A naturally occurring bile acid, chenodiol inhibits production of cholesterol and cholic acid by the liver.

Government-Approved Uses for This Drug
To treat certain gallstones in unsuitable candidates for surgery.

Unofficial Uses
As an appetite suppressant.

When Not to Use This Drug
In certain liver or bile-duct abnormalities; in women who are or may become pregnant; in nursing mothers; if allergic to this drug or to any related drug.

Side Effects From Use of This Drug
Constipation or diarrhea (more common); cramps; nausea; vomiting; gas; gastrointestinal upset; heartburn; various liver and gallbladder abnormalities; changes in cholesterol levels.

Effects on Appetite and Body Weight as Disclosed by the Drug's Manufacturer
Loss of appetite.

Detailed Effects on Appetite and Body Weight
Decreased appetite: In a small-scale study comparing chenodiol with several other bile acids, chenodiol caused decreased appetite in 3 of 5 patients.

Dosage Levels at Which Effects Occur
Decreased appetite: Reported at 1,200mg. daily.

Remedies
Not applicable.

How Long It Takes Till Reversal of Drug Effects
Not applicable.

Source
Bray, G.A., Gallagher, T.F., Jr. "Suppression of appetite by bile acids." *Lancet*, 1968, 1(551): 1066–67.

DEOXYCHOLIC ACID

Brand Names
Note: Several bile acids have similar names and uses; among them are:
U.S.A.: Atrocholin (Glaxo), Cholan-DH (Penwalt), Cholan-HMB (Penwalt), Decholin (Miles).
Canada: Dehydrocholic acid (Stanley), Dycholium (Rhône-Poulenc).
Great Britain: Marketed as "dehydrocholic acid" by various manufacturers.

What This Drug Does
Digestive aid.

How This Drug Affects Body Weight
Deoxycholic acid and other related bile salts (such as dehydrocholic acid) increase the solubility of cholesterol. This aids in preventing its buildup in the bile duct, a condition that could cause various blockages and other complications. These drugs also promote normal digestion and absorption of fats and cholesterol from the diet by stimulating bile flow from the liver.

Government-Approved Uses for This Drug
To temporarily relieve constipation; as an adjunct in treating various biliary tract complications and conditions.

Unofficial Uses
None.

When Not to Use This Drug
In the presence of gallstones; in severe liver problems; if there is complete obstruction of the bile ducts; if there is obstruction of the gastrointestinal or genitourinary tracts; in the presence of abdominal pain, nausea, or vomiting; do not use as a diuretic; if allergic to this drug or to any related drug.

Side Effects from Use of This Drug
Diarrhea; weakness.

Effects on Appetite and Body Weight as Disclosed by the Drug's Manufacturer
None.

Detailed Effects on Appetite and Body Weight
Loss of appetite: In a 3-month study of 6 obese patients, 4 reported decreased appetite during periods of deoxycholic acid use but not when given a placebo.

Dosage Levels at Which Effects Occur
Loss of appetite: Reported at a daily dose of 1,200mg.

Remedies
Loss of appetite: The maintenance of adequate fluid intake and the avoidance of excessive alcohol use may aid in reversing appetite loss.

How Long It Takes Till Reversal of Drug Effects
Unknown.

Source
Bray, G.A., Gallagher, T.F., Jr. "Suppression of appetite by bile salts." *Lancet*, 1968, 1(551): 1066–67.

METOCLOPRAMIDE

Brand Names
U.S.A.: Clopra (Quantum), Maxolon (Beecham), Octamide (Adria), Reclomide (Major), Reglan (Robins).
Canada: Maxeran (Nordic), Reglan (Robins).
Great Britain: Maxolon (Beecham), Primperan (Berk).

What This Drug Does
Gastrointestinal stimulant.

How This Drug Affects Body Weight
By speeding up emptying of the stomach contents, metoclopramide relieves some after-meal discomfort reported by sufferers of anorexia nervosa (such as fullness and bloating).

Government-Approved Uses for This Drug
To treat delayed gastric emptying; to prevent nausea and vomiting associated with cancer chemotherapy.

Unofficial Uses
To improve lactation; to treat nausea and vomiting due to a variety of causes; to treat hiccups.

When Not to Use This Drug
In presence of gastrointestinal hemorrhage, obstruction, or perforation; in patients with pheochromacytoma (adrenal gland tumor); in epileptics; if taking any other drug likely to cause extrapyramidal reactions (trembling hands, legs, and arms; stiff arm and leg movements); if allergic to this drug or to any related drug.

Side Effects From Use of This Drug
Restlessness; drowsiness; fatigue; lassitude; insomnia; headache; dizziness; nausea; extrapyramidal reactions; Parkinson-like reactions (fixed mask-like facial expression; trembling hands, legs, and arms; stiff arm and leg movements); anxiety; diarrhea; depression.

Effects on Appetite and Body Weight as Disclosed by the Drug's Manufacturer
None.

Detailed Effects on Appetite and Body Weight
Treatment of anorexia nervosa: Patients suffering from anorexia nervosa often complain of flatulent dyspepsia. This syndrome of stomach discomfort, fullness, and bloating after meals prevents many anorexics from finishing their food. Metoclopramide, a drug that accelerates the emptying of the stomach contents, has been successfully used with these patients. In a 4-week study of 5 anorexia nervosa patients (4 women and 1 man),

administration of metoclopramide allowed all subjects to complete their meals.

Dosage Levels at Which Effects Occur
Treatment of anorexia nervosa: Reported effective at a daily dose of 30mg. (10mg. given 3 times daily after meals).

Remedies
Treatment of anorexia nervosa: Not applicable.

How Long It Takes Till Reversal of Drug Effects
Half the dose of metoclopramide is cleared from the blood within 3–6 hours, with up to 80% eliminated from the body in about 1 day.

Sources
Moldofsky, H., et al. "Preliminary report on metoclopramide in anorexia nervosa." In R.A. Vigersky, ed., *Anorexia Nervosa*. New York: Raven Press, 1977, 373–75.

Silverstone, T., ed. *Drugs and Appetite*. London and New York: Academic Press, 1982.

MINERAL OIL

Brand Names
U.S.A.: †Agoral Plain (Parke-Davis),†Kondremul Plain (Fisons), †Milkinol (Kremers-Urban), †Neo-Cultol (Fisons), †Zymenol (Houser).
Canada: Marketed under its generic name (mineral oil) by various manufacturers.
Great Britain: *Agarol (Warner), Astrolene (Astor), Petrolagar Emulsion [Blue Label] (Wyeth), *Petrolagar Emulsion [Red Label] (Wyeth).

What This Drug Does
Laxative.

How This Drug Affects Body Weight
By lubricating the gastrointestinal tract, mineral oil may decrease by several hours the transit time of food moving through

---

†Denotes over-the-counter availability in the U.S.A.
*Combination drug.

the intestines. This could result in incomplete digestion, with decreased absorption of nutrients and accompanying weight loss. Mineral oil may also inhibit the absorption of fat-soluble vitamins, such as A and D. By its intestinal coating action, mineral oil may also inhibit gastric secretions, further compromising the digestive process.

Government-Approved Uses for This Drug
As a laxative.

Unofficial Uses:
None.

When Not to Use This Drug
In the presence of nausea, vomiting, or other symptoms of appendicitis; if there is rapid onset of acute abdominal pain or other undiagnosed abdominal pain; in fecal impaction; with intestinal obstruction; if pregnant (may inhibit vitamin absorption); if allergic to this drug or to any related drug.

Side Effects from Use of This Drug
Nausea; vomiting; diarrhea; abdominal cramps; laxative dependence (if used long-term or excessively); anal seepage (with large doses).

Effects on Appetite and Body Weight as Disclosed by the Drug's Manufacturer
Decreased absorption of food and fat-soluble vitamins.

Detailed Effects on Appetite and Body Weight
Weight loss: In a report detailing 34 adult females, all of whom complained of gradual weight loss and decreased appetite, the cause was narrowed down to overuse of the laxative mineral oil. Some took it 3 times daily and others used 1 or 2 large tablespoonfuls at bedtime. When mineral oil was discontinued, gradual weight gain occurred. One woman who weighed 98 pounds when using mineral oil attained a weight of 134 pounds 2 months after its withdrawal.

In an article in the *Journal of the American Medical Association* (*JAMA*), mineral oil's harmful effects were detailed. Among them were loss of appetite and weight loss of from 10–60 pounds. In one case, over a 100-pound drop in body weight is alleged to have occurred. This "mineral oil poisoning" was usually reversed rapidly after withdrawal of the substance.

Several researchers have reported weight loss in children given mineral oil. This may be partially explained by the substance's ability to inhibit absorption of the fat-soluble vitamins A and D. Mineral oil also speeds up the passage of food through the small intestine, causing incomplete digestion.

Three case reports describe children given mineral oil with a resultant, although unspecified degree of, weight loss. A 26-month-old girl had a fairly normal history of weight gain until given 1 tablespoon of mineral oil daily for 2 weeks. A 15-month-old boy also showed normal physical development until receiving 2 teaspoons daily for 3 weeks. A girl aged 4 years and 1 month showed normal development until given 1 and sometimes 2 tablespoons of mineral oil daily for 2 months.

Dosage Levels at Which Effects Occur
Weight loss: Reported to occur as low as 15ml. (1 tablespoon) daily.

Remedies
Weight loss: It has been suggested that mineral oil be taken at least 2 hours before or after eating. Some studies have shown malabsorption and weight loss to occur even when mineral oil is taken at bedtime. In these cases, discontinuation of mineral oil is the only known method of restoring normal digestion.

How Long It Takes Till Reversal of Drug Effects
Weight loss: In one study cited above, weight loss was reversed within 2 weeks of withdrawal of mineral oil. In another case, this did not occur until 2–3 months after stopping the use of this substance.

Sources
Becker, G.L. "The case against mineral oil." *American Journal of Digestive Diseases*, 1952, 19: 344.

Christakis, G., Miridjanian, A. "Diet, drugs and their interrelationship." *Journal of the American Dietetic Association*, 1968, 52: 21–24.

Dunley-Owen, A. "The indiscriminate use of liquid paraffin." *South African Medical Journal*, 1932, 6: 87.

Morgan, J.W. "Misgivings on mineral oil as a laxative." *American Journal of Surgery*, 1938, 42: 360–64.

Morgan, J.W. "The harmful effects of mineral oil (liquid petrolatum) purgatives." *Journal of the American Medical Association*, 1941, 117(2): 1335–56.

Smith, C.H., Bidlack, W.R. "Dietary concerns associated with the use of medications." *Journal of the American Dietetic Association*, 1984, 84: 901–14.
Till, J. "Liquid paraffin: A cause of loss in weight in children?" *Journal of State Medicine*, 1934, 42: 363–65.

SCOPOLAMINE

Brand Names
U.S.A.: Dallergy (Laser),*Ru-Tuss (Boots), Transderm-Scop (Ciba), Triptone (Commerce).
Canada: Transderm-V (Ciba).
Great Britain: Buscopan (Boehringer Ingelheim), Hyscine (various manufacturers).

What This Drug Does:
Anticholinergic.

How This Drug Affects Body Weight
Scopolamine exerts an anticholinergic effect in the body. This is thought to cause a decrease in the neurotransmitter (chemical messenger) acetylcholine. Acetylcholine controls the parasympathetic (involuntary) nervous system and use of scopolamine may cause an inhibition of salivary secretions.

Government-Approved Uses for This Drug
To prevent nausea and vomiting associated with motion sickness.

Unofficial Uses
None.

When Not to Use This Drug
In glaucoma; in children; if allergic to this drug or to any related drug.

*Combination drug.

Side Effects From Use of This Drug

Disorientation; restlessness; incoherence; headache; palpitations; dilated pupils; blurred vision and various other eye problems; difficult swallowing; constipation; dry mouth; nausea; vomiting; stomach upset; difficulty in urinating; flushing; dry skin; breathing difficulties; fever.

Effects on Appetite and Body Weight as Disclosed by the Drug's Manufacturer

None.

Detailed Effects on Appetite and Body Weight

Loss of appetite; weight loss: A case report describes an unusual reaction to scopolamine in a 71-year-old female. The use of transdermal scopolamine patches has recently gained popularity as a treatment for motion sickness. The subject complained of a marked decrease in appetite following treatment with transdermal scopolamine for vertigo and nausea associated with a middle ear infection. This resulted in a 30-pound weight loss over a 3-month period. She remarked that after chewing food for a few seconds, it grew into a "big tasteless wad" which she was unable to swallow. All medical tests proved negative and it was only upon physical examination that her physician noticed a scopolamine patch behind her left ear. Although originally prescribed short-term, she had continued its use on her own initiative. Upon withdrawal of the medication, the patient developed a voracious appetite accompanied by rapid weight gain.

Dosage Levels at Which Effects Occur

Loss of appetite; weight loss: Noted at 0.5mg. daily (as a 1.5mg. transdermal patch delivering 0.5mg. daily over 3 days).

Remedies

Loss of appetite; weight loss: The maintenance of adequate fluid intake and the avoidance of excessive alcohol use may aid in reversing appetite loss.

A switch to a different agent in the same therapeutic category could accomplish similar benefits while minimizing undesirable dietary influences. Consult your physician.

How Long It Takes Till Reversal of Drug Effects

Taken orally, scopolamine's duration of action is 4–6 hours, with effects of large doses lasting for up to 24 hours. When given as a transdermal patch, duration of action is 72 hours.

Source

Gonzalez, J.J. "You better look behind the ears." *North Carolina Medical Journal*, 1984, 45(10): 649.

Heart Drugs

DIGOXIN

Brand Names
U.S.A.: Lanoxicaps (Burroughs Wellcome), Lanoxin (Burroughs Wellcome).
Canada: Lanoxin (Burroughs Wellcome), Natigoxine (Sabex), Novo digoxin (Novopharm).
Great Britain: Digoxin Nativelle (Wilcox; Lewis), Lanoxin (Wellcome).

What This Drug Does
   Cardiotonic. It acts directly on the heart muscle to increase the force of its contractions.

How This Drug Affects Body Weight
   Unknown.

Government-Approved Uses for This Drug
   To treat congestive heart failure; to treat various heart-rhythm irregularities.

Unofficial Uses
   To treat obesity.
   Warning: This drug is hazardous and may result in dangerous side effects or death.

When Not to Use This Drug
   In certain rapid heartbeat conditions; if allergic to this drug or to any related drug.

Side Effects From Use of This Drug
Nausea; vomiting; diarrhea; fatigue; muscle weakness; agitation; hallucinations; headache; dizziness; vertigo; numbness or tingling; various heart irregularities, some of which may be life-threatening; low blood pressure; visual disturbance; gynecomastia (enlargement of the male breasts, often accompanied by tenderness) in both adults and children.

Effects on Appetite and Body Weight as Disclosed by the Drug's Manufacturer
Loss of appetite.

Detailed Effects on Appetite and Body Weight
Loss of appetite: Although no specific studies have been done measuring digoxin's effect on appetite loss or its implications for body weight, this phenomenon is quite common. In fact, loss of appetite is a primary indicator of digitalis toxicity and is a valuable tool in determining the proper dosage level for each patient. Gastrointestinal disturbances, of which loss of appetite is one, account for about 25% of all adverse effects from digoxin.

Dosage Levels at Which Effects Occur
Loss of appetite: May occur within the usual daily dosage range of 0.125–0.25mg.

Remedies
Loss of appetite: Since anorexia may be an indication of drug toxicity, consult your physician immediately. Do not attempt to alter the dose of digoxin on your own.

How Long It Takes Till Reversal of Drug Effects
Although half the dose of digoxin is cleared from the blood within 30–40 hours, 6 to 8 days may elapse before its effects are reversed.

Sources
Olin, B.R. (ed.). *Facts and Comparisons*. St. Louis: Facts and Comparisons, 1988.
Physicians' Desk Reference. Oradell, NJ: Medical Economics, 1988.
USP DI. Rockville, MD: The United States Pharmacopeial Convention, Inc., 1989.

High-Blood-Pressure Drugs

ATENOLOL

Brand Names
U.S.A: ★Tenoretic (Stuart), Tenormin (Stuart).
Canada: None.
Great Britain: ★Tenoret 50 (Stuart), ★Tenoretic (Stuart), Tenormin (Stuart).

What This Drug Does
Antihypertensive.

How This Drug Affects Body Weight
Atenolol's beta-adrenergic blocking activity may cause inhibited breakdown of fat-tissue stores, an effect that may be potentiated by the actions of the hypothalamus.

Government-Approved Uses for This Drug
To control high blood pressure; to treat angina pectoris (chest pain caused by coronary artery spasm).

Unofficial Uses
To prevent migraine headaches; to decrease mortality following myocardial infarction (damage to the heart muscle due to loss of its blood supply); to treat alcohol-withdrawal syndrome; to treat certain anxiety.

★Combination drug.

When Not to Use This Drug

In certain heart conditions; if allergic to this drug or to any related drug.

Side Effects From Use of This Drug

Fatigue; slowed heartbeat; low blood pressure; congestive heart failure; dizziness or dizziness on standing; diarrhea; nausea; vomiting; breathing difficulties; skin rash; fever.

Effects on Appetite and Body Weight as Disclosed by the Drug's Manufacturer

Edema; anorexia; weight gain or loss.

Detailed Effects on Appetite and Body Weight

Detailed manufacturer's disclosure: Although atenolol's official literature lists water retention, loss of appetite, and weight changes as potential side effects, more detailed information from independent sources is unavailable.

A related drug, propranolol, is well documented for its potential to cause weight gain and that information appears in this book.

Dosage Levels at Which Effects Occur

May occur within the normal daily dosage range of 50–100mg.

Remedies

Weight gain: Substitution of low-calorie foods, beverages, and snacks for normal dietary intake may aid in reversing some atenolol-induced weight gain.

Loss of appetite; weight loss: The maintenance of adequate fluid intake and the avoidance of excessive alcohol use may aid in reversing appetite loss.

Water retention: Possible use of a diuretic may help rid the body of excess water. This should only be attempted under the supervision of a doctor.

How Long It Takes Till Reversal of Drug Effects

With half the dose of atenolol being cleared from the blood within 6–7 hours, its therapeutic effects have been found to persist up to 24 hours after a single dose.

Sources

Olin, B.R. (ed.). *Facts and Comparisons*. St. Louis: Facts and Comparisons, 1988.

Physicians' Desk Reference. Oradell, NJ: Medical Economics, 1988.
USP DI. Rockville, MD: The United States Pharmacopeial Convention, Inc., 1989.

CAPTOPRIL

Brand Names
U.S.A.: Capoten (Squibb), *Capozide (Squibb).
Canada: Capoten (Squibb).
Great Britain: Capoten (Squibb).

What This Drug Does:
Antihypertensive.

How This Drug Affects Body Weight
It has been speculated that captopril may bind zinc ions at its site of action in the body. Decreased zinc levels may cause loss of taste sensation.

Government-Approved Uses for This Drug
To control high blood pressure; in combination with other drugs to treat heart failure.

Unofficial Uses
To manage hypertensive crisis; to treat rheumatoid arthritis.

When Not to Use This Drug
If allergic to this drug or to any related drug.

Side Effects From Use of This Drug
Various blood abnormalities; dizziness; fainting; fast heartbeat; low blood pressure; angina pectoris; congestive heart failure; protein in the urine; various kidney dysfunctions; frequent urination; high blood potassium levels; skin rash; various other skin reactions; itching; fever; liver dysfunction.

Effects on Appetite and Body Weight as Disclosed by the Drug's Manufacturer
Loss of appetite; loss of taste.

*Combination drug.

Detailed Effects on Appetite and Body Weight

Altered taste: In a study of 11 patients with high blood pressure and treated with captopril and a diuretic, 2 patients reported a marked loss of taste. Since their hypertension was deemed too severe to discontinue drug therapy, medication was continued, with normal taste sensation returning spontaneously.

Another report describing 10 subjects treated with captopril and a diuretic claimed one of them was forced to discontinue the drug due in part to loss of taste.

A case report describes a 56-year-old male with severe high blood pressure who had captopril added to a multiple drug regimen. After using captopril for about 1 month, another drug, propranolol, was added. Within 24 hours, the patient reported loss of taste, which continued for over 6 weeks. This was accompanied by weight loss of more than 5 pounds. Through trial and error, the possible offending agents were narrowed down, with all evidence finally pointing to captopril.

Three case reports are described by one researcher: In the first instance, a 55-year-old female taking captopril noted that by the fifth week of use, sweet foods tasted salty and a bitter taste remained in the mouth. This was followed by a steady loss of ability to discriminate among various tastes.

The second case involved a 65-year-old male who complained of loss of taste sensation after 3 weeks of captopril use. He also reported a persistent salty taste in the mouth. After the drug was discontinued, normal taste returned. Upon rechallenge with captopril, loss of taste recurred after only 5 days.

The third case describes a 43-year-old female receiving captopril who, after 4 weeks, complained of taste disturbance affecting all types of food. Normal taste returned after discontinuation of captopril.

In a Swiss study of 51 subjects treated with captopril for high blood pressure, 1 patient reported a partial loss of taste sensation, while another complained of complete taste loss. The first patient regained normal taste within 3 weeks without stopping captopril. The second regained taste sensation only after discontinuing the drug.

In a 1986 study of 4,445 patients taking captopril, 2.2% reported a loss of taste sensation. In a 1984 survey of 6,737 patients on captopril, 2.7% experienced altered taste. Of 1,146 patients taking captopril and polled in 1980, 6–7% complained of taste loss.

In a survey of 292 patients treated with captopril, over 30% reported some changes in taste perception. The highest incidence (15.1%) involved loss of taste; 9.3% reported a metallic taste, 4.5% reported salty taste, and 1.7% reported sweet taste. Of all those experiencing alterations in taste, two-thirds felt this was minor, one-quarter judged it moderate, and 13% severe; 23% had a return to normal taste in spite of continued captopril use.

Water retention: In a Swiss study of 51 patients treated with captopril for high blood pressure, 2 gained weight from fluid retention immediately after starting the drug. In 1 subject, a weight gain of about 10 pounds was recorded within 3 days, while in the second case, the increase was 3.3 pounds within 2 days.

Dosage Levels at Which Effects Occur
Altered taste: Reported as low as 20mg. daily, although the average daily dose in the numerous cases cited was about 350mg.
Water retention: Reported as low as 75mg. daily.

Remedies
Altered taste: Captopril-induced taste disturbance may be countered in several ways. Taking the drug with an adequate fluid intake, chewing sugarless gum or using a mouthwash of water and lemon juice, and practicing good oral hygiene may help restore normal taste sensation.

In one study cited above, a switch to enalapril, a different drug in the same chemical family, restored normal taste sensation to 95% of the patients.
Water retention: In the study cited above, the addition of a diuretic drug reversed water retention and consequent weight gain.

How Long It Takes Till Reversal of Drug Effects
Altered taste: Reversal was variable in the many examples cited above. In one case, normal taste returned 2 days after captopril was discontinued; in another it took 4 weeks. One patient who was put on and then taken off the drug twice regained normal taste acuity in 10 days the first time and in 3 days the second. In one study, a switch to a different drug restored normal taste

after 2 weeks. Of 8 patients who developed taste loss while on captopril and discontinued its use, 3 still had partial taste loss for up to 23 months. Finally, in a study where captopril was continued despite altered taste, normal taste returned after 2–5 weeks.

Water retention: It takes up to 2 hours for half the dose of captopril to be cleared from the blood, assuming normal kidney function. Duration of action of captopril's therapeutic effects can be up to 12 hours. In 24 hours, 95% of the drug has been eliminated from the body.

Sources

Atkinson, A.B., et al. "Combined treatment of severe intractable hypertension with captopril and diuretic." *Lancet*, 1980, ii: 105–8.

Edwards, I.R., et al. "Captopril: 4 years of post marketing surveillance of all patients in New Zealand." *British Journal of Clinical Pharmacology*, 1987, 23(5): 529–36.

Irvin, J.D., Viau, J.M. "Safety profiles of the angiotensin converting enzyme inhibitors captopril and enalapril." *American Journal of Medicine*, 1986, 81(4C): 46–50.

MacGregor, G.A., et al. "Captopril in essential hypertension; contrasting effects of adding hydrochlorothiazide or propranolol." *British Medical Journal*, 1982, 284(6317): 693–96.

McNeil, J.J., et al. "Taste loss associated with oral captopril treatment." *British Medical Journal*, 1979, 2: 1555–56.

Studer, A., et al. "Captopril in various forms of severe therapy-resistant hypertension." *Klinische Wochen-Schrift*, 1981, 59(2): 59–67.

Vlasses, P.H., Ferguson, R.K. "Temporary ageusia related to captopril." *Lancet*, 1979, ii: 526.

White, N.J., et al. "Captopril and frusemide in severe drug-resistant hypertension." *Lancet*, 1980, ii: 108–10.

CLONIDINE

Brand Names

U.S.A.: Catapres (Boehringer Ingelheim), Catatpres-TTS (Boehringer Ingelheim), *Combipres (Boehringer Ingelheim).
Canada: Catapres (Boehringer Ingelheim), *Combipres (Boehringer Ingelheim), Dixarit (Boehringer Ingelheim).

*Combination drug.

Great Britain Catapres (Boehringer Ingelheim), Catapres PL (Boehringer Ingelheim), Dixarit (WB) (Boehringer Ingelheim).

What This Drug Does
Antihypertensive.

How This Drug Affects Body Weight
Transient weight gain seen in those taking clonidine may result from sodium retention and adjustments by the kidneys to decreased blood pressure. The weight loss observed after discontinuation of clonidine may be attributable to sodium and fluid loss. The sedative effects of clonidine help counter the hyperactivity seen in those suffering from anorexia nervosa.

Government-Approved Uses for This Drug
To control high blood pressure.

Unofficial Uses
To treat Tourette's disorder (a condition characterized by facial twitches, uncontrolled arm and shoulder motions, and spontaneous and often obscene vocalizations); to treat migraine headaches; to control menopausal flushing; as an adjunct to detoxification in those addicted to methadone and other opiates, alcohol, and benzodiazepine drugs (such as Valium and related substances).

When Not to Use This Drug
If pregnant; if allergic to this drug or to any related drug.

Side Effects From Use of This Drug
Drowsiness; dizziness or dizziness upon standing; sedation; headache; slowed heartbeat; nervousness; dry mouth; constipation; difficulty in urinating; impotence; gynecomastia (enlargement of the male breasts).

Effects on Appetite and Body Weight as Disclosed by the Drug's Manufacturer
Anorexia; weight gain; water retention.

Detailed Effects on Appetite and Body Weight
Treatment of anorexia nervosa: The administration of clonidine to 4 female anorexics over an 8-week trial period (4 weeks on active drug and 4 weeks on placebo) failed to promote appreciable weight gains. However, there was a small but significant

weight increase at the time of crossover from placebo to clonidine and a similar reverse shift in body weight when placebo was substituted for clonidine. This observation has led researchers to speculate that clonidine may have some value in the treatment of anorexia nervosa at higher dosage levels than those used in this trial.

Water retention: In a study evaluating clonidine's effectiveness in lowering blood pressure, it was noted that the drug caused a weight gain of 10 pounds in 1 patient within the first 3 weeks of use. This was explained as sodium retention, causing water to be retained in the body.

Dosage Levels at Which Effects Occur
Treatment of anorexia nervosa: Reported as low as 500mcg. daily.
Water retention: Reported at 225mcg. daily.

Remedies
Treatment of anorexia nervosa: Not applicable.
Water retention: Use of a thiazide diuretic caused a 13-pound weight loss in the study cited.

How Long It Takes Till Reversal of Drug Effects
Clonidine's duration of action is from 6–8 hours following a single dose. It takes from 12–16 hours for half the drug dose to be cleared from the blood.

Sources
Casper, R.C., et al. "A placebo-controlled crossover study of oral clonidine in acute anorexia nervosa." *Psychiatry Research*, 1987, 20(3): 249–50.
Davidson, M., et al. "The antihypertensive effects of an imidazoline compound." *Clinical Pharmacology and Therapeutics*, 1967, 8: 810–16.

DILTIAZEM

Brand Names
U.S.A.: Cardizem (Marion).
Canada: Cardizem (Nordic).
Great Britain: None.

What This Drug Does
Antianginal.

How This Drug Affects Body Weight

Unknown. Calcium channel blocker drugs inhibit the movement of calcium ions across cell membranes. The migration of calcium ions is intrinsic to the contraction of smooth muscle in the heart.

Government-Approved Uses for This Drug

To treat angina pectoris (chest pain caused by coronary artery spasm).

Unofficial Uses

To treat certain types of high blood pressure; to treat certain myocardial infarction (heart artery blockage).

When Not to Use This Drug

In certain cases of low blood pressure; if certain heart block or heart-rhythm irregularities are present; if breast-feeding; if allergic to this drug or any related drug.

Side Effects From Use of This Drug

Headache; drowsiness; fatigue; dizziness; depression; insomnia; mental confusion; heart-rhythm irregularities; flushing; low blood pressure; nausea; vomiting; diarrhea or constipation (reported with equal frequency); excessive urination; liver dysfunction; skin rash or itching; sensitivity to sunlight.

Effects on Appetite and Body Weight as Disclosed by the Drug's Manufacturer

Water retention; weight gain; anorexia.

Detailed Effects on Appetite and Body Weight

Loss of taste: A case report describes a 73-year-old male who, when switched from a previous medication to diltiazem, reported profound loss of taste. In addition, he also complained of a loss of smell. Since the patient refused to change medication a second time, diltiazem was continued, with taste sensation returning over a 10-week period.

Dosage Levels at Which Effects Occur

Loss of taste: Reported at 270mg. daily.

Remedies

Loss of taste: Diltiazem-induced taste disturbance may be countered in several ways. Taking the drug with an adequate fluid intake, chewing sugarless gum or using a mouthwash of water and lemon juice, and practicing good oral hygiene may help restore normal taste sensation.

How Long It Takes Till Reversal of Drug Effects
Loss of taste: In the case report cited above, normal taste sensation was restored within 10 weeks while diltiazem was continued.

Half the dose of diltiazem is cleared from the blood in 3–5 hours.

Source
Berman, J.L. "Dysomia, dysgeusia, and diltiazem." *Annals of Internal Medicine*, 1985, 102(5): 717.

ENALAPRIL

Brand Names
U.S.A.: *Vaseretic (MSD), Vasotec (MSD).
Canada: None.
Great Britain Innovace (MSD).

What This Drug Does
Antihypertensive.

How This Drug Affects Body Weight
Enalapril inhibits conversion of mostly inactive angiotensin I to angiotensin II, a potent vasoconstrictor. This leads to decreased levels of aldosterone (a hormone secreted by the adrenal cortex), which in turn causes sodium and fluid loss. This diuretic effect may cause significant water-weight loss.

Government-Approved Uses for This Drug
To control high blood pressure.

Unofficial Uses
To treat congestive heart failure.

*Combination drug.

When Not to Use This Drug
If breast-feeding; if allergic to this drug or to any related drug.

Side Effects From Use of This Drug
Chest pain; low blood pressure; heart palpitations; insomnia; numbness or tingling sensation; headache; dizziness; fainting; fatigue; abdominal pain; nausea; vomiting; diarrhea; breathing difficulties; liver dysfunction; muscle cramps; cough; skin rash or itching; various blood abnormalities; impotence.

Effects on Appetite and Body Weight as Disclosed by the Drug's Manufacturer
Altered taste.

Detailed Effects on Appetite and Body Weight
Weight loss: In a 16-week study of 28 patients treated with enalapril (12 weeks on the active drug and 4 weeks on a placebo), an average weight loss of over 3 pounds was recorded. The maximum individual weight loss seen was about 7.5 pounds.

Dosage Levels at Which Effects Occur
Weight loss: Reported at 20mg. daily.

Remedies
Weight loss: A decrease in daily dosage could help alleviate enalapril's effects on body weight. But this must be carefully balanced against maintaining adequate therapeutic blood levels.

A switch to a different agent in the same therapeutic category could accomplish similar benefits while minimizing undesirable dietary influences. Consult your physician.

How Long It Takes Till Reversal of Drug Effects
Weight loss: Although half the dose of enalapril is cleared from the blood in 11 hours, its therapeutic effects persist for at least 24 hours.

Source
Enalapril in Hypertension Study Group (U.K.). "Enalapril in essential hypertension: A comparative study with propranolol." *British Journal of Clinical Pharmacology*, 1984, 18(1): 51–56.

LABETALOL

Brand Names
U.S.A.: Normodyne (Schering), Trandate (Glaxo).
Canada: None.
Great Britain: Trandate (Allen & Hanburys).

What This Drug Does
Antihypertensive.

How This Drug Affects Body Weight
Labetalol's beta-adrenergic blocking activity may cause inhibited breakdown of fat-tissue stores, an effect that may be potentiated by the actions of the hypothalamus.

Government-Approved Uses for This Drug
To treat high blood pressure.

Unofficial Uses
None.

When Not to Use This Drug
In bronchial asthma; in certain heart problems; if allergic to this drug or to any related drug.

Side Effects From Use of This Drug
Fatigue; headache; drowsiness; difficulty in urinating; diarrhea; liver dysfunction; breathing difficulties; weakness; muscle cramps; eye problems; various skin reactions; systemic lupus erythematosus; nasal congestion; nausea; vomiting; stomach upset; dizziness or dizziness upon standing; scalp and/or skin tingling; vertigo; sweating; ejaculation failure; impotence; Peyronie's disease (a fibrous growth on the penis causing deflection and possible pain when erect).

Effects on Appetite and Body Weight as Disclosed by the Drug's Manufacturer
Taste distortion; water retention.

Detailed Effects on Appetite and Body Weight
Weight gain: In a 6-week trial of labetalol in 18 subjects, the

average weight gain after 4 weeks was 1.32 pounds. After 6 weeks, this figure was 5.5 pounds. Most of the weight gain was seen in the last 2 weeks of the study.

In a 14-week study of labetalol's use in controlling high blood pressure, 24 patients who completed the study went from an average pretrial weight of 147.4 pounds to a final weight of 156.2 pounds. This was almost a 9-pound gain.

Dosage Levels at Which Effects Occur
Weight gain: Reported as low as 300mg. daily.

Remedies
Weight gain: A decrease in daily dosage could help alleviate labetalol's effects on appetite and body weight. But this must be carefully balanced against maintaining adequate therapeutic blood levels.

A switch to a different agent in the same therapeutic category could accomplish similar benefits while minimizing undesirable dietary influences. Consult your physician.

How Long It Takes Till Reversal of Drug Effects
Weight gain: Although half the dose of labetalol is eliminated from the body within 6–8 hours, its effects may persist for 8–12 hours.

Sources
Dux, S., et al. "Labetalol in the treatment of essential hypertension: A single-blind dose ranging study." *Journal of Clinical Pharmacology*, 1986, 26(5): 346–50.

Weidman, P., et al. "Alpha and Beta adrenergic blockade with orally administered labetalol in hypertension." *American Journal of Cardiology*, 1978, 41(3): 570–76.

METHYLDOPA

Brand Names
U.S.A.: ★Aldochlor (MSD), Aldomet (MSD), ★Aldoril (MSD).
Canada: Aldomet (MSD), ★Aldoril (MSD), Apo-Methyldopa

★Combination drug.

(Apotex), Dopamet (ICN), Medimet-250 (Medic), Melopa (Riva), Novomedopa (Novopharm).
Great Britain: Aldomet (MSD), Co-Caps Methyldopa (DDSA), Dopamet (Berk), *Hydromet (MSD), Medomet (DDSA).

What This Drug Does
Lowers blood pressure.

How This Drug Affects Body Weight
By virtue of its close similarity to one of the body's neurotransmitters, norepinephrine, methyldopa substitutes for it in the nervous system as a false neurotransmitter. This inhibits the passage of nerve impulses to areas responsible for maintaining blood pressure. The effect is to relax blood vessels, lowering pressure. Methyldopa also reduces tissue concentrations of serotonin, a substance that inhibits appetite.

Government-Approved Uses for This Drug
To control high blood pressure.

Unofficial Uses
None.

When Not to Use This Drug
In cases of active liver disease (hepatitis, cirrhosis); if previous therapy with this drug has caused liver disorders; if allergic to this drug or to any related drug.

Side Effects From Use of This Drug
Sedation, drowsiness, headache, and weakness may occur temporarily during the first few weeks of therapy or can continue longer; light-headedness; tingling or burning sensations of the skin; Parkinsonism; Bell's palsy (facial paralysis); mental confusion; nightmares; mild psychosis (reversible); depression; slowed heartbeat; aggravation of angina pectoris (chest pain caused by coronary artery spasm); dizziness upon standing; nausea; vomiting; constipation or diarrhea (reported with equal frequency); dry mouth; nasal stuffiness; irritation of the tongue; inflammation of the pancreas; liver dysfunction (jaundice); abnormal liver-function tests; bone-marrow depression; various anemias; various allergic reactions such as fever, lupus-like

*Combination drug.

symptoms (a long-term swelling disease affecting many body systems), and inflammation of the heart; various skin reactions; muscle and joint pain; impotence; failure to ejaculate; decreased libido; breast enlargement; gynecomastia (enlargement of the male breasts); lactation (breast-milk flow); galactorrhea (breast-milk flow unrelated to childbirth or nursing); amenorrhea (cessation of menstruation).

Effects on Appetite and Body Weight as Disclosed by the Drug's Manufacturer
Water retention; weight gain.

Detailed Effects on Appetite and Body Weight
Water retention; weight gain: A clinical study of methyldopa involving 9 patients with high blood pressure showed the most troublesome side effect to be water retention and weight gain. One of the symptoms this presented was as edema (water swelling). In one patient, weight gain was 13.2 pounds within 10 days of starting the drug. This phenomenon appears more prevalent in those with severe hypertension or kidney failure.

In a group of 20 patients studied for the effects of methyldopa on high blood pressure, 6 showed gradual weight gain during the first week of treatment. This gain did not exceed 5 pounds in any subject. It was attributed to water retention and responded to diuretic use.

Eleven of 15 patients taking methyldopa reported fluid retention, with 2 developing peripheral edema. Weight gain was noted but the authors of the report did not elaborate.

Malabsorption; weight loss: A 58-year-old male treated with methyldopa for 6 months reported severe diarrhea for half that time, as well as a 33-pound weight loss. After withdrawal of the drug, diarrhea ceased in 1 month. Four months later, he was restarted on methyldopa and diarrhea returned, gradually increasing in severity. Within 10 months, the patient had lost 70 pounds and methyldopa was again discontinued. When the drug was again given 3 months later, diarrhea occurred within a few days. Intestinal biopsy showed damage to the mucosal lining of the small intestine and was attributed to the use of methyldopa.

Dosage Levels at Which Effects Occur
Water retention; weight gain: Reported as low as 500mg. daily.
Malabsorption; weight loss: Reported as low as 750mg. daily.

Remedies
Water retention; weight gain: In one case cited above, a diuretic, chlorothiazide, was successful in reversing water retention in 1 patient. Four others, however, did not respond to this and withdrawal of methyldopa was necessary. In another report, use of a similar diuretic, hydrochlorothiazide, was successful in all cases.
Malabsorption; weight loss: A decrease in daily dosage could help alleviate methyldopa's effects on absorption and body weight. But this must be carefully balanced against maintaining adequate therapeutic blood levels.

A switch to a different agent in the same therapeutic category could accomplish similar benefits while minimizing undesirable dietary influences. Consult your physician.

How Long It Takes Till Reversal of Drug Effects
Water retention; weight gain: In one of the studies cited above, adverse drug effects were reversed within 3–4 days after withdrawal of methyldopa.
Malabsorption; weight loss: Methyldopa's duration of action is 12–24 hours.

Sources
Bayliss, R.I.S., Harvey-Smith, E.A. "Methyldopa in the treatment of hypertension." *Lancet*, 1962, 1: 763–68.
Beck, B. "Methyldopum i behandling af hypertensio arterialis isaer med henblik på vaeskeretention og blodvolumen." *Ugeskrift for Laeger*, 1965, 125: 1472.
Dollery, C.T., Harrington, M. "Methyldopa in hypertension, clinical and pharmacological studies." *Lancet*, 1962, 1: 759–63.
Hansen, J. "Alpha-methyl-dopa (Aldomet) in the treatment of hypertension. The effects on blood volume, exchangeable sodium, body weight, and blood pressure." *Acta Medica Scandinavica*, 1968, 183(4): 323–27.
Shneerson, J.M., Gazzard, D.G. "Reversible malabsorption caused by methyldopa." *British Medical Journal*, 1977, 2: 1456–57.

METOPROLOL

Brand Names
U.S.A.: Lopressor (Geigy), *Lopressor HCT (Geigy).
Canada: Betaloc (Astra), Lopressor (Geigy).
Great Britain Betaloc (Astra), Betaloc-SA (Astra), *Co-Betaloc (Astra), *Lopresoretic (Geigy), Lopressor (Geigy), Lopresor SR (Geigy).

What This Drug Does
Antihypertensive.

How This Drug Affects Body Weight
Metoprolol's beta-adrenergic blocking activity may cause inhibited breakdown of fat-tissue stores, an effect that may be potentiated by the actions of the hypothalamus.

Government-Approved Uses for This Drug
To control high blood pressure; to treat myocardial infarction (damage to the heart muscle due to loss of its blood supply).

Unofficial Uses
By intravenous injection to suppress certain heart-rhythm irregularities.

When Not to Use This Drug
In certain heart conditions; if allergic to this drug or to any related drug.

Side Effects From Use of This Drug
Nausea; vomiting; diarrhea; fatigue; slowed heartbeat; low blood pressure; congestive heart failure; skin rash; fever; Peyronie's disease (a fibrous growth, causing a hardening of part of the penis with pain and deflection when erect); reduced libido.

Effects on Appetite and Body Weight as Disclosed by the Drug's Manufacturer
Edema; anorexia; weight gain or loss.

*Combination drug.

Detailed Effects on Appetite and Body Weight

Detailed manufacturer's disclosure: Although metoprolol's official literature lists water retention, loss of appetite, and weight change as potential side effects, more detailed information from independent sources is unavailable.

A related drug, propranolol, is well documented for its potential to cause weight gain and that information appears in this book.

Dosage Levels at Which Effects Occur

May occur within the normal daily dosage range of 100–450mg.

Remedies

Water retention: Use of a diuretic may help rid the body of excess water. This should only be attempted under the supervision of a doctor.

Loss of appetite; weight loss: The maintenance of adequate fluid intake and the avoidance of excessive alcohol use may aid in restoring normal appetite.

Weight gain: Substitution of low-calorie foods, beverages, and snacks for normal dietary intake may aid in reversing some metoprolol-induced weight gain.

How Long It Takes Till Reversal of Drug Effects

Half the dose of metoprolol is cleared from the blood within 3–7 hours. However, significant drug effects may still be evident as long as 12 hours after the last drug dose.

Sources

Olin, B.R. (ed.). *Facts and Comparisons*. St. Louis: Facts and Comparisons, 1988.

Physicians' Desk Reference. Oradell, NJ: Medical Economics, 1988.

USP DI. Rockville, MD: The United States Pharmacopeial Convention, Inc., 1989.

NIFEDIPINE

Brand Names

U.S.A.: Adalat (Miles), Procardia (Pfizer).
Canada Adalat (Miles).

Great Britain: Adalat (Bayer).

What This Drug Does
Antianginal.

How This Drug Affects Body Weight
Inhibits the movement of calcium ions (charged particles) across cell membranes. Since calcium is involved in the transmission of nerve impulses, its antagonism slows the action of vascular smooth muscle.

Government-Approved Uses for This Drug
To treat angina pectoris (chest pain caused by coronary artery spasm).

Unofficial Uses
To lower blood pressure in hypertensive emergencies; to treat Raynaud's phenomenon (sporadic constriction and spasm of the blood vessels of the fingers, toes, ears, and nose); to treat pulmonary hypertension (abnormally high pressure within the veins and arteries of the lungs); to treat asthma; to stop premature labor.

When Not to Use This Drug
If allergic to this drug or to any related drug.

Side Effects From Use of This Drug
Dizziness; light-headedness; flushing; headache; weakness; fainting; low blood pressure; heart palpitations; nasal congestion; nausea; diarrhea or constipation (reported with equal frequency); abdominal cramps; gas; muscle cramps; breathing difficulties; skin rash and itching; fever or chills (reported with equal frequency); sexual difficulties.

Effects on Appetite and Body Weight as Disclosed by the Drug's Manufacturer
Water retention; altered taste.

Detailed Effects on Appetite and Body Weight
Altered taste: In a survey of 770 patients treated with nifedipine, almost 20% reported some abnormality of taste sensation; 9.1% reported loss of taste, 6.2% complained of a metallic taste, 3% had a salty taste, and 1.6% had a sweet taste.

In a case report, a physician described a 71-year-old female receiving nifedipine for more than 13 months who had a weight loss of almost 60 pounds. Questioning of the patient revealed a severe loss of taste and smell, starting 1 year before (and 1 month after beginning the drug). Claiming an intense revulsion for food, the patient complained that food tasted and smelled like coffee.

In another report, a 45-year-old female is described who, after 4 days of nifedipine use, began refusing food, characterizing its taste as "awful." Withdrawal of nifedipine caused a reversal of these symptoms.

Water retention: Of 23 patients over 60 years old being treated with nifedipine to control high blood pressure, 43% (10) complained of fluid retention in the legs. Of these reports, 4 cases were considered mild and transient, 3 were moderate and transient, and 3 were severe enough to cause the patients to be taken off nifedipine. Since body weight did not change in those suffering from nifedipine-induced edema, the fluid in the legs was probably redistributed from other areas of the body.

Dosage Levels at Which Effects Occur
Altered taste: Reported as low as 30mg. daily.
Water retention: Reported as low as 40mg. daily.

Remedies
Altered taste: Nifedipine-induced taste disturbance may be countered in several ways. Taking the drug with an adequate fluid intake, chewing sugarless gum or using a mouthwash of water and lemon juice, and practicing good oral hygiene may help restore normal taste sensation.

In one case cited above, a switch to a related drug, diltiazem, restored normal taste in as little as 2 days. At a 2-month follow-up, taste was still normal.

Water retention: A decrease in daily dosage could help alleviate nifedipine's effects on water retention. But this must be carefully balanced against maintaining adequate therapeutic blood levels.

A switch to a different agent in the same therapeutic category or the addition of a diuretic drug could minimize edema. Consult your physician.

How Long It Takes Till Reversal of Drug Effects
Altered taste: In one case cited above, normal taste sensation

returned within 2 days after withdrawal of nifedipine. In another instance, this occurred within 24 hours.

Water retention: Half the dose of nifedipine is cleared from the blood in 2–5 hours. Its duration of action persists about 4 hours.

Sources

Edwards, I.R., et al. "Captopril: 4 years of post marketing surveillance of all patients in New Zealand." *British Journal of Clinical Pharmacology*, 1987, 23(5): 529–36.

Levinson, J.L., Kennedy, K. "Dysomia, dysgeusia, and nifedipine." *Annals of Internal Medicine*, 1985, 102(1): 135–36.

Schnapp, P., et al. "Nifedipine monotherapy in the hypertensive elderly; a placebo-controlled clinical trial." *Current Medical Research and Opinion*, 1987, 10(6): 407–13.

PHENOXYBENZAMINE

Brand Names:
U.S.A.: Dibenzyline (SKF).
Canada: None.
Great Britain: Dibenyline (SKF).

What This Drug Does
Antihypertensive.

How This Drug Affects Body Weight
By blocking alpha-adrenergic nerve receptors (located in smooth muscle), phenoxybenzamine may decrease levels of noradrenaline (a body hormone). Excessive noradrenaline activity may be associated with some human appetite disorders.

Government-Approved Uses for This Drug
To treat pheochromacytoma (adrenal gland tumor).

Unofficial Uses
To treat premature ejaculation; to treat certain difficulties in urination.

When Not to Use This Drug
If a fall in blood pressure is unwanted; if allergic to this drug or to any related drug.

Side Effects From Use of This Drug

Sedation; fatigue; fast heartbeat; dizziness upon standing; constriction of the pupil; nasal congestion; gastrointestinal irritation; inhibition of ejaculation.

Effects on Appetite and Body Weight as Disclosed by the Drug's Manufacturer

None.

Detailed Effects on Appetite and Body Weight

Treatment of anorexia nervosa: A case report describes a 123-pound, 21-year-old female anorexic who when first seen was losing weight. Her history included a previous weight loss greater than 25% of her body weight. She also reported loss of menstruation and some bulimic symptoms (binge-eating followed by forced vomiting). During an evaluation period, she was observed to drop an average of about a third of a pound per day. After unsuccessful treatment with propranolol (a beta-blocker drug), she was started on phenoxybenzamine. Weight gain commenced and continued until unwanted side effects forced the drug's withdrawal for a 2-day period. During this time, weight loss resumed. When phenoxybenzamine was restarted at a lower daily dosage for 11 days, weight gain was steady at 0.6 pounds daily.

Weight gain: In a 6-week trial of 11 subjects given phenoxybenzamine and several other antihypertensive medications, phenoxybenzamine caused an average weight gain of slightly over 6 pounds.

Dosage Levels at Which Effects Occur

Treatment of anorexia nervosa: Reported effective at 20mg. daily.

Weight gain: Reported as low as 5mg. daily.

Remedies

Treatment of anorexia nervosa: Not applicable.

Weight gain: Substitution of low-calorie foods, beverages, and snacks for normal dietary intake may aid in reversing some drug-induced weight gain.

How Long It Takes Till Reversal of Drug Effects

Phenoxybenzamine is a long-acting drug, with half the dose taking 24 hours or more to be cleared from the blood. Its duration of action may extend to 3–4 days.

Sources

Beilin, L.J., Juel-Jensen, B.E. "Alpha- and beta-adrenergic blockade in hypertension." *Lancet*, 1972, 1(758): 979–82.

Redmond, D.E., et al. "Phenoxybenzamine in anorexia nervosa." *Lancet*, 1976, 2(7980): 307.

PINDOLOL

Brand Names
U.S.A.: Visken (Sandoz).
Canada: Visken (Sandoz).
Great Britain *Viskaldix (Sandoz), Visken (Sandoz).

What This Drug Does
Antihypertensive.

How This Drug Affects Body Weight
Pindolol's beta-adrenergic blocking activity may cause inhibited breakdown of fat-tissue stores, an effect that may be potentiated by the actions of the hypothalamus.

Government-Approved Uses for This Drug
To control high blood pressure.

Unofficial Uses
None.

When Not to Use This Drug
In bronchial asthma; in various heart abnormalities; if breastfeeding; if allergic to this drug or to any related drug.

Side Effects From Use of This Drug
Nausea; vomiting; diarrhea; insomnia; fatigue; dizziness; hallucinations; slow heartbeat; congestive heart failure; low blood pressure; visual disturbances; low blood sugar; skin rash; breathing difficulties; muscle and joint pain; chest pain; impotence.

Effects on Appetite and Body Weight as Disclosed by the Drug's Manufacturer
Water retention; weight gain.

*Combination drug.

Detailed Effects on Appetite and Body Weight
Weight gain: In a comprehensive New Zealand study of 46 hypertensive patients given pindolol by several different protocols, weight gain was seen in various phases of the trial. Over several weeks, and with varying dosages, pindolol caused weight gains of from 0.84–9.2 pounds. In those kept on the drug for an average of 4.5 months, a mean weight gain of 2.3 pounds was recorded.

Dosage Levels at Which Effects Occur
Weight gain: Reported to occur at 2.5–55mg. daily (average 15mg.).

Remedies
Weight gain: Substitution of low-calorie foods, beverages, and snacks for normal dietary intake may aid in reversing some pindolol-induced weight gain.

How Long It Takes Till Reversal of Drug Effects
Half the dose of pindolol is cleared from the blood within 3–4 hours. In elderly patients, this may require up to 15 hours.

Source
Waal-Manning, H.J., Simpson, F.O. "Pindolol: A comparison with other antihypertensive drugs and a double-blind placebo trial." *New Zealand Medical Journal*, 1974, 80(522): 151–57.

PRAZOSIN

Brand Names
U.S.A.: Minipres (Pfizer), *Minizide (Pfizer).
Canada: Minipres (Pfizer).
Great Britain: Hypovase (Pfizer).

What This Drug Does
Antihypertensive.

How This Drug Affects Body Weight
By blocking alpha-receptors in the blood vessels, prazosin exerts a dilating (opening) effect on both arteries and veins. Pra-

*Combination drug.

zosin-induced water retention may be due to decreased venous blood return from the lower extremities or from reduced renal blood flow relative to cardiac output.

Government-Approved Uses for This Drug
To control high blood pressure.

Unofficial Uses
To treat congestive heart failure; to manage Raynaud's vasospasm (sporadic constriction and spasm of the blood vessels of the fingers, toes, ears, and nose).

When Not to Use This Drug
If allergic to this drug or to any related drug.

Side Effects From Use of This Drug
Dizziness or dizziness upon standing; headache; drowsiness; weakness; fainting (often associated with the first dose taken); depression; palpitations; blurred vision; dry mouth; vomiting; diarrhea or constipation (reported with equal frequency); abdominal cramps; nausea; impotence; priapism (prolonged, often painful erection unrelated to sexual desire).

Effects on Appetite and Body Weight as Disclosed by the Drug's Manufacturer
Water retention; weight gain.

Detailed Effects on Appetite and Body Weight
Water retention; weight gain: A study of 10 patients with congestive heart failure who were treated with prazosin showed an average increase in body weight of 6.6 pounds after 6 weeks. This occurred despite the use of diuretics to control its cause, water retention. Edema was evidenced by swelling of the ankles and lower legs.

Dosage Levels at Which Effects Occur
Water retention; weight gain: Reported to occur as low as 3mg. daily.

Remedies
A decrease in daily dosage could help alleviate prazosin's effects on water retention and body weight. But this must be carefully balanced against maintaining adequate therapeutic blood levels.

A switch to a different agent in the same therapeutic category could accomplish similar benefits while minimizing undesirable influences. Consult your physician.

How Long It Takes Till Reversal of Drug Effects
Half the dose of prazosin is cleared from the blood within 2–3 hours, but its effects may persist for about 10 hours.

Source
Riegger, G.A., et al. "Contribution of the renin-angiotensin-aldosterone system to development of tolerance and fluid retention in chronic congestive heart failure during prazosin treatment." *American Journal of Cardiology*, 1987, 59(8): 906–10.

PROPRANOLOL

Brand Names
U.S.A.: Inderal (Ayerst), *Inderide (Ayerst).
Canada: Apo-Propranolol (Apotex), Detensol (Desbergers), Inderal (Ayerst), *Inderide (Ayerst), Novopranol (Novopharm).
Great Britain: Angilol (DDSA), Apsolol (Approved Prescription Services), Berkolol (Berk), Inderal (ICI), Inderal LA (ICI), *Inderetic (ICI).

What This Drug Does
Antihypertensive; antiarrhythmic.

How This Drug Affects Body Weight
Propranolol's beta-adrenergic blocking activity may cause inhibited breakdown of fat-tissue stores, an effect that may be potentiated by the actions of the hypothalamus.

Government-Approved Uses for This Drug
To control heart-rhythm irregularities and various other cardiac problems; to control high blood pressure; to prevent migraine headache.

Unofficial Uses
To treat gastrointestinal bleeding in cirrhotic (liver destruction) patients; to treat schizophrenia; to control essential tremor;

*Combination drug.

to treat tardive dyskinesia (a drug-induced condition); to control panic reactions (such as stage fright); of possible value as a vaginal contraceptive.

When Not to Use This Drug

In bronchial asthma; if experiencing seasonal hay fever; in the presence of cardiogenic shock (caused when the heart fails to supply enough blood to the body); if suffering from certain heart block or slowed heartbeat; in the presence of overt congestive heart failure; if allergic to this drug or to any related drug.

Side Effects From Use of This Drug

Fatigue; hallucinations; slowed heartbeat; low blood pressure; congestive heart failure; nausea; vomiting; diarrhea; low blood sugar; skin rash; breathing difficulties; fever; burning or tingling sensation of the hands; mental depression; insomnia; visual disturbances; increased risk of asthma; reversible hair loss; impotence; Peyronie's disease (a fibrous growth on the penis causing deflection and possible pain when erect).

Effects on Appetite and Body Weight as Disclosed by the Drug's Manufacturer

Anorexia; weight gain or loss.

Detailed Effects on Appetite and Body Weight

Weight gain: In a 24-week study of 19 hypertensive patients treated with propranolol, an average weight gain of 4.84 pounds was seen.

In a group of 25 patients with overactive thyroid who were treated with propranolol for 1–2 weeks, some showed marked weight gain (in one case 7.7 pounds). When untreated, an overactive thyroid gland often results in weight loss. It is interesting to note that propranolol overcame this tendency, actually causing weight gain in some subjects.

In a 16-week trial of propranolol in which 26 patients received the active drug for 12 weeks, average weight gain was about 2 pounds. One patient showed a 5.5-pound increase.

In a study of 63 obese patients treated at a hospital nutrition clinic, weight loss results of nonmedicated individuals were compared with those given various medications, propranolol among them. While the group as a whole lost an average of 2.45 pounds per month by diet alone, those taking propranolol either continued to gain weight until the drug was discontinued or lost only at a very discouraging rate of 2–3 pounds per year.

Dosage Levels at Which Effects Occur
Weight gain: May occur within propranolol's normal daily dosage range of 30–240mg.

Remedies
Weight gain: Substitution of low-calorie foods, beverages, and snacks for normal dietary intake may aid in reversing some propranolol-induced weight gain.

How Long It Takes Till Reversal of Drug Effects
Half the dose of propranolol is cleared from the blood within 3–5 hours.

Sources
Enalapril in Hypertension Study Group (U.K.) "Enalapril in essential hypertension: A comparative study with propranolol." *British Journal of Clinical Pharmacology*, 1984, 18(1): 51–56.

Feely, J., et al. "Propranolol dynamics in thyrotoxicosis." *Clinical Pharmacology and Therapeutics*, 1980, 28(1): 40–44.

Naukkarinen, V.A., et al. "Comparison of nicardipine and propranolol in the treatment of mild and moderate hypertension." *European Journal of Clinical Pharmacology*, 1987, 33(2): 119–26.

Stein, P.M., et al. "Predicting weight loss success among obese clients in a hospital nutrition clinic." *American Journal of Clinical Nutrition*, 1981, 34(10): 2039–44.

TERAZOSIN

Brand Names
U.S.A.: Hytrin (Abbott/Burroughs Wellcome).
Canada: None.
Great Britain: None.

What This Drug Does
Antihypertensive.

How This Drug Affects Body Weight
By blocking alpha-receptors in the blood vessels, terazosin exerts a dilating (opening) effect on both arteries and veins. Ter-

azosin-induced water retention may be due to decreased venous blood return from the lower extremities or from reduced renal blood flow relative to cardiac output.

Government-Approved Uses for This Drug
To control high blood pressure.

Unofficial Uses
None.

When Not to Use This Drug
If allergic to this drug or to any related drug.

Side Effects From Use of This Drug
Heart palpitations; fast heartbeat; dizziness or dizziness upon standing; light-headedness; nausea; vomiting; dry mouth; diarrhea or constipation (reported with equal frequency); gas; difficult breathing; nasal congestion; sinus inflammation; cold or flu symptoms; nosebleed; pain of the back or extremities; joint, muscle, or neck pain; gout; blurred vision or other eye problems; ringing in the ears; nervousness; burning or tingling sensation of the arms or legs; drowsiness; weakness or loss of energy; headache; fever; decreased libido; impotence.

Effects on Appetite and Body Weight as Disclosed by the Drug's Manufacturer
Water retention; weight gain.

Detailed Effects on Appetite and Body Weight
Weight gain: During clinical trials of terazosin, males gained an average of 1.7 pounds and females gained an average of 2.2 pounds. Among those taking a placebo, males lost 0.2 pounds and females lost 1.2 pounds.

In a 10-week study of 43 patients (29 men and 14 women) receiving terazosin to control high blood pressure, females showed an average weight gain of about 1.8 pounds. This compared unfavorably with women given a placebo, who lost an average of 1.1 pounds. Males given the drug also tended to gain weight but the difference was not considered statistically significant from those taking a placebo. The authors of the study speculate that the weight gain seen in the females was caused by water retention in the body.

In a study of 874 patients (205 females and 669 males), some were given terazosin and some a placebo for 4–13 weeks. Males taking terazosin gained an average of 2 pounds versus a loss of 0.1 pounds for those on a placebo. Females gained an average of 1.9 pounds on terazosin as compared to a 0.5-pound loss with placebo. The physicians conducting this study state that those on long-term terazosin monotherapy (no other drugs given simultaneously) also tend to gain weight but no relationship between the amount of gain and length of therapy can be determined.

Dosage Levels at Which Effects Occur
Weight gain: Reported as low as 1mg. daily.

Remedies
Weight gain: Substitution of low-calorie foods, beverages, and snacks for normal dietary intake may aid in reversing some drug-induced weight gain.

How Long It Takes Till Reversal of Drug Effects
Half the dose of terazosin is cleared from the blood in 9–12 hours.

Sources
Holtzman, J.L., et al. "Concomitant administration of terazosin and atenolol for the treatment of essential hypertension." *Archives of Internal Medicine*, 1988, 148(3): 539–43.

Kastrup, E.K., ed. *Facts and Comparisons*. St. Louis: Facts and Comparisons, 1988.

Sperzel, W.D., et al. "Overall safety of terazosin as an antihypertensive agent." *American Journal of Medicine*, 1986, 80(suppl. 5B): 77–81.

TIMOLOL

Brand Names
U.S.A.: Blocadren (MSD), *Timolide (MSD), Timoptic (MSD).
Canada: Blocadren (Frosst), *Timolide (Frosst), Timoptic (MSD).
Great Britain Betim (Burgess), Blocadren (MSD), *Moducren (Morson), *Prestim (Leo), Timoptol (MSD).

What This Drug Does
Antihypertensive (oral form); antiglaucoma (ophthalmic form).

*Combination drug.

How This Drug Affects Body Weight
Timolol's beta-adrenergic blocking activity may cause inhibited breakdown of fat-tissue stores, an effect that may be potentiated by the actions of the hypothalamus.

Government-Approved Uses for This Drug
Oral dosage form: To control high blood pressure; to prevent myocardial infarction (damage to the heart muscle due to loss of its blood supply).
Ophthalmic: To treat glaucoma.

Unofficial Uses
To prevent migraine headaches (oral dosage form).

When Not to Use This Drug
In bronchial asthma (or a history of it); if there is a history of chronic obstructive pulmonary disease; in various heart conditions; if breast-feeding; if allergic to this drug or to any related drug.

Side Effects From Use of This Drug
Nausea; vomiting; diarrhea; fatigue; vivid dreams; slowed heartbeat; low blood pressure; congestive heart failure; certain circulatory disease; low blood sugar; skin rash; breathing difficulties; fever; decreased libido; impotence.

Effects on Appetite and Body Weight as Disclosed by the Drug's Manufacturer
Edema; anorexia; weight gain or loss.

Detailed Effects on Appetite and Body Weight
Detailed manufacturer's disclosure: Although timolol's official literature lists water retention, loss of appetite, and weight changes as potential side effects, more detailed information from independent sources is unavailable.

A related drug, propranolol, is well documented for its potential to cause weight gain and that information appears in this book.

Dosage Levels at Which Effects Occur
Oral dosage form: May occur within the usual daily dosage range of 20–60mg.
Ophthalmic: May occur at the usual daily dosage of 2 drops per eye (of either 0.25% or 0.5% solution).

Remedies
Weight gain: Substitution of low-calorie foods, beverages, and snacks for normal dietary intake may aid in reversing some timolol-induced weight gain.

Loss of appetite; weight loss: The maintenance of adequate fluid intake and the avoidance of excessive alcohol use may aid in reversing appetite loss.

Water retention: Possible use of a diuretic may help rid the body of excess water. This should only be attempted under the supervision of a doctor.

How Long It Takes Till Reversal of Drug Effects
Oral: Half the dose of oral timolol is cleared from the blood in about 4 hours.

Ophthalmic: Adverse influences usually disappear promptly after discontinuing use of timolol as an eyedrop.

Sources
Olin, B.R. (ed.). *Facts and Comparisons*. St. Louis: Facts and Comparisons, 1988.

Physicians' Desk Reference. Oradell, NJ: Medical Economics, 1988.

USP DI. Rockville, MD: The United States Pharmacopeial Convention, Inc., 1989.

Hormones/Hormone Antagonists (Fertility Agents, Sex Hormones, Contraceptives, Thyroid Drugs)

DANAZOL

Brand Names
U.S.A.: Danocrine (Winthrop-Breon).
Canada: Cyclomen (Winthrop).
Great Britain: Danol (Winthrop).

What This Drug Does
Synthetic male hormone.

How This Drug Affects Body Weight
Danazol may cause weight gain through its anabolic (tissue-building) effects. It may have weak mineralocorticoid and glucocorticoid properties that result in water retention and weight gain.

Government-Approved Uses for This Drug
To treat endometriosis (abnormal growth of uterine cells); to treat fibrocystic breast disease; to treat hereditary angioedema (localized swelling) in both sexes.

Unofficial Uses
To control precocious puberty; to treat gynecomastia (enlargement of the male breasts); to control excessive menstrual blood loss; as a female contraceptive; as a male contraceptive; to treat alpha-1-

antitrypsin deficiency; to treat systemic lupus erythematosis (a long-term inflammatory disease affecting many body systems).

When Not to Use This Drug

In undiagnosed abnormal vaginal bleeding; in impaired liver, kidney, or heart function; if pregnant; if breast-feeding; if allergic to this drug or to any related drug.

Side Effects From Use of This Drug

Acne; swelling; hoarseness; male-pattern baldness; oily skin or hair; dizziness; headache; fatigue; tremor; irritability; mental depression; sleep disorders; chills; burning sensations of the skin; high blood pressure; stomach irritation; nausea; vomiting; diarrhea or constipation (reported with equal frequency); blood in the urine; liver dysfunction; flushing; sweating; muscle cramps or spasms; mild hirsutism (male-type hair growth in females); decrease in breast size; deepening of the voice (in females); clitoral enlargement; decrease in testicle size; vaginitis including itching, dryness, burning, and vaginal bleeding; changes in libido; pelvic pain; changes in semen volume and viscosity; changes in sperm count and sperm motility.

Effects on Appetite and Body Weight as Disclosed by the Drug's Manufacturer

Weight gain; appetite change; water retention.

Detailed Effects on Appetite and Body Weight

Weight gain: In a 6-month study of 20 females treated with danazol, a steady increase in body weight was recorded. In fact, this was the most common side effect observed with use of this drug. Average total weight gain was 6.6 pounds during the course of the trial.

In a group of 25 patients treated with danazol for 6 months, average weight gain was 7 pounds, with a maximum reported increase of 13 pounds. This occurred despite advance mention of this possibility and a caution from doctors to exercise dietary restriction while taking this drug.

In a 6-month study of 20 females receiving danazol, 25% reported weight gain, with one subject reporting an increase of 13.2 pounds.

Thirty patients took part in a 6-month study using danazol as an oral contraceptive. Although daily dosages were lower than those generally used to treat endometriosis (the drug's primary indication), weight gain was the most common side effect but only became significant at the upper end of the dosage scale (200mg. daily). At this dose, weight gain averaged 8.5 pounds.

In a study of 32 females given danazol to treat endometriosis, 6 months of drug therapy revealed weight gain as the most frequent side effect. Half the study population showed gains of 10 pounds or more, with an average increase of 13.2 pounds (the range was 10–31 pounds). Ninety-five percent of all weight gained occurred within the first 2 months of danazol use, with gains leveling off after the fourth month.

In a study of 100 women treated with danazol for an average of 17.3 weeks, 55 reported weight gains.

In a 3-month study of 15 females given danazol, average weight gain was 16.3 pounds.

In a study of 18 women treated for mennorhagia (abnormally heavy or long menstrual periods) with danazol for 3 months, average weight gain was about 10 pounds.

Water retention: In a 6-month study of 20 women taking danazol, half reported water retention.

Of 30 females taking danazol as an oral contraceptive for 6 months, 10% exhibited water retention, with more patients affected at the higher end of the dosage scale (200mg. daily).

In a group of 32 females given danazol for the treatment of endometriosis, 6 months of drug therapy saw over 13% reporting water retention. In 2 patients, this effect was severe enough to cause discontinuation of the drug.

In a study of 100 females treated with danazol for 17.3 weeks, 55 subjects complained of water retention.

Dosage Levels at Which Effects Occur
Weight gain: Reported as low as 100mg. daily.
Water retention: Reported as low as 50mg. daily.

Remedies
Weight gain: In one study cited above, a decrease in daily dosage resulted in lessening of all side effects including weight gain.

Substitution of low-calorie foods, beverages, and snacks for normal dietary intake may aid in reversing some drug-induced weight gain.

How Long It Takes Till Reversal of Drug Effects

It may take about 2–3 months for danazol's effects to dissipate after its discontinuation.

Weight gain: In one study cited above, normal body weight returned within 2–3 weeks after discontinuation of danazol. In another study, this took 2 months.

Sources

Barbieri, R.L., et al. "Danazol in the treatment of endometriosis: Analysis of 100 cases with a 4-year follow-up." *Fertility and Sterility*, 1982, 37(6): 737–46.

Biberoglu, K.O., Behrman, S.J. "Dosage aspects of danazol therapy in endometriosis: Short-term and long-term effectiveness." *American Journal of Obstetrics and Gynecology*, 1981, 139(6): 645–54.

Chalmers, J.A., Shervington, P.C. "Follow-up of patients with endometriosis treated with danazol." *Postgraduate Medical Journal*, 1979, 55(suppl. 5): 44–47.

Chimbira, T.H., et al. "The effects of danazol on menorrhagia, coagulation mechanisms, haematological indices, and body weight." *British Journal of Obstetrics and Gynaecology*, 1979, 86(1): 46–50.

Guoth, J., et al. "Endocrine consequences of danazol treatment in menorrhagia." *European Journal of Obstetrics, Gynecology, and Reproductive Biology*, 1986, 23(1–2): 79–83.

Lauersen, N.H., Wilson, K.H. "Evaluation of danazol as an oral contraceptive." *Obstetrics and Gynecology*, 1977, 50(1): 91–96.

Noble, A.D., Letchworth, A.T. "Medical treatment of endometriosis: A comparative trial." *Postgraduate Medical Journal*, 1979, 55(suppl. 5): 37–39.

Ronnberg, L., et al. "Effects of danazol in the treatment of severe endometriosis." *Postgraduate Medical Journal*, 1979, 55(suppl. 5): 21–26.

ESTROGEN

Brand Names

U.S.A.: Amnestrogen (Squibb), Estraderm (Ciba), Estratab (Reid-Provident), *Estratest (Reid-Rowell), Estrocon (Savage), Evex (Syntex), Femogen (Private Formulations), Menest (Beecham), *Menrium (Roche), *Milprem (Wallace), *PMB (Ayerst), Premarin (Ayerst), Progens (Major).

Canada: Estrace (Bristol), Femogen (Stickley), *Menrium (Roche).

Great Britain: Premarin (Ayerst), Prempak (Ayerst).

*Combination drug.

What This Drug Does
Female hormone.

How This Drug Affects Body Weight
Estrogen is the hormone responsible for development and maintenance of the female reproductive system as well as secondary sex characteristics. Its metabolic effects include protein-building and promotion of sodium and water retention.

Government-Approved Uses for This Drug
To treat various menopausal symptoms; to treat shrinkage, dryness and itching of the vagina; to supplement low levels of natural estrogen; to treat osteoporosis (bone loss); to treat certain breast cancers; to treat prostate cancer; to prevent breast enlargement after giving birth.

Unofficial Uses
As a postcoital (after sex) contraceptive.

When Not to Use This Drug
In impaired liver function; in most breast cancers and certain other cancers; in blood-clot disorders; in undiagnosed abnormal genital bleeding; in pregnancy; in certain circulatory disorders; if allergic to this drug or to any related drug.

Side Effects From Use of This Drug
Nausea; vomiting; cramping; bloating; liver dysfunction (jaundice); various skin reactions; changes in hair growth; various eye problems; headache; dizziness; depression; possible cancer of the breast, cervix, vagina, uterus, and liver; gallbladder disease (postmenopausal); widespread blood clots and diseases associated with them; lesions of the liver; high blood pressure; decreased tolerance to glucose; high blood calcium levels (in patients with breast or bone cancers); breakthrough bleeding (bleeding at abnormal times of the menstrual cycle); spotting; changes in menstrual flow; dysmenorrhea (painful menstruation); premenstrual-like syndrome; amenorrhea (cessation of menstruation) during and after treatment; increase in size of uterine fibromyomas; vaginal candidiasis; changes in cervical erosion and degree of cervical secretions; breast tenderness, enlargement, and secretion; hirsutism (male-type hair growth in females); changes in libido.

Effects on Appetite and Body Weight as Disclosed by the Drug's Manufacturer

Loss of appetite; increased appetite; weight gain or loss; retention of water.

Detailed Effects on Appetite and Body Weight

Weight gain: In a study of 63 obese patients treated at a hospital nutrition clinic, results of nonmedicated individuals were compared with those on various medications, estrogen among them. While the group as a whole lost an average of 2.45 pounds per month through diet alone, those taking estrogen (in the conjugated form) either continued to gain weight until the drug was discontinued or lost at a very discouraging rate of 2–3 pounds over the entire year of the study.

Dosage Levels at Which Effects Occur

Weight gain: May occur within the normal daily dosage range of 0.3–30mg.

Remedies

Weight gain: Substitution of low-calorie foods, beverages, and snacks for normal dietary intake may aid in reversing some drug-induced weight gain.

How Long It Takes Till Reversal of Drug Effects

Oral estrogens have a short duration of action, with daily doses usually needed to maintain their effectiveness.

Source

Stein, P.M., et al. "Predicting weight loss success among obese clients in a hospital nutrition clinic." *American Journal of Clinical Nutrition*, 1981, 34(10): 2039–44.

ETIDRONATE

Brand Names

U.S.A.: Didronel (Norwich Eaton).
Canada: Didronel (Norwich Eaton).
Great Britain: Didronel Tablets (Brocades).

What This Drug Does

Lowers blood calcium levels.

How This Drug Affects Body Weight
Unknown. Inhibits breakdown of bone as well as retarding new bone formation.

Government-Approved Uses for This Drug
To treat Paget's disease (bone-tissue breakdown) of oral bone; to treat various states of high blood calcium.

Unofficial Uses
None.

When Not to Use This Drug
If certain kidney dysfunction exists; if allergic to this drug or to any related drug.

Side Effects From Use of This Drug
Diarrhea; increased frequency of bowel movements; nausea; increased or persistent bone pain; enhanced risk of bone fracture; high blood phosphate levels.

Effects on Appetite and Body Weight as Disclosed by the Drug's Manufacturer
Metallic or altered taste; loss of taste.

Detailed Effects on Appetite and Body Weight
Loss of taste: In a survey of 48 patients receiving etidronate by mouth, 4% complained of taste loss. When a group of 44 patients was given the drug by intravenous infusion, 52% had this complaint. It usually was evident after the first or second dose. Some subjects noted a metallic taste but further questioning by researchers revealed this to be an inability to discriminate between various flavors.

Dosage Levels at Which Effects Occur
Loss of taste: Reported at a daily dose of 20mg. per kilogram of body weight when taken orally and at 7.5mg. per kilogram daily when given by intravenous infusion.

Remedies
Loss of taste: Etidronate-induced taste disturbance may be countered in several ways. Taking the drug with an adequate fluid intake, chewing sugarless gum or using a mouthwash of water and lemon juice, and practicing good oral hygiene may help restore normal taste sensation.

How Long It Takes Till Reversal of Drug Effects
Loss of taste: This resolved spontaneously in all cases cited above. Normal taste usually is restored within hours whether or not etidronate is continued.

Source
Jones, P.B., et al. "Transient taste-loss during treatment with etidronate [letter]." *Lancet*, 1987, 2(8559): 637.

GLUCAGON

Brand Names
U.S.A.: Glucagon (Lilly).
Canada: Glucagon (Lilly).
Great Britain: Glucagon (Lilly), Glucagon Novo (Novo; Farillon).

What This Drug Does
Glucose elevating agent.

How This Drug Affects Body Weight
Glucagon is a hormone produced by the pancreas that raises blood-sugar levels and generally acts in opposition to insulin, another pancreatic hormone. Glucagon relaxes the smooth muscles of the gastrointestinal tract. It also decreases stomach secretions as well as inhibits gastric movement in the fasting stomach. Glucagon may exert a direct effect on the central nervous system, a process thought to be mediated by the effects of glucose in the brain.

Government-Approved Uses for This Drug
To raise blood-sugar levels in suitable diabetics or during insulin shock therapy; as a diagnostic aid in certain x-ray exams of the gastrointestinal tract.

Unofficial Uses
To treat propranolol overdose; to treat certain cardiovascular emergencies; to treat certain gastrointestinal spasms.

When Not to Use This Drug
If allergic to this drug or to any related drug.

Side Effects From Use of This Drug

Nausea; vomiting; various allergic responses such as rash, breathing difficulties, and low blood pressure.

Effects on Appetite and Body Weight as Disclosed by the Drug's Manufacturer

None.

Detailed Effects on Appetite and Body Weight

Decreased appetite: Ten male patients from 16 to 45 years of age were studied for 5 weeks in a hospital setting while taking glucagon and a placebo. All subjects were permitted an unlimited supply of food, provided it was consumed only at meal time. Glucagon was administered by intramuscular injection 10 minutes prior to each meal. Almost all subjects reported decreased appetite when receiving the active drug. Several claimed to be very hungry when they sat down to eat (about 5 minutes after the injection) but suddenly lost their desire for food. Nine of the 10 showed lower caloric intake when on glucagon than when given placebo, with an average daily decrease of 440 calories. In 6 of 10 cases, a small weight loss occurred as well when taking glucagon.

In a study design similar to the one above, 4 male volunteers were given glucagon by intramuscular injection. It caused previously hungry subjects to rate themselves as "not hungry" 2 hours later.

In an experiment comparing response to a single dose of glucagon versus chronic administration over a 25-day period, both regimens inhibited appetite. The single-dose protocol caused significantly decreased food intake at test meals as soon as 1 hour after injection. The drug's effect peaked at 2 hours but effects continued for 5 hours. The drug decreased the average caloric intake by 30%. With long-term drug administration, subjects consistently reduced eating and lost weight.

Seven healthy adult males received intravenous glucagon for a total of 16 separate doses. Hunger contractions in the stomach ceased within 3 minutes of receiving the drug on every occasion. Sensation of hunger was decreased or absent shortly thereafter.

Dosage Levels at Which Effects Occur

Decreased appetite: Reported at 1–2mg. by intramuscular injection either as a single dose or 3 times daily prior to meals.

Remedies
Not applicable.

How Long It Takes Till Reversal of Drug Effects
Decreased appetite: When given by intramuscular injection, glucagon's duration of action is from 12–27 minutes at a 1mg. dose, and from 22–25 minutes at a 2mg. dose.

Sources
Penick, S.B., Hinkle L.E., Jr. "Depression of food intake induced in healthy subjects by glucagon." *New England Journal of Medicine*, 1961, 264: 893–97.

Penick, S.B., Hinkle, L.E., Jr. "The effect of glucagon, phenmetrazine and epinephrine on hunger, food intake and plasma NEFA." *American Journal of Clinical Nutrition*, 1963, 13: 110–14.

Schulman, J.L., et al. "Effect of glucagon on food intake and body weight in man." *Journal of Applied Physiology*, 1957, 11: 419–21.

Stunkard, A.J., et al. "The mechanism of satiety: Effect of glucagon on gastric hunger contractions in man." *Proceedings of the Society of Experimental Biology and Medicine*, 1955, 89: 258–61.

HUMAN CHORIONIC GONADOTROPIN (HCG)

Brand Names
U.S.A. Android-HCG (Brown), A.P.L. Secules (Ayerst), Chorex (Hyrex), Corgonject-5 (Mayrand), Follutein (Squibb), Glukor (Hyrex), Gonic (Hauck), Libigen (Savage), Pregnyl (Organon), Profasi HP (Serono).
Canada: Antuitrin (Parke-Davis), A.P.L. (Ayerst), Profasi HP (Pharmascience).
Great Britain: Gonadotropin LH (Paines & Byrne), Pregnyl (Organon), Profasi (Serono).

What This Drug Does
Fertility agent; gonadal stimulant.

How This Drug Affects Body Weight
Human chorionic gonadotropin may partly deactivate hypothalamic control. This portion of the brain determines equilibrium set point for body mass and composition. Some evidence suggests that HCG may have thyroid-stimulating activity.

Government-Approved Uses for This Drug

To help the testicles descend in prepubertal males; to treat certain pituitary deficiency in males; to induce ovulation in infertile females.

Unofficial Uses

As an aid in weight loss.

CAUTION: The FDA and the American Medical Association do not officially condone use of HCG for weight loss. The FDA requires all product labeling to disclose that safety and effectiveness has not been demonstrated for the drug's use in the treatment of obesity.

When Not to Use This Drug

In precocious (early) puberty; in prostate cancer or certain other androgen (male hormone)-dependent cancers; if pregnant; if allergic to this drug or to any related drug.

Side Effects From Use of This Drug

Headache; fatigue; irritability; depression; voice change; growth of body hair; precocious puberty; gynecomastia (enlargement of the male breasts).

Effects on Appetite and Body Weight as Disclosed by the Drug's Manufacturer

Water retention.

Detailed Effects on Appetite and Body Weight

Weight loss: HCG use for weight control is controversial, with studies reporting conflicting results. One of the originators of its use, A.T. Simeons, maintains that the substance itself has no weight-reducing activity. Its primary value is claimed to be its ability to cause preferential loss of fat from areas of abnormal fat deposit, as opposed to depleting normal fat reserves when diet is attempted alone.

HCG has been shown to be of greatest value as an adjunct to a 500-calorie-per-day diet. While almost no one can maintain this level of dieting by sheer willpower, Simeons claims 80% of those attempting this while taking HCG are successful.

In a South African study of 23 obese subjects given HCG, the 20 who completed the program lost an average of 90 pounds in 7 months. Once their "normal" weight was attained, a follow-up 1 year later showed only 2 subjects regaining any weight at all.

Forty overweight adult females were divided into two equal groups. One group received HCG and the other placebo. Both groups were placed on a 500- to 550-calorie-per-day diet and were given daily injections 6 days per week for 6 weeks. At the end of this time, the average weight loss for those taking the active drug was almost 20 pounds, compared with about 11 pounds for the placebo group.

Sixty-four patients were treated by a variety of protocols using HCG or placebo. The average weight loss after 34 days of active drug use was 18.7 pounds in one group and 14.1 pounds after 23 days in another. Those receiving inactive medication for an average of 27 days lost an average 12.3 pounds. All subjects in the project were maintained on a 500-calorie daily diet.

Although not conducted in a strictly scientific manner, one report from the 1950's describes HCG's action on obese patients. It was said to decrease measurements taken around the hips and waist without any corresponding decrease in body weight. The significance of this was interpreted as a dispersal of fat away from traditional deposit sites to be utilized for metabolic purposes. HCG was thought to allow patients to exist comfortably on a diet of only 500 calories per day. After about 40 days of treatment with diet and HCG, a loss of 20–30 pounds was claimed in more than 500 cases treated over a 20-year period. After 40 days, despite continued HCG injections, weight loss ceased. However, after a 6-week drug-free period, the course of therapy could be repeated with equal effectiveness.

Dosage Levels at Which Effects Occur
Weight loss: Reported at 125 I.U. (international units) daily by intramuscular injection.

Remedies
Not applicable.

How Long It Takes Till Reversal of Drug Effects
Eighty percent of injected HCG is inactivated by the body within 24 hours.

Sources
Asher, W.L., Harper, H.W. "Effects of human chorionic gonadotropin on

weight loss, hunger, and feeling of well-being." *American Journal of Clinical Nutrition*, 1973, 26: 211–18.

Brady, P.J. "Human chorionic gonadotropin: A new role?" *Obesity and Bariatric Medicine*, 1979, 8(2): 60–61.

Lebon, P. "Treatment of overweight patients with chorionic gonadotropin: Follow-up study." *Journal of the American Geriatric Society*, 1966, 14: 116.

Simeons, A.T.W. "Actions of chorionic gonadotropin in the obese." *Lancet*, 1954, 2: 946–47.

Simeons, A.T.W. "Chorionic gonadotropin in the treatment of obese women." *American Journal of Clinical Nutrition*, 1963, 13: 197–98.

Simeons, A.T.W. "Chorionic gonadotropin in the treatment of obesity." *American Journal of Clinical Nutrition*, 1964, 15: 188.

Willis, J. "About body wraps, pills and other magic wands for losing weight." *FDA Consumer*, 1982, 16: 18–20.

HUMAN GROWTH HORMONE

Brand Names
U.S.A.: Humatrope [somatropin] (Lilly), Protropin [somatrem] (Genentech).
Canada: Crescormon (Pharmacia).
Great Britain: Crescormon (KabiVitrum), Nanormon (Nordisk-UK).

What This Drug Does
Growth hormone.

How This Drug Affects Body Weight
A purified product of recombinant DNA technology, synthetic human growth hormone (somatrem and somatropin) mimic almost exactly the sequence of amino acids that form the body's natural human growth hormone secreted by the pituitary gland. In growth-hormone-deficient individuals, long-term administration of this synthetic substance often results in reduction of body fat. Human growth hormone may also stimulate thyroid gland activity.

Government-Approved Uses for This Drug
For long-term treatment of children with growth failure due to lack of adequate levels of natural growth hormone.

Unofficial Uses
None.

When Not to Use This Drug
If bone growth has ceased; in the presence of active intracranial (brain) lesion; if allergic to benzyl alcohol (applies only to somatrem); if allergic to m-cresol or glycerin (applies only to somatropin); if allergic to human growth hormone or to any related drug.

Side Effects From Use of This Drug
Possible development of antibodies to growth hormone; headache; muscle pain; weakness; high blood sugar.

Effects on Appetite and Body Weight as Disclosed by the Drug's Manufacturer
Water retention.

Detailed Effects on Appetite and Body Weight
Weight loss: Eighty grossly obese female subjects weighing from 298 to 470 pounds and ranging in age from 29 to 51 were studied in a hospital setting for the effects of human growth hormone on weight loss. By measuring oxygen consumption, a correlation to fat oxidation (elimination) was drawn. During one 4-day period of growth hormone use, oxygen consumption increased by 60 liters per day. This translated to a daily oxidation of an additional 30 grams of fat. The significance of this effect is unknown and the use of human growth hormone for this purpose is extremely controversial.

Dosage Levels at Which Effects Occur
Weight loss: Reported to occur at a dose of 8mg. daily.

Remedies
Weight loss: Not applicable.

How Long It Takes Till Reversal of Drug Effects
Unknown.

Source
Bray, G.A, "Calorigenic effect of growth hormone in obesity." *Journal of Clinical Endocrinology and Metabolism*, 1969, 29: 119.

LEVOTHYROXINE (T4)

Brand Names
U.S.A.: Levothroid (USV), Synthroid (Flint), Syroxine (Major).
Canada: Eltroxin (Glaxo), Synthroid (Flint).
Great Britain: Eltroxin (Glaxo).

What This Drug Does
Thyroid hormone.

How This Drug Affects Body Weight
Thyroid hormone alters the body's basal metabolic rate (the amount of energy needed to maintain the body's essential functions such as breathing, temperature, circulation). This affects how the body utilizes oxygen. The effect of taking in additional thyroid hormone may exaggerate energy expenditure, increasing oxygen consumption to cause accelerated protein breakdown. The greater weight loss seen with the use of thyroid hormones as compared with other diet drugs is believed to derive not from fat loss, but mainly from the breakdown of lean muscle tissue.

Natural thyroid hormone is composed of two components, T3 (liothyronine) and T4 (levothyroxine). Twenty times as much T4 is present than T3 in the body's natural thyroid secretion. T3, however, is 3–5 times more active and works more rapidly. Most of the effect of thyroid hormone comes from T3.

Commercially available thyroid supplements include natural products extracted from beef or pork that approximate the balance of T3 and T4 found in human thyroid hormone. Synthetic derivatives are available as pure T3, pure T4, and liotrix, a mixture of T3 and T4 (4 to 1).

Government-Approved Uses for This Drug
As a thyroid hormone replacement; to treat certain goiters; to treat thyroid cancer; as a diagnostic aid in detecting certain thyroid abnormalities.

Unofficial Uses
As an aid to weight loss.

When Not to Use This Drug

In the presence of an overactive thyroid gland; in certain heart disease; with certain adrenal gland insufficiency; if allergic to this drug or to any related drug.

Side Effects From Use of This Drug

Side effects would result from overdosage, since proper dosing should restore the body to its normal level of thyroid hormone. Signs of overdosage include rapid or irregular heartbeat; tremors; headache; diarrhea; insomnia; sweating; heat and fever intolerance; anginal pain (chest pain caused by coronary artery spasm); menstrual irregularities.

Effects on Appetite and Body Weight as Disclosed by the Drug's Manufacturer

Changes in appetite; weight loss.

Detailed Effects on Appetite and Body Weight

Weight loss: *Note: The treatment of obese individuals with thyroid hormones tends to cause a preferential loss of lean body mass, as opposed to body fat. One study showed only 20% of the weight lost with use of thyroid hormones attributable to fat loss.*

In a study of 7 obese patients given levothyroxine for 30 weeks, average weekly weight loss was 1.04 pounds for a total loss of over 31 pounds.

Dosage Levels at Which Effects Occur

Weight loss: Reported at 800–2,400mcg. daily.

Remedies

Not applicable.

How Long It Takes Till Reversal of Drug Effects

Weight loss: *Note: Those treated for obesity with thyroid hormone show a tendency to regain lost weight rapidly after withdrawal of the drug.*

In normal individuals, half the dose of levothyroxine is cleared from the blood in 6–7 days.

Sources

Garrow, J.S. *Treat Obesity Seriously*. Edinburgh: Churchill Livingstone, 1981.
Gwinup, G., Poucher, R. "A controlled study of thyroid analogs in the therapy of obesity." *American Journal of Medical Science*, 1967, 254:416–20.

LIOTHYRONINE (T3)

Brand Names
U.S.A.: Cyronine (Major), Cytomel (SKF).
Canada: Cytomel (SKF).
Great Britain: Tertroxin (Glaxo).

What This Drug Does
Thyroid hormone.

How This Drug Affects Body Weight
Thyroid hormone alters the body's basal metabolic rate (the amount of energy needed to maintain the body's essential functions such as breathing, temperature, circulation). This affects how the body utilizes oxygen. The effect of taking in additional thyroid hormone may exaggerate energy expenditure, increasing oxygen consumption to cause accelerated protein breakdown. The greater weight loss seen with the use of thyroid hormones as compared with other diet drugs is believed to derive not from fat loss, but mainly from the breakdown of lean muscle tissue.

Natural thyroid hormone is composed of two components, T3 (liothyronine) and T4 (levothyroxine). Twenty times as much T4 is present than T3 in the body's natural thyroid secretion. T3, however, is 3–5 times more active and works more rapidly. Most of the effect of thyroid hormone comes from T3.

Commercially available thyroid supplements include natural products extracted from beef or pork that approximate the balance of T3 and T4 found in human thyroid hormone. Synthetic derivatives are available as pure T3, pure T4, and liotrix, a mixture of T3 and T4 (4 to 1).

Government-Approved Uses for This Drug
As a thyroid hormone replacement; to treat certain goiters; to treat thyroid cancer; as a diagnostic aid in detecting certain thyroid abnormalities.

Unofficial Uses
As an aid to weight loss.

When Not to Use This Drug
In the presence of an overactive thyroid gland; in certain heart disease; with certain adrenal gland insufficiency; if allergic to this drug or to any related drug.

Side Effects From Use of This Drug
Side effects would result from overdosage, since proper dosing should restore the body to its normal level of thyroid hormone. Signs of overdosage include rapid or irregular heartbeat; weight loss; tremors; headache; diarrhea; insomnia; sweating; heat and fever intolerance; anginal pain (chest pain caused by coronary artery spasm); menstrual irregularities.

Effects on Appetite and Body Weight as Disclosed by the Drug's Manufacturer
Changes in appetite; weight loss.

Detailed Effects on Appetite and Body Weight
Weight loss: *Note: The treatment of obese individuals with thyroid hormones tends to cause a preferential loss of lean body mass, as opposed to body fat. One study showed only 20% of the weight lost by use of thyroid hormones attributable to fat loss.*

In a 16-week study, 55 obese patients were given both a combination of amphetamine and amobarbital, and liothyronine. Greatest weight loss was found to occur after 8 weeks of the amphetamine-amobarbital preparation when this preceded the addition of liothyronine. Average weight loss was about 1 pound per week during both the amphetamine and liothyronine phases of the study, provided amphetamine was given first. When liothyronine was the first drug given, weight loss during that time was about the same, but switching to amphetamine alone produced no additional loss.

In a study of 8 obese patients given liothyronine for 12 weeks, weight loss was significantly greater than that for a group given a placebo. Average weight loss for those taking the active drug was almost 40 pounds by the end of the 3 months.

In a group of 6 obese patients given liothyronine for 30 weeks, an average weekly weight loss of 0.85 pounds was recorded. Total average loss was 25.5 pounds.

Seventeen patients who were more than 100 pounds over their ideal weight were enrolled in a 12-week study to determine the effects of liothyronine. One group took the drug while sticking to a weight-loss diet; the others relied on diet alone. After 8 weeks, average weight loss in the liothyronine group was about 29 pounds. Diet alone caused an average loss of about 17 pounds. After 12 weeks, those taking the drug lost an average 37 pounds versus 23.3 pounds for the others.

Dosage Levels at Which Effects Occur
Weight loss: Reported as low as 25mcg. daily.

Remedies
Weight loss: Not applicable.

How Long It Takes Till Reversal of Drug Effects
Weight loss: *Note: Those treated for obesity loss with thyroid hormone show a tendency to regain lost weight rapidly after withdrawal of the drug.*

While half the dose of liothyronine is cleared from the blood in about 2 days, its duration of action lasts about 2.5 hours after the last dose.

Sources
Garrow, J.S. *Treat Obesity Seriously*. Edinburgh: Churchill Livingstone, 1981.
Gelvin, E.P., et al. "Results of addition of liothyronine to a weight-reduction regimen." *Journal of the American Medical Association*, 1959, 170: 1507–12.
Gwinup, G., Poucher, R. "A controlled study of thyroid analogs in the therapy of obesity." *American Journal of Medical Science*, 1967, 254: 416–20.
Hollingsworth, D.R., et al. "Quantitative and qualitative effects of triiodothyronine in massive obesity." *Metabolism*, 1970, 19: 934–39.
Moore, R., et al. "The treatment of obesity with triiodothyronine in conjunction with a very low calorie formula diet." *Lancet*, 1980, i(8162): 223.
Rivlin, R.S. "Therapy of obesity with hormones." *New England Journal of Medicine*, 1975, 292: 26–29.
Weidenhamer, J.E. "L-triiodothyronine as administrative therapy in the management of obesity: Preliminary report." *American Practitioner and Digest of Treatment*, 1957, 8: 419–23.

METHIMAZOLE

Brand Names
U.S.A.: Tapazole (Lilly).
Canada: Tapazole (Lilly).

Great Britain: None.

What This Drug Does
Antithyroid agent.

How This Drug Affects Body Weight
Prevents the synthesis of thyroid hormone in the thyroid gland. Methimazole may remove zinc from the taste cells. Zinc deficiency has been linked to taste disturbance.

Government-Approved Uses for This Drug
To treat overactive thyroid gland.

Unofficial Uses
None.

When Not To Use This Drug
If a nursing mother; if allergic to this drug or to any related drug.

Side Effects From Use Of This Drug
Headache; drowsiness; vertigo; nausea; diarrhea; vomiting; various blood abnormalities; liver dysfunction (jaundice); various skin reactions; joint or muscle pain; enlargement of the salivary glands.

Effects on Appetite and Body Weight as Disclosed by the Drug's Manufacturer
Loss of taste; water retention.

Detailed Effects on Appetite and Body Weight
Loss of taste; loss of smell: A 55-year-old male lost the ability to taste after 4 weeks of methimazole use. Smell remained intact. When the drug was withdrawn, taste sensation gradually returned.

A 31-year-old female lost all sense of taste 31 days after starting methimazole. Sense of smell remained unaffected and taste was restored gradually after the drug's withdrawal.

A 30-year-old housewife reported sudden and complete loss of all sense of taste and smell 3 weeks after starting methimazole. After being switched to a different drug, both senses began to return 10 days later. Sweet and salt sensation were the first to be restored and a few days after that, all affected senses returned to normal.

Dosage Levels at Which Effects Occur
Loss of taste; loss of smell: Reported as low as 30mg. daily.

Remedies
Loss of taste; loss of smell: Methimazole-induced taste disturbance may be countered in several ways. Taking the drug with an adequate fluid intake, chewing sugarless gum or using a mouthwash of water and lemon juice, and practicing good oral hygiene may help restore normal taste sensation.

In one case cited above, switching to a different drug, propylthiouracil, reversed taste loss.

How Long It Takes Till Reversal of Drug Effects
Loss of taste; loss of smell: In the cases reported above, restoration of taste and smell took anywhere from 10 days to 3 weeks after withdrawal of methimazole.

It takes 3–5 hours for half the dose of methimazole to clear the blood.

Sources
Erikssen, J., et al. "Side-effect of thiocarbamides." *Lancet*, 1975, 1, 231–32.
Hallman, B.L., Hurst, J.W. "Loss of taste as toxic effect of methimazole (Tapazole) therapy." *Journal of the American Medical Association*, 1953, 152, 322.

ORAL CONTRACEPTIVES— COMBINATION DRUGS

Brand Names
U.S.A.: *Brevicon (Syntex), *Demulen (Searle), *Enovid (Searle), *Genora (Rugby), *Gynex (Searle), *Levlen (Berlex), *Loestrin (Parke-Davis), *Lo/Ovral (Wyeth), *Modicon (Ortho), *Nordette (Wyeth), *Norinyl (Syntex), *Norlestrin (Parke-Davis), *Ortho-Novum (Ortho), *Ovcon (Mead Johnson), *Ovral (Wyeth), *Ovulen (Searle), *Tri-Norinyl (Syntex), *Triphasil (Wyeth).
Canada: *Brevicon (Syntex), *Demulen (Searle), *Enovid-E (Searle), *Loestrin (Parke-Davis), *Minestrin (Parke-Davis), *Min-Ovral (Wyeth), *Norinyl (Syntex), *Norlestrin (Parke-Davis), *Ortho-Novum (Ortho), *Ovral (Wyeth), *Ovulen (Searle).

*Combination drug.

Great Britain: ★Anovlar 21 (Schering), ★Binovum (Ortho-Cilag), ★Brevinor (Syntex), ★Conova 30 (Searle), ★Controvlar (Schering), ★Demulen 50 (Searle), ★Eugynon 30 (Schering), ★Eugynon 50 (Schering), ★Gynovlar 21 (Schering), ★Loestrin 20 (Parke-Davis), ★Logynon (Schering), ★Logynon ED (Schering), ★Microgynon 30 (Schering), ★Minilyn (Organon), ★Minovlar (Schering), ★Minovlar ED (Schering), ★Norinyl-1 (Syntex), ★Norlestrin (Parke-Davis), ★Normin (Syntex), ★Orlest 21 (Parke-Davis), ★Ortho-Novin 1/50 (Ortho-Cilag), ★Ovran (Wyeth), ★Ovranette (Wyeth), ★Ovulen 50 (Searle), ★Ovysmen (Ortho-Cilag), ★Trinordiol (Wyeth).

What This Drug Does
Prevents conception.

How This Drug Affects Body Weight
The mechanism by which oral contraceptives affect body weight is unknown. They inhibit ovulation by suppressing follicle-stimulating hormone and leutinizing hormone. The estrogen component of oral contraceptives blocks ovarian follicular development and ovulation. The progestin ingredient ensures that even if the follicle develops, ovulation will not occur.

Government-Approved Uses for This Drug:
To prevent pregnancy.

Unofficial Uses
Ovral (a brand-name product by Wyeth) has been given in high doses as a postcoital contraceptive ("morning-after pill").

When Not to Use This Drug
In the presence of various blood-clot abnormalities; in certain heart and circulatory disease; in certain breast cancers; in liver tumors (past or present); if there is undiagnosed abnormal vaginal bleeding; if pregnant or plan to become pregnant within 3 months; if breast-feeding; if allergic to this product or to any related drug.

Side Effects From Use of This Drug
Headache or migraine headache; dizziness; depression; blood clots; high blood pressure; worsening of certain eye problems; nausea; vomiting; abdominal cramps; inflammation of the pancreas; gallbladder disease; liver dysfunction; high blood sugar;

★Combination drug.

high blood calcium levels; folic acid deficiency; rash; acne; oily skin; changes in skin pigmentation; breakthrough bleeding (bleeding at abnormal times of the menstrual cycle); spotting; change in menstrual flow; dysmenorrhea (painful menstruation); amenorrhea (cessation of menstruation) during and after oral contraceptive use; temporary infertility after discontinuation of oral contraceptive; changes in cervical erosion and cervical secretions; vaginal candidiasis (fungal infection); breast tenderness, enlargement, and secretions; premenstrual-like syndrome; changes in libido; hirsutism (male-type hair growth in females); vaginitis.

Effects on Appetite and Body Weight as Disclosed by the Drug's Manufacturer

Loss or changes of appetite; water retention; weight gain.

Detailed Effects on Appetite and Body Weight

Weight change: Specific investigations detailing the effects that oral contraceptives exert on body weight are few. Those more general studies that mention this phenomenon tend to attribute greater body weight changes to high-dose oral contraceptives. Women taking the newer low-dose combinations tend to have weight profiles similar to those of women who do not use this form of birth control.

Cyclic weight gains commonly seen in those taking oral contraceptives may be due to fluid retention. In other cases, when weight gains occur steadily, the cause may be an increased appetite from the androgenic (male-like) effects of the progestin component of some combination oral contraceptives.

A patient population of 50 women given two different strengths of oral contraceptives for 3 months or longer was followed for the effects on weight and body measurements. Weight changes for the two groups were comparable, with about 60% reporting weight gains and about 20% claiming weight loss. Chest measurements increased in about 40% of cases, while about 20% noted a reduction. Waist size increased for about one-third, while 32–46% showed a decrease. Hip measurements increased for 30–50%, as opposed to a loss in about 40% of cases.

Twenty-one women taking oral contraceptives were evaluated for weight and figure changes over an average of 7.2 months; 52% gained weight, while 28.5% lost. The average weight fluctuation was plus 16.5 pounds (range 4–52 pounds). Chest measurements increased in 66.5% of the women and decreased in 28.5%. Breast-cup size became larger in 24% of cases and smaller in 33.5% of subjects. Waist measurements increased in 33% and decreased in 62%. Hips increased in size in 28.5% and decreased in 47.5% of cases.

In a study of 63 obese patients treated at a hospital nutrition clinic, results in nonmedicated subjects were compared with those in patients taking various drugs, oral contraceptives among them. While the group as a whole lost an average of 2.45 pounds per month through a diet program alone, those taking oral contraceptives either continued to gain weight until the Pill was discontinued, or lost weight at a very discouraging rate of 2–3 pounds yearly while continuing with this method of birth control.

Dosage Levels at Which Effects Occur
Weight change: May occur while taking any combination oral contraceptives, regardless of the dose of each ingredient.

Remedies
Weight change: Substitution of low-calorie foods, beverages, and snacks for normal dietary intake may aid in reversing some oral-contraceptive-induced weight gain.

When cyclic weight gains due to fluid retention occur, a salt-restricted diet may help restore more normal weight parameters.

How Long It Takes Till Reversal of Drug Effects
Half the dose of combination oral contraceptives is cleared from the blood in 6–45 hours.

Sources
Block, M., Rulin, M.C. "Managing patients on oral contraceptives." *American Family Physician*, 1985, 32(2): 154–68.
Cooper, W.H., et al, "A preliminary report on 'The Pill' and figure changes." *Virginia Medical Monthly*, 1968, 95: 283–85.
Gravlee, L.C. "Clinical evaluation of oral contraceptives in respect to weight change and body measurements." *Journal of the Medical Association of the State of Alabama*, 1969, 38(7): 620–21.
Shearman, R.P. "Oral contraceptive agents." *Medical Journal of Australia*, 1986, 144(4): 201–5.
Stein, P.M., et al. "Predicting weight loss success among obese clients at a

hospital nutrition clinic." *American Journal of Clinical Nutrition*, 1981, 34(10): 2039–44.

TESTOSTERONE

Brand Names
U.S.A.: *Andrest 90-4 (Seatrace), Andro 100 (Forest), Andro-Cyp (Keene), *Andro-Estro 90-4 (Rugby), *Andro/Fem (Pasadena), *Androgyn L.A. (Forest), Android (Brown), Android-T (Brown), Andro L.A. 200 (Forest), Andronaq (Central), Andronate (Pasadena), Andropository 100 (Rugby), Andryl 200 (Keene), Anthatest (Kay), dDepotest (Hyrex), *De-Comberol (Schein), *Deladumone (Squibb), Delatest (Dunhall), *Delatestadiol (Dunhall), *Delatestryl (Squibb), depAndro (Forest), *depAndrogyn (Forest), Depo-Testadiol (Upjohn), *Depotestogen (Hyrex), Depo-Testosterone (Upjohn), *Dilate-DS (Savage), Ditate-DS (Savage), *Duo-Cyp (Keene), *Duo-Gen L.A. (Vortech), *Duoval PA (Reid-Rowell), Duratest (Hauck), *Duratestrin (Hauck), Durathate-200 (Hauck), *Estratest (Reid-Rowell), *Estra-Testrin (Pasadena), Everone (Hyrex), Histerone (Hauck), *Menoject-LA (Mayrand), Metandren (Ciba), Oreton Methyl (Schering), *Premarin with Methyltestosterone (Ayerst), T-Cypionate (Legere), T-E-Cypionate (Legere), *Teev (Keene), Testa-C (Vortech), *Testadiate (Kay), Testadiate-Depo (Kay), Testamone 100 (Dunhall), Testaqua (Kay), Testate (Savage), Testaval 90/4 (Legere), *Test-Estra-C (Vortech), *Test-Estro Cypionates (Rugby), Testex (Pasadena), Testoject (Mayrand), Testone LA (Ortega), *Testradiol 90/4 (Schein), Testred (ICN), Testred Cypionate 200 (ICN), Testrin PA (Pasadena), Testroval-P.A. (Reid-Provident), T-Ionate P.A. (Reid-Provident), *Tylosterone (Lilly), *Valertest No. 1 (Hyrex), Virilon (Star).
Canada: Delatestryl (Squibb), Depo-Testosterone (Upjohn), Malogen (Stickley), Malogex (Stickley).
Great Britain: Andromar Retard (Marshall's), Femalone 25 (Marshall's), *Plex-Hormone Injection (Consolidated Chem.), Primoteston-Depot 250mg. (Schering), Restandol (Organon),

*Combination drugs

Sustanon (Organon), Testoral Sublings (Organon), Virormone
(Paines & Byrne).

What This Drug Does
Androgen.

How This Drug Affects Body Weight
Weight gain in those taking testosterone may be due to the
drug's anabolic (tissue-building) effects.

Government-Approved Uses for This Drug
In males: To treat testosterone (male hormone) deficiency.
In females: To treat certain breast cancers; to treat breast pain
and engorgement in non-nursing mothers.

Unofficial Uses
To increase muscle mass and improve strength and power in
competitive athletes.

When Not to Use This Drug
In men with breast or prostate cancer; if pregnant; if allergic
to this drug or to any related drug.

Side Effects From Use of This Drug
Acne and oily skin (in females); hirsutism (male-type hair growth
in females); flushing and sweating (in females); nausea; vomiting;
gastroenteritis; irritable bladder; jaundice (reversible); high blood
calcium levels. In preadolescent males: phallic (penis) enlargement; increased frequency of erections.

Effects on Appetite and Body Weight as Disclosed by the Drug's Manufacturer
Change in appetite; weight gain; water retention.

Detailed Effects on Appetite and Body Weight
Weight gain: In a study of 4 males given testosterone by intramuscular injection for an average of about 11 days, mean weight
gain was 4.4 pounds.

A case report describes a man given testosterone for 8 days
and gaining 2.2 pounds.

In another report, a male receiving testosterone weekly for
about 3 months showed a weight gain of 6.6 pounds and a lean
body mass (nonfat) increase of 13.64 pounds.

A male receiving intramuscular injections of testosterone weekly for about 3 months gained about 2.5 pounds in weight but 18.7 pounds in lean body mass (nonfat).

Dosage Levels at Which Effects Occur
Weight gain: Reported to occur at 25mg. daily by intramuscular injection and as low as 300mg. per week by the same route of administration.

Remedies
Weight gain: Weight gain associated with testosterone use may be a desired effect in some users. In those not seeking this end, substitution of low-calorie foods, beverages, and snacks for normal dietary intake may aid in reversing some testosterone-induced weight gain.

How Long It Takes Till Reversal of Drug Effects
Although testosterone's half-life (the time it takes for 50% of a dose to be cleared from the blood) is relatively short (10–100 minutes), use of long-acting injectable dosage forms will prolong its effects for up to several weeks.

Source
Forbes, G.B. "The effect of anabolic steroids on lean body mass: The dose response curve." *Metabolism, Clinical and Experimental*, 1985, 34(6): 571–73.

THYROID (T3; T4)

Brand Names
U.S.A.: Armour Thyroid (USV), Euthroid (Parke-Davis), Proloid (Parke-Davis), S-P-T (Fleming), Thyrar (USV), Thyrolar (USV), Thyro-Teric (Mallard).
Canada: Proloid (Parke-Davis).
Great Britain: Thyroid tablets (various manufacturers).

What This Drug Does
Thyroid hormone.

How This Drug Affects Body Weight
This hormone is a natural product secreted by the thyroid gland, although some brand names listed above are synthetic

analogs. Thyroid hormone alters the basal metabolism (the amount of energy needed to maintain the body's essential functions such as breathing, temperature, circulation), which affects how the body utilizes oxygen. The effect of taking in additional thyroid hormone may act to increase oxygen consumption and cause increased protein breakdown.

Although weight loss does occur from the use of thyroid hormone, its greater efficacy over other drugs such as anorectics (amphetamine, etc.) comes mostly from the loss of lean tissue, not body fat.

Natural thyroid hormone is composed of two components, T3 (liothyronine) and T4 (levothyroxine). Twenty times as much T4 is present than T3 in the body's natural hormone secretion. T3, however, is 3–5 times more active and works more rapidly than T4. Most of the effect of thyroid hormone comes from T3.

Commercially available thyroid supplements include natural products extracted from beef or pork that approximate the mixture of T3 and T4 found in humans, while synthetic derivatives are available as pure T3, pure T4, and liotrix, a mixture of T3 and T4 (4 to 1).

Government-Approved Uses for This Drug

As a thyroid hormone replacement; to treat certain goiters; to treat thyroid cancer; as a diagnostic aid in detecting certain thyroid abnormalities.

Unofficial Uses

As an aid to weight loss.

When Not To Use This Drug

In overactive thyroid gland; in certain heart disease; in certain adrenal gland insufficiency; if allergic to this drug or to any related drug.

Side Effects From Use of This Drug

Side effects would result from overdosing, since proper dosing should restore the body to its normal level of thyroid hormone. Signs of overdosing include rapid or irregular heartbeat; weight loss; tremors; headache; diarrhea; insomnia; sweating; heat and fever intolerance; anginal pain (chest pain caused by coronary artery spasm); menstrual irregularities.

Effects on Appetite and Body Weight as Disclosed by the Drug's Manufacturer

Changes in appetite; weight loss.

Detailed Effects on Appetite and Body Weight

Weight loss: *Note: The treatment of obese individuals with thyroid hormone tends to cause a preferential loss of lean body mass, as opposed to body fat. One study showed only 20% of the weight lost by use of thyroid hormones attributable to fat loss.*

In a 12-week study of 101 subjects, mostly females who were at least 10 pounds overweight, 48 were given a combination of dextroamphetamine and thyroid, and 53 received dextroamphetamine alone. The dextroamphetamine group lost an average of 10.9 pounds during the study, while the thyroid group averaged a 14.7-pound loss.

In a study of 106 obese subjects, the effect of thyroid hormone was evaluated after an initial weight loss was achieved by diet alone. Average weight lost by diet was 16 pounds during a 6-month period. When thyroid was added to this regimen, an additional 13 pounds on average was lost in 5 months.

A report describes a group of 21 formerly obese subjects who had recently lost an average of 93 pounds in 4 months. They accomplished this through a combination of fasting and a 500-calorie-per-day diet. All were then treated with high doses of thyroid or a placebo in alternating 2-month cycles. This study was designed to test thyroid's effectiveness in controlling weight gain after major weight loss had occurred. Thyroid use resulted in an average additional weight loss of 12 pounds versus an average gain of 32 pounds during the periods of placebo use. Thyroid dosages were higher than those normally used and this could account for the study's better than usual results.

In one pioneer study, 35 obese individuals were observed for weight loss by diet alone and by administration of thyroid extract. While on a 1,000-calorie-per-day diet, average daily weight loss was about a third of a pound daily. Thyroid use, however, caused a loss of from 0.5–0.9 pounds daily, depending on the dose. The author of the study calculated that each grain (60mg.) of thyroid added to the daily dose produced an additional daily weight loss of 17.67 grams (0.04 pounds). It was also estimated that a daily dose of 9 grains of thyroid is necessary to equal the weight-reducing effect of a 1,000-calorie-per-day diet. Weight loss from a low-calorie diet alone is due initially mostly to the removal of water from the body. This is followed by a period in which about 80% of weight loss is attributable to fat loss (the other 20% is still water loss). When thyroid is given, fat loss decreases while water loss increases.

Dosage Levels at Which Effects Occur
Weight loss: Reported to occur from 0.01–15 grains daily.

Remedies
Weight loss: Not applicable.

How Long It Takes Till Reversal of Drug Effects
Weight loss: *Note: Those treated for obesity with thyroid hormone show a tendency to regain lost weight rapidly after withdrawal of the drug.*

In one study cited above, the effects of thyroid hormone persisted for several days after its withdrawal, at which time a slowing of weight loss occurred (provided a low-calorie diet was maintained).

It may take up to 10 days for half the dose of thyroid supplement to be cleared from the blood.

Sources
Asher, W.L., Dietz, R.E. "Effectiveness of weight reduction involving 'Diet Pills.'" *Current Therapeutic Research, Clinical and Experimental*, 1972, 14: 510–24.

Drenick, E.J., Fisler, J.L. "Prevention of recurrent weight gain with large doses of synthetic thyroid hormones." *Current Therapeutic Research, Clinical and Experimental*, 1970, 12: 570–76.

Garrow, J.S. *Treat Obesity Seriously*. Edinburgh: Churchill Livingston, 1981: 198.

Gray, H., Kallenbach, D.E. "Obesity treatment: Results on 212 outpatients." *Journal of the American Dietetic Association*, 1939, 15: 239–45.

Kaplan, N.M., Jose, A. "Thyroid as an adjuvant to amphetamine therapy of obesity. A controlled double-blind study." *American Journal of Medical Science*, 1970, 260: 105–11.

Lyon, D.M., Dunlop, D.M. "The treatment of obesity. A comparison of the effects of diet and of thyroid extract." *Quarterly Journal of Medicine*, 1932, 25: 331–51.

Muscle Relaxant Drugs

CYCLOBENZAPRINE

Brand Names
U.S.A: Flexeril (MSD).
Canada: Flexeril (MSD).
Great Britain: None.

What This Drug Does
  Skeletal muscle relaxant.

How This Drug Affects Body Weight
  Unknown. Acts on the central nervous system to reduce muscle activity.

Government-Approved Uses for This Drug
  To relieve muscle spasm.

Unofficial Uses
  None.

When Not to Use This Drug
  If taking or have taken within the last 14 days any monoamine oxidase inhibitor drug; immediately following myocardial infarction (damage to the heart muscle due to loss of its blood supply); in various heart conditions; in presence of overactive thyroid gland; in children under 15 years of age; if allergic to this drug or to any related drug.

Side Effects From Use of This Drug

Drowsiness; weakness; headache; insomnia; nightmares; numbness or tingling sensations; euphoria; dizziness; fast heartbeat; blurred vision; abdominal pain; upset stomach; constipation; dry mouth; skin rash or itching; difficulty in urinating; decreased or increased libido; impotence; testicular swelling; breast enlargement in males and females; galactorrhea (breast-milk flow).

Effects on Appetite and Body Weight as Disclosed by the Drug's Manufacturer

Unpleasant taste; anorexia; edema; weight gain or loss.

Detailed Effects on Appetite and Body Weight

Detailed manufacturer's disclosure: Although cyclobenzaprine's official literature lists altered taste, loss of appetite, water retention, and body-weight changes as potential side effects, more detailed information from independent sources is unavailable.

Unpleasant taste has occurred in 1–3% of patients taking this drug, while effects on appetite, body weight, and water retention occur in less than 1% of cases.

Dosage Levels at Which Effects Occur

May occur within the usual daily dosage range of 30–60mg.

Remedies

Taste change: Cyclobenzaprine-induced taste disturbance may be countered in several ways. Taking the drug with an adequate fluid intake, chewing sugarless gum or using a mouthwash of water and lemon juice, and practicing good oral hygiene may help restore normal taste sensation.

Water retention: Use of a diuretic may help rid the body of excess water. This should only be attempted under the supervision of a doctor.

Weight gain: Substitution of low-calorie foods, beverages, and snacks for normal dietary intake may aid in reversing some cyclobenzaprine-induced weight gain.

Loss of appetite; weight loss: The maintenance of adequate fluid intake and the avoidance of excessive alcohol use may aid in restoring normal appetite.

How Long It Takes Till Reversal of Drug Effects

Half the dose of cyclobenzaprine is eliminated from the body in 1–3 days, with its duration of action persisting 12–24 hours.

Sources

Olin, B.R. (ed.). *Facts and Comparisons*. St. Louis: Facts and Comparisons, 1988.
Physicians' Desk Reference. Oradell, NJ: Medical Economics, 1988.
USP DI. Rockville, MD: The United States Pharmacopeial Convention, Inc., 1989.

Narcotic Antagonists

NALOXONE

Brand Names
U.S.A.: Narcan (DuPont).
Canada: Narcan (DuPont).
Great Britain: Narcan (DuPont).

What This Drug Does
Blocks the action of opioid narcotics.

How This Drug Affects Body Weight
Naloxone blocks the effects of opium-derived drugs by binding at opioid receptors (cells that have an affinity for that specific drug). Drugs of this chemical family have experimentally blocked insulin secretion from the pancreas in response to intravenous administration of glucose. In this way, naloxone could interfere with insulin's physiologic role in storing glucose as fat.

Naloxone may counter the effects of some endorphins. These natural body substances with morphine-like effects may be related to appetite control.

Binging and purging activity, a characteristic of bulimia, may be regulated by opioid reward or enhanced central nervous system opioid activity. Naloxone is thought to interrupt this process and so have value as a treatment for bulimia.

Government-Approved Uses for This Drug

To partially or completely reverse the depressant effects of opioids and related drugs; to diagnose suspected opioid overdosage.

Unofficial Uses

To improve circulation in certain shock; to reverse alcoholic coma, Alzheimer-type dementia, and schizophrenia.

When Not to Use This Drug

If allergic to this drug or to any related drug.

Side Effects From Use of This Drug

When abrupt reversal of narcotic depression has taken place: Nausea; vomiting; sweating; fast heartbeat; elevated blood pressure; muscle tremors.

Effects on Appetite and Body Weight as Disclosed by the Drug's Manufacturer

None.

Detailed Effects on Appetite and Body Weight

Decreased appetite: Twelve healthy subjects of normal weight were given naloxone and placebo by injection and allowed to eat freely for 4 hours. Two hours after the naloxone dose, there was a significantly lower food intake as compared with a placebo. By 2.5 hours, naloxone had decreased food intake by about 25%.

Six obese female volunteers were given either intravenous naloxone or a placebo in order to compare their effects on appetite. Five of the 6 showed considerably lowered food intake with naloxone, recording a net decrease in caloric consumption of about 25%. Even though they ate less food, subjects given naloxone reported feeling fuller after their meal.

Seven normal subjects were given naloxone by intravenous infusion in a laboratory on two separate days in order to evaluate its effects on food consumption. A 28% average decrease in food intake was recorded. While protein and fat ingestion were significantly suppressed, little effect was seen on carbohydrate intake.

Weight loss: In a trial involving 14 obese subjects (all 88–247% above their ideal body weight) and 9 lean individuals (within 15%

of their ideal body weight) all were given naloxone by injection. There was a significantly decreased food intake in 7 obese subjects given high-dose infusions of naloxone (15mg.). Low doses (2mg.) had little effect on these overweight individuals and no effect on the appetite of lean subjects.

Treatment of anorexia nervosa: A study of 12 hospitalized females suffering from anorexia nervosa detailed their treatment with intravenous naloxone. During an average treatment period of 5 weeks, about a 4-pound-per-week weight gain was recorded.

Treatment of bulimia: In a small-scale study of 5 bulimic females, the amount of calories consumed during binge-eating episodes was compared when the subjects were treated with naloxone and with a placebo. On average, 23% less calories were consumed during naloxone use as compared to placebo.

Dosage Levels at Which Effects Occur

Decreased appetite: Reported as low as 0.8mg. by intravenous infusion. Also effective at 0.5–2mg. per kilogram of body weight by intravenous infusion. In a 200-pound individual, this would translate to a dose range of 45.5–182mg.

Weight loss: Weight loss occurred at the high dose (15mg.) but not at the low dose (2mg.).

Treatment of anorexia nervosa: Reported at 3.2–4.8 mg. daily by intravenous infusion.

Treatment of bulimia: Reported at 6mg. by intravenous infusion over a 2-minute period, administered 5–7 minutes before onset of binge-eating episodes. This is followed by 0.1mg. per minute over 120 minutes (maximum 12mg. in total).

Remedies
Not applicable.

How Long It Takes Till Reversal of Drug Effects
When given by intravenous infusion, half the dose of naloxone is cleared from the blood in 60 minutes.

Sources
Atkinson, R.L. "Decreased food intake after naloxone." *Obesity and Bariatric Medicine*, 1983, 12(3): 76.
Cohen, M.R., et al. "Naloxone reduces food intake in humans." *Psychosomatic Medicine*, 1985, 47: 132–38.

Mitchell, J.E., et al. "Naloxone but not CCK-8 may attenuate binge-eating behavior in patients with the bulimia syndrome." *Biological Psychiatry*, 1986, 21(14): 1399–1406.

Moore, R., et al. "Naloxone in the treatment of anorexia nervosa: Effect on weight gain and lipolysis." *Journal of the Royal Society of Medicine*, 1981, 74: 129–31.

Trenchard, E., Silverstone, T. "Naloxone reduces the food intake of normal human volunteers." *Appetite*, 1983, 4: 43–50.

Wolkowitz, O., et al. "Effect of naloxone on food consumption in obesity." *New England Journal of Medicine*, 1985, 313: 327.

NALTREXONE

Brand Names
U.S.A.: Trexan (DuPont).
Canada: None.
Great Britain: None.

What This Drug Does
Blocks the action of opioid narcotics.

How This Drug Affects Body Weight
Naltrexone blocks the effects of opium-derived drugs by binding at opioid receptors (cells that have an affinity for that specific drug). Drugs of this chemical family have experimentally blocked insulin secretion from the pancreas in response to intravenous administration of glucose. In this way, naltrexone could interfere with insulin's physiologic role in storing glucose as fat.

Naltrexone may counter the effects of some endorphins. These natural body substances with morphine-like effects may be related to appetite control.

Binging and purging activity, a characteristic of bulimia, may be regulated by opioid reward or enhanced central nervous system opioid activity. Naltrexone is thought to interrupt this process and so have value as a treatment for bulimia.

Government-Approved Uses for This Drug
To assist in maintaining an opioid-free state in former addicts.

Unofficial Uses
To treat certain complications arising from concussion; to treat certain eating disorders.

When Not to Use This Drug

If receiving an opioid analgesic; if dependent on an opioid drug; if undergoing acute opioid withdrawal; if determined to be unsuitable for naltrexone therapy by prior screening methods; in certain liver dysfunction; in children under 18 years of age; if allergic to this drug or to any related drug.

Side Effects From Use of This Drug

Insomnia; anxiety; headache; irritability; dizziness; mental depression; drowsiness; confusion; hallucinations; nightmares; nosebleed; increased blood pressure; fast heartbeat; palpitations; abdominal cramps or pain; nausea; vomiting; diarrhea or constipation (reported with equal frequency); gas; hemorrhoids; dry mouth; liver dysfunction; nasal congestion; breathing difficulties; sore throat; cough; joint and muscle pain; difficulties in urinating; skin rash or itching; acne; athlete's foot; cold sores; hair loss; visual disturbances; ringing in the ears; chills; yawning; delayed ejaculation; decreased potency; increased or decreased sexual interest (reported with equal frequency).

Effects on Appetite and Body Weight as Disclosed by the Drug's Manufacturer

Water retention; loss of appetite; increased thirst; weight loss or gain.

Detailed Effects on Appetite and Body Weight

Decreased appetite: A case report describes a 24-year-old male heroin and cocaine addict who, after detoxification, was started on naltrexone. He soon complained of diminished appetite and a loss of 11 pounds over a 3-week period was documented. In light of continued weight loss, naltrexone was discontinued. Appetite returned to normal and when the drug was later reintroduced, this phenomenon promptly returned.

Among 10 subjects given naltrexone in a 3-week study, 6 reported decreased food intake. None of the subjects was a narcotics addict and the appetite effects of the drug was not the principal aim of the study.

A case report describes a patient who was formerly addicted to oxycodone (a form of codeine). The 18-year-old male was started on naltrexone and within 3 weeks lost 6 pounds due to severe appetite loss.

Seventeen obese men were given naltrexone in increasing doses in a 4-day laboratory protocol. Its effect on lunch meal consumption showed an average decrease of 30%. Food intake was lowered on day 2 of naltrexone administration and remained depressed for the duration of the study.

Weight loss: In an 8-week study of 60 obese patients given a placebo and naltrexone, weight loss with the active drug was not significant for the group as a whole. However, when results were broken down by sex, females given naltrexone had an average weight loss of 3.74 pounds as compared with no change for the men.

Treatment of bulimia: In a study of 5 bulimic patients given naltrexone over a 6-week period, significant reduction of binging-purging activity was seen. By the end of the trial, average binging days per week went from 7 to 1.4. Average purging days went from 4.4 to 1.2 weekly. The average duration of binges dropped from 59 minutes to 12 minutes.

Dosage Levels at Which Effects Occur

Decreased appetite: Reported as low as 10mg. daily.
Weight loss: Reported as low as 50mg. daily.
Treatment of bulimia: Reported effective at an average dose of 200mg. daily.

Remedies

Decreased appetite; weight loss: The maintenance of adequate fluid intake and the avoidance of excessive alcohol use may aid in reversing appetite loss.

A decrease in daily dosage could help alleviate naltrexone's effects on appetite and body weight. But this must be carefully balanced against maintaining adequate therapeutic blood levels.

A switch to a different agent in the same therapeutic category could accomplish similar benefits while minimizing undesirable dietary influences. Consult your physician.

Treatment of bulimia: Not applicable.

How Long It Takes Till Reversal of Drug Effect

Naltrexone's major active metabolite (product of biotransformation in the liver) is 50% eliminated from the body in 12.9 hours. The drug's duration of action may persist from 24–72 hours.

Decreased appetite: In one study cited above, appetite was still suppressed for 1 week after withdrawal of naltrexone. In some cases, this effect lingered for up to 6 months.

Sources

Atkinson, R.L., et al. "Effects of long-term therapy with naltrexone on body weight in obesity." *Clinical Pharmacology and Therapeutics*, 1985, 38: 419–22.

Hollister, L.E., et al. "Adverse effects of naltrexone in subjects not dependent on opiates." *Drug and Alcohol Dependence*, 1981, 8: 37–41.

Jonas, J.M., Gold, M.S. "Naltrexone reverses bulimic symptoms." *Lancet*, 1986, 1: 807.

Spiegel, T.A., et al. "Effect of naltrexone on food intake, hunger, and satiety in obese men." *Physiology and Behavior*, 1987, 40(2): 135–41.

Sternbach, H.A., et al. "Anorexic effects of naltrexone in man." *Lancet*, 1982, 1: 388–89.

Tranquilizers/Sleep Aids

ALPRAZOLAM

Brand Names
U.S.A.: Xanax (Upjohn).
Canada: Xanax (Upjohn).
Great Britain: None.

What This Drug Does
Antianxiety agent.

How This Drug Affects Body Weight
Acts on the limbic system (a portion of the midbrain associated with various emotions and feelings) and certain spinal-cord nerves.

Government-Approved Uses for This Drug
To relieve anxiety.

Unofficial Uses
None.

When Not to Use This Drug
If pregnant; if breast-feeding; with narrow-angle glaucoma; if allergic to this or any related drug.

Side Effects From Use of This Drug
Drowsiness; light-headedness; depression; headache; confusion; insomnia; nervousness; fainting; dizziness; dry mouth; constipation or diarrhea (reported with equal frequency); nausea; vomiting; increased salivation; fast heartbeat; palpitations; low

blood pressure; blurred vision; muscle rigidity; tremor; various skin reactions; nasal congestion; changes in libido; menstrual irregularities.

Effects on Appetite and Body Weight as Disclosed by the Drug's Manufacturer
Anorexia; change in appetite; fluid retention; increase or decrease in weight.

Detailed Effects on Appetite and Body Weight
Treatment of bulimia: A 25-year-old female bulimic suffering from daily binging, vomiting, and laxative abuse was treated with a series of drugs, none of which proved satisfactory. Finally alprazolam was tried over a 3-month period. It proved effective in markedly decreasing all symptoms to a frequency of once or twice a month.

Dosage Levels at Which Effects Occur
Treatment of bulimia: Successfully treated at 6mg. daily.

Remedies
Not applicable.

How Long It Takes Till Reversal of Drug Effects
Half the dose of alprazolam is cleared from the body within 12–15 hours.

Source
Opler, L.A., Mickley, D. "Alprazolam in the treatment of bulimia." *Journal of Clinical Psychiatry*, 1986, 47, 49.

DIAZEPAM

Brand Names
U.S.A.: Q-Pam (Quantum), Valium (Roche), Valrelease (Roche).
Canada: Apo-Diazepam (Apotex), E-Pam (ICN), Meval (Medic), Neo-Calme (Neolab), Novodipam (Novopharm), Rival (Riva), Stress-Pam (Sabex), Valium (Roche), Vivol (Horner).
Great Britain: Atensine (Berk), Diazemuls (KabiVitrum), Evacalm (Unimed), Salis (Galen), Tensium (DDSA), Valium (Roche), Valrelease (Roche).

What This Drug Does
Antianxiety agent.

How This Drug Affects Body Weight
Acts on the limbic system (a portion of the midbrain associated with various emotions and feelings) and certain spinal-cord nerves.

Government-Approved Uses for This Drug
To relieve anxiety; to treat symptoms of alcohol withdrawal; as a muscle relaxant; as an anticonvulsant; to relieve anxiety prior to surgery.

Unofficial Uses
To treat tension headache.

When Not to Use This Drug
In children under 6 months old; in acute narrow-angle glaucoma; during the first 3 months of pregnancy; if allergic to this drug or to any related drug.

Side Effects From Use of This Drug
Drowsiness; lack of coordination; mental confusion; constipation; visual disturbances; depression; headache; low blood pressure; liver dysfunction (jaundice); nausea; various skin reactions; slurred speech; muscle tremor; difficulty in urinating; dizziness; anxiety; hallucinations; insomnia; rage; changes in libido.

Effects on Appetite and Body Weight as Disclosed by the Drug's Manufacturer
Anorexia; change in appetite; edema; increase or decrease in body weight.

Detailed Effects on Appetite and Body Weight
Detailed manufacturer's disclosure: Although diazepam's official literature lists loss or change of appetite, water retention, and body-weight changes as potential side effects, more detailed information from independent sources is unavailable.

Many animal studies exist, but their relationship to human responses to diazepam cannot be assumed.

Dosage Levels at Which Effects Occur
May occur within diazepam's normal therapeutic range of 6–40mg. daily.

Remedies

Loss of appetite; weight loss: The maintenance of adequate fluid intake and the avoidance of excessive alcohol use may aid in restoring normal appetite.

Water retention: Possible use of a diuretic may help rid the body of excess water. This should only be attempted under the supervision of a doctor.

Weight gain: Substitution of low-calorie foods, beverages, and snacks for normal dietary intake may aid in reversing some diazepam-induced weight gain.

How Long It Takes Till Reversal of Drug Effects

It takes from 20 to 50 hours for half the dose of diazepam to be eliminated from the body.

Sources

Olin, B.R. (ed.). *Facts and Comparisons*. St. Louis: Facts and Comparisons, 1988.
Physicians' Desk Reference. Oradell, NJ: Medical Economics, 1988.
USP DI. Rockville, MD: The United States Pharmacopeial Convention, Inc., 1989.

FLURAZEPAM

Brand Names

U.S.A.: Dalmane (Roche).
Canada: Dalmane (Roche).
Great Britain: Dalmane (Roche).

What This Drug Does

Hypnotic (sleep aid).

How This Drug Affects Body Weight

Acts on the limbic system (a portion of the midbrain associated with various emotions and feelings) and certain spinal-cord nerves.

Government-Approved Uses for This Drug

To treat insomnia.

Unofficial Uses

None.

When Not to Use This Drug

If pregnant; if breast-feeding; if allergic to this or any related drug.

Side Effects From Use of This Drug

Drowsiness; light-headedness; depression; headache; confusion; sleep disturbance; nervousness; dizziness; dry mouth; constipation or diarrhea (reported with equal frequency); nausea; vomiting; fast heartbeat; visual disturbance; muscle rigidity; tremor; various skin reactions; nasal congestion; changes in libido; menstrual irregularities.

Effects on Appetite and Body Weight as Disclosed by the Drug's Manufacturer

Anorexia; taste alterations.

Detailed Effects on Appetite and Body Weight

Detailed manufacturer's disclosure: Although flurazepam's official literature lists loss of appetite and taste changes as potential side effects, more detailed information from independent sources is unavailable.

Dosage Levels at Which Effects Occur

May occur within the usual daily dosage range of 15–30mg. taken at bedtime.

Remedies

Loss of appetite: The maintenance of adequate fluid intake and the avoidance of excessive alcohol use may aid in restoring normal appetite.

Taste change: Flurazepam-induced taste disturbance may be countered in several ways. Taking the drug with an adequate fluid intake, chewing sugarless gum or using a mouthwash of water and lemon juice, and practicing good oral hygiene may help restore normal taste sensation.

How Long It Takes Till Reversal of Drug Effects

Flurazepam has a duration of action of 7–8 hours. Half the dose is cleared from the blood in 50–100 hours.

Sources

Olin, B.R. (ed.). *Facts and Comparisons*. St. Louis: Facts and Comparisons, 1988.

Physicians' Desk Reference. Oradell, NJ: Medical Economics, 1988.
USP DI. Rockville, MD: The United States Pharmacopeial Convention, Inc.,
1989.

LORAZEPAM

Brand Names
U.S.A: Ativan (Wyeth), Loraz (Quantum).
Canada: Ativan (Wyeth).
Great Britain: Ativan (Wyeth).

What This Drug Does
Antianxiety agent.

How This Drug Affects Body Weight
Acts on the limbic system (a portion of the midbrain associated
with various emotions and feelings) and certain spinal-cord nerves.

Government-Approved Uses for This Drug
To treat anxiety; as an injection to produce sedation and relieve
anxiety prior to surgery.

Unofficial Uses
As an injection to treat status epilepticus (rapid epileptic seizures).

When Not to Use This Drug
In acute narrow-angle glaucoma; in certain states of mental
depression or psychosis; during the first 3 months of pregnancy;
if allergic to this drug or to any related drug.

Side Effects From Use of This Drug
Drowsiness; dizziness; unsteadiness upon standing or walking;
disorientation; mental depression; indigestion; headache; sleeping difficulties; agitation; various skin reactions; blurred vision
or other disturbances of eye function.

Effects on Appetite and Body Weight as Disclosed by the Drug's Manufacturer
Anorexia; change in appetite; edema; increase or decrease in
body weight.

Detailed Effects on Appetite and Body Weight

Detailed manufacturer's disclosure: Although lorazepam's official literature lists loss or change of appetite, water retention, and body-weight changes as potential side effects, more detailed information from independent sources is unavailable.

Dosage Levels at Which Effects Occur

May occur within the usual daily dosage range of 2–6mg.

Remedies

Loss of appetite; weight loss: The maintenance of adequate fluid intake and the avoidance of excessive alcohol use may aid in restoring normal appetite.

Water retention: Use of a diuretic may help rid the body of excess water. This should only be attempted under the supervision of a doctor.

Weight gain: Substitution of low-calorie foods, beverages, and snacks for normal dietary intake may aid in reversing some lorazepam-induced weight gain.

How Long It Takes Till Reversal of Drug Effects

Half the dose of lorazepam is cleared from the blood within 10–18 hours.

Sources

Olin, B.R. (ed.). *Facts and Comparisons*. St. Louis: Facts and Comparisons, 1988.

Physicians' Desk Reference. Oradell, NJ: Medical Economics, 1988.

USP DI. Rockville, MD: The United States Pharmacopeial Convention, Inc., 1989.

NITRAZEPAM

Brand Names

U.S.A.: None.

Canada: Mogadon (Roche).

Great Britain: Mogadon (Roche), Nitrados (Berk), Remnos (DDSA), Somnite (Norgine), Surem (Galen), Unisomnia (Unigreg).

What This Drug Does
Sedative/hypnotic.

How This Drug Affects Body Weight
Acts on the limbic system (a portion of the midbrain associated with various emotions and feelings) and certain spinal-cord nerves.

Government-Approved Uses for This Drug
None. Nitrazepam has been used widely in Europe and Canada for many years as a sedative/hypnotic, and to treat certain seizures in childhood epilepsy.

Unofficial Uses
None.

When Not to Use This Drug
If pregnant; if breast-feeding; with narrow-angle glaucoma; if allergic to this or any related drug.

Side Effects From Use of This Drug
Drowsiness; light-headedness; depression; headache; hangover; mental confusion; insomnia; nightmares; nervousness; fainting; dizziness; dry mouth; constipation or diarrhea (reported with equal frequency); nausea; vomiting; increased salivation; fast heartbeat; palpitations; low blood pressure; blurred vision; muscle rigidity; tremor; various skin reactions; nasal congestion; changes in libido; menstrual irregularities.

Effects on Appetite and Body Weight as Disclosed by the Drug's Manufacturer
Anorexia; change in appetite; water retention; increase or decrease in weight.

Detailed Effects on Appetite and Body Weight
Weight loss: Although drugs of the benzodiazepine class (nitrazepam is one) are most commonly thought to cause weight gain, a study of 25 subjects given nitrazepam nightly for 28 weeks showed significantly greater weight loss than that produced in a group given a placebo. The nitrazepam group, composed of 18 females and 7 males, showed no sex-based difference in weight loss. Of the 25 subjects given nitrazepam, 4 gained weight, 3 showed no change, and 18 lost weight.

Dosage Levels at Which Effects Occur
Weight loss: Reported to occur at a daily dose of 5mg.

Remedies
Weight loss: A decrease in daily dosage could help alleviate nitrazepam's effects on body weight. But this must be carefully balanced against maintaining adequate therapeutic blood levels.

A switch to a different agent in the same therapeutic category could accomplish similar benefits while minimizing undesirable weight change. Consult your physician.

How Long It Takes Till Reversal of Drug Effects
Weight loss: Half the dose of nitrazepam is eliminated from the body in about 30 hours.

Source
Oswald, I., Adam, K. "Benzodiazepines cause small loss of body weight." *British Medical Journal*, 1980, 281(6247): 1039–40.

TEMAZEPAM

Brand Names
U.S.A.: Restoril (Sandoz).
Canada: Restoril (Anca).
Great Britain: Normison (Wyeth).

What This Drug Does
Hypnotic (sleep aid).

How This Drug Affects Body Weight
Acts on the limbic system (a portion of the midbrain associated with various emotions and feelings) and certain spinal-cord nerves.

Government-Approved Uses for This Drug
To treat insomnia.

Unofficial Uses
None.

When Not to Use This Drug
If pregnant; if breast-feeding; if allergic to this or any related drug.

Side Effects From Use of This Drug
Drowsiness; light-headedness; depression; headache; confusion; sleep disturbance; nervousness; dizziness; dry mouth; constipation or diarrhea (reported with equal frequency); nausea; vomiting; fast heartbeat; visual disturbance; muscle rigidity; tremor; various skin reactions; nasal congestion; changes in libido; menstrual irregularities.

Effects on Appetite and Body Weight as Disclosed by the Drug's Manufacturer
Anorexia; taste alterations.

Detailed Effects on Appetite and Body Weight
Detailed manufacturer's disclosure: Although temazepam's official literature lists loss of appetite and taste changes as potential side effects, more detailed information from independent sources is unavailable.

Dosage Levels at Which Effects Occur
May occur within the usual daily dosage range of 15–30mg. taken at bedtime.

Remedies
Loss of appetite: The maintenance of adequate fluid intake and the avoidance of excessive alcohol use may aid in restoring normal appetite.
Taste change: Temazepam-induced taste disturbance may be countered in several ways. Taking the drug with an adequate fluid intake, chewing sugarless gum or using a mouthwash of water and lemon juice, and practicing good oral hygiene may help restore normal taste sensation.

How Long It Takes Till Reversal of Drug Effects
Half the dose of temazepam is cleared from the blood in 10–17 hours.

Sources
Olin, B.R. (ed.). *Facts and Comparisons*. St. Louis: Facts and Comparisons, 1988.
Physicians' Desk Reference. Oradell, NJ: Medical Economics, 1988.
USP DI. Rockville, MD: The United States Pharmacopeial Convention, Inc., 1989.

TRIAZOLAM

Brand Names
U.S.A.: Halcion (Upjohn).
Canada: Halcion (Upjohn).
Great Britain: Halcion (Upjohn).

What This Drug Does
Hypnotic (sleep aid).

How This Drug Affects Body Weight
Acts on the limbic system (a portion of the midbrain associated with various emotions and feelings) and certain spinal-cord nerves.

Government-Approved Uses for This Drug
To treat insomnia.

Unofficial Uses
None.

When Not to Use This Drug
If pregnant; if breast-feeding; if allergic to this or any related drug.

Side Effects From Use of This Drug
Drowsiness; light-headedness; depression; headache; confusion; sleep disturbance; nervousness; dizziness; dry mouth; constipation or diarrhea (reported with equal frequency); nausea; vomiting; fast heartbeat; visual disturbance; muscle rigidity; tremor; various skin reactions; nasal congestion; changes in libido; menstrual irregularities.

Effects on Appetite and Body Weight as Disclosed by the Drug's Manufacturer
Anorexia; taste alterations.

Detailed Effects on Appetite and Body Weight
Detailed manufacturer's disclosure: Although triazolam's official literature lists loss of appetite and taste changes as potential side effects, more detailed information from independent sources is unavailable.

Dosage Levels at Which Effects Occur

May occur within the usual daily dosage range of 0.25–0.5mg. taken at bedtime.

Remedies

Loss of appetite: The maintenance of adequate fluid intake and the avoidance of excessive alcohol use may aid in restoring normal appetite.

Taste change: Triazolam-induced taste disturbance may be countered in several ways. Taking the drug with an adequate fluid intake, chewing sugarless gum or using a mouthwash of water and lemon juice, and practicing good oral hygiene may help restore normal taste sensation.

How Long It Takes Till Reversal of Drug Effects

Half the dose of triazolam is cleared from the blood within 1.5–5.4 hours.

Source

Olin, B.R. (ed.). *Facts and Comparisons*. St. Louis: Facts and Comparisons, 1988.

Physicians' Desk Reference. Oradell, NJ: Medical Economics, 1988.

USP DI. Rockville, MD: The United States Pharmacopeial Convention, Inc., 1989.

Vitamins/Nutritionals

ARGININE

Brand Names
U.S.A.: *†Alpha Plus (Tyson), *†Aminolete (Tyson), *†Amino-plex (Tyson), *†Aminostasis (Tyson), *†Aminotate (Tyson), ‡R-Gene 10 (KabiVitrum).
Canada: None.
Great Britain: Arginine-Sorbitol (EGIC; Servier; was produced under this brand name by these two companies but has since been withdrawn from the market).

What This Drug Does
Arginine is an amino acid used as a diagnostic aid.

How This Drug Affects Body Weight
Arginine stimulates human growth hormone production by the pituitary gland. When given by intravenous infusion, it may promote a rise in the plasma level of human growth hormone, a substance associated with decreased fat storage.

Government-Approved Uses for This Drug
As an aid in diagnosing various abnormalities of the pituitary gland.

*Combination drug.
†Denotes over-the-counter availability in the U.S.A.
‡Denotes prescription-only status in the U.S.A.

Unofficial Uses
None.

When Not to Use This Drug
If allergic to this substance or to any related substance.

Side Effects From Use of This Drug
Nausea; vomiting; headache; flushing; numbness; skin rash; decreased blood platelet count.

Effects on Appetite and Body Weight as Disclosed by the Drug's Manufacturer
None.

Detailed Effects on Appetite and Body Weight
Weight loss: Arginine may promote the secretion of human growth hormone. Levels of these secretions in the body usually decrease after age 30. This may result in increased fat accumulation. Arginine, by stimulating growth hormone secretions, may decrease fat storage, resulting in leaner body mass.

Five normal, healthy male volunteers, all within 10% of their ideal body weight, were given an intravenous infusion of arginine after an overnight fast. All subjects experienced a significant rise in growth hormone release, with its peak reached 45–60 minutes after receiving the drug.

Taking a skeptical view of arginine's value as a weight-loss aid, one medical writer looked upon its use in endocrinologic testing as a tenuous link to the highly exaggerated claims made of this amino acid by various promoters. One huckster, referring to arginine as "Growth Factor," advertised the product as follows: "Growth Factor has been discovered to have the remarkable ability to speed wound healing, increase the body's ability to ward off disease, increase muscle tone, and help rid the body of excess fat. As you grow older, the normal flow of Growth Factor keeps slowing down. This may be the reason that a youthful body is slim and trim, but grows flabby with age."

While it is often difficult to know when an advertised weight-loss product actually contains arginine, the tip-off is the mention of growth hormone. Many of these products use the misleading come-on of "losing weight while you sleep."

Dosage Levels at Which Effects Occur
Weight loss: Most arginine-containing products that are pro-

moted for weight loss are sold as tablets, with a suggested oral daily dose of 700 mg. However 20–30 grams (25,000–30,000mg.) given as an intravenous infusion is actually necessary to achieve any human growth hormone release from the pituitary gland.

Remedies
Not applicable.

How Long It Takes Till Reversal of Drug Effects
Unknown.

Sources

Bratusch-Marrain, P., Waldhäusl, W. "The influences of amino acids and somatostatin on prolactin and growth hormone release in man." *Acta Endocrinologica* (Copenhagen), 1979, 90:403–8.

Ghadimi, H. "Amino acids and obesity." *Pediatric Annals*, 1984, 13(7): 557–63.

Uretsky, S.D. "A pharmacists' guide to quack weight products." *American Pharmacy*, 1985, NS25(2): 24–29.

EVENING PRIMROSE OIL

Brand Names
U.S.A.: †Efamol (Murdock), Evening Primrose Oil (marketed by various manufacturers).
Canada: Efamol (Efamol).
Great Britain: Efamol (Agricultural Holdings), Evening Primrose Oil Capsules (Evening Primrose Oil Co.), Naudicelle (Bio-Oil Research).

What This Drug Does
Source of unsaturated fatty acids.

How This Drug Affects Body Weight
Evening primrose oil is an extremely rich source of unsaturated fatty acids. Fatty acids aid in fat transport and metabolism. Since these substances form prostaglandins (which help organ muscles contract, regulate stomach acid, lower blood pressure, and regulate body temperature), evening primrose oil may help increase their synthesis.

---

†Denotes over-the-counter availability in the U.S.A.

Government-Approved Uses for This Drug
None.

Unofficial Uses
To reduce serum cholesterol levels; to treat rheumatoid arthritis; to treat multiple sclerosis.

When Not to Use This Drug
If allergic to this drug or to any related drug.

Side Effects From Use of This Drug
None.

Effects on Appetite and Body Weight as Disclosed by the Drug's Manufacturer
None.

Detailed Effects on Appetite and Body Weight
Weight loss: In a group of 38 subjects of normal weight and given evening primrose oil for 6–8 weeks, significant weight loss occurred in some; 22 of the subjects within 10% of their ideal body weight showed no gain or loss greater than 4.4 pounds. Of the other 16, all more than 10% over their ideal weight, 5 showed no change while 11 lost an average of 9 pounds. Four subjects who took double the normal daily dose (4.8ml.) showed the highest weight loss (18–28 pounds).

Dosage Levels at Which Effects Occur
Weight loss: Reported to occur within a range of 2.4–4.8ml. daily.

Remedies
Weight loss: Not applicable.

How Long It Takes Till Reversal of Drug Effects
Unknown.

Sources
Douglas, J.G., Munro, J.F. "Drug treatment and obesity." *Pharmacology and Therapeutics*, 1982, 18: 351.
Vaddadi, K.S., Horrobin, D.F. "Weight loss produced by Evening Primrose Oil administration in normal and schizophrenic individuals." *I.R.C.S. Journal of Medical Science*, 1979, 7: 52.

GLYCINE

Brand Names
U.S.A.: *†Alka-2 (Miles) *†Aminolete (Tyson), *†Aminomine (Tyson), *†Aminoplex (Tyson), *†Aminosine (Tyson), *†Aminostasis (Tyson), *†Aminotate (Tyson), *†Calcilac (Schein), *†Calglycine (Rugby), *†Equilet (Mission), *†Genalac (Goldline), *†Glycate (Forest), *†Pama No. 1 (Vortech), *†Titracid (Trimen), *†Titralac (3M).
Canada: None.
Great Britain: *Paynocil (Beecham Research), *Titralac (Riker).

What This Drug Does
Amino acid.

How This Drug Works
Glycine, the simplest of all the amino acids, when given by intravenous infusion may promote a rise in the plasma level of human growth hormone. Human growth hormone is a substance associated with decreased fat storage in the body.

Government-Approved Uses for This Drug
In combination with calcium carbonate and other antacids to treat gastric hyperacidity; as an ingredient in some aspirin tablets to relieve gastric irritation; as a sterile solution of 15% glycine in water for bladder irrigation during genitourinary surgery.

Unofficial Uses
None.

When Not to Use This Drug
If allergic to this substance or to any related substance.

Side Effects From Use of This Drug
None.

Effects on Appetite and Body Weight as Disclosed by the Drug's Manufacturer
None.

*Combination drug.
†Denotes over-the-counter availability in the U.S.A.

Detailed Effects on Appetite and Body Weight

Growth hormone release: Glycine may promote the secretion of human growth hormone. Levels of these secretions in the body usually decrease after age 30. This may result in increased fat accumulation. Glycine, by stimulating growth hormone secretions, may decrease fat storage, resulting in leaner body mass.

In a Japanese study of 25 normal-weight subjects (13 males and 12 females), all were given an intravenous infusion of glycine in the morning after fasting overnight. Blood levels of growth hormone were measured before and after the dose. At doses of 4 and 8 grams of glycine, a significant increase in growth hormone release was recorded. At 12 grams, an even greater release took place.

Dosage Levels at Which Effects Occur

Growth hormone release: Occurred at doses of 4, 8, and 12 grams of glycine in normal saline solution administered by intravenous infusion over 15-30 minutes.

Remedies

Growth hormone release: Not applicable.

How Long It Takes Till Reversal of Drug Effects

Half the dose of glycine is cleared from the blood in 240 hours.

Source

Kasai, K., et al. "Glycine stimulates growth hormone release in man." *Acta Endocrinologica* (Copenhagen), 1980, 93(3): 283–86.

L-HISTIDINE

Brand Names

U.S.A.: *†Aminolete (Tyson), *†Aminomine (Tyson), *†Aminoplex (Tyson), *†Aminosine (Tyson), *†Aminostasis (Tyson), *†Aminotate (Tyson). Also marketed as "L-histadine" by various manufacturers.
Canada: None.

*Combination drug.
†Denotes over-the-counter availability in the U.S.A.

Great Britain: Histacaps (Geistlich; no longer marketed).

What This Drug Does
Essential amino acid (in infants and growing children).

How This Drug Affects Body Weight
L-histidine has been observed to increase urinary excretion of zinc, resulting in lowered levels of this metal in the body. Mild zinc deficiency has been shown to cause loss of appetite.

Government-Approved Uses for This Drug
As a dietary supplement.

Unofficial Uses
To investigate folic acid deficiency.

When Not to Use This Drug
If allergic to this drug or to any related drug.

Side Effects From Use of This Drug
None.

Effects on Appetite and Body Weight as Disclosed by the Drug's Manufacturer
None.

Detailed Effects on Appetite and Body Weight
Decreased appetite; weight loss; altered taste: Twenty-one subjects who were 20% above their ideal body weight were enrolled in a 9-week study to test the effects of L-histidine. Eleven were given active drug and 10 were given maltose, a sugar. The dosage regimen of L-histidine was 8 grams daily for 3 weeks; 16 grams daily for 3 weeks; and 24 grams daily for 2 weeks. Average weight loss using L-histidine was almost 6 pounds. Six of the 11 patients on active medication reported a loss of appetite when taking 16 grams or more of L-histidine daily. The study's author felt that potential side effects outweighed benefits of L-histidine use. One subject had a psychotic episode lasting 12 hours and other researchers have reported altered sense of taste and smell.

In a study of 8 adult males of normal weight, L-histidine given in lower daily doses than described above showed no effect on appetite, taste, smell, or body weight.

Six patients treated with L-histidine for progressive systemic sclerosis (a degenerative disease affecting many body systems) all developed loss of appetite, as well as taste and smell dysfunction. Length of drug administration ranged from 2–12 days. Researchers involved in this study speculated that an L-histidine–induced drop in zinc blood levels was at fault. The first and most severe symptom was bitter taste perception, with ability to taste sweets the least affected.

In a study of 8 patients, the effects of L-histidine were analyzed during short-term administration. A 32-gram dose resulted in a 5- to 80-fold increase in the taste thresholds of salt, sucrose, hydrochloric acid, and urea. Loss of appetite was also reported by all participants.

Dosage Levels at Which Effects Occur
Decreased appetite; weight loss; altered taste: Reported as low as 8 grams daily.

Remedies
Decreased appetite; altered taste: In one study cited above, administration of zinc sulfate, 110mg. by mouth given 4 times daily, reversed loss of taste and appetite, whether or not L-histidine was continued.

How Long It Takes Till Reversal of Drug Effects
Decreased appetite; altered taste: In one case described above, use of zinc returned taste to normal within 8 hours.

In another instance, zinc use restored normal taste sense and appetite within 24–48 hours.

Sources
Haymes, D.A. "Psychosis during use of L-histidine as an anorectic agent." *Obesity and Bariatric Medicine*, 1983, 12(4): 88–89.

Henkin, R.I., et al. "Histidine-dependent zinc loss, hypogeusia, anorexia, and hyposmia." *Journal of Clinical Investigation*, 1972, 51(suppl.): 44a.

Henkin, R.I., et al. "A syndrome of acute zinc loss: Cerebellar dysfunction, mental changes, anorexia, and taste and smell dysfunction." *Archives of Neurology*, 1975, 32: 745–51.

Schechter, P.J., Prakash, N.J. "L-histidine and anorexia." *Obesity and Bariatric Medicine*, 1979, 8(6): 198.

NICOTINIC ACID

Brand Names
U.S.A.: †Niac (Forest), †Niacels (Hauck), †Nico-400 (Jones Medical), †Nicobid (Armour), ‡Nicolar (Armour), †Nicotinex (Fleming), ‡Span-Niacin-150 (Scrip).
Canada: Novoniacin (Novopharm).
Great Britain: Marketed as "nicotinic acid" by various manufacturers. *Chilblain Treatment Dellipsoids D 27 (Pilsworth), *Pernivit (Duncan, Flockhart).

What This Drug Does
Vitamin.

How This Drug Affects Body Weight
Unknown. Also known as vitamin B_3, nicotinic acid produces peripheral vasodilation, causing blood to suffuse the face, neck, and chest. In large doses, it also lowers cholesterol and triglyceride blood levels.

Government-Approved Uses for This Drug
To correct niacin deficiency; to treat or prevent pellagra; to treat high blood lipid levels.

Unofficial Uses
To treat schizophrenia.
Caution: Megadoses of nicotinic acid used in "orthomolecular psychiatry" to treat schizophrenia may be associated with various toxicities including liver damage, peptic ulcer, heart irregularities, and gastrointestinal upset.

When Not to Use This Drug
In liver dysfunction; in active peptic ulcer; with severe low blood pressure; in certain bleeding; if allergic to this substance or to any related substance.

---

†Denotes over-the-counter availability in the U.S.A.
‡Denotes prescription-only status in the U.S.A.
*Combination drug.

Side Effects From Use of This Drug
Activation of peptic ulcer; liver dysfunction (jaundice); nausea; vomiting; abdominal pain; diarrhea; flushing; itching; various skin reactions; visual disturbance; low blood pressure; transient headache; high blood uric acid levels.

Effects on Appetite and Body Weight as Disclosed by the Drug's Manufacturer
None.

Detailed Effects on Appetite and Body Weight
Weight loss: In a study of 63 obese patients treated at a hospital nutrition clinic, results of nonmedicated individuals were compared to those on various drugs, nicotinic acid among them. While the group as a whole lost an average of 2.45 pounds per month by diet alone, those taking nicotinic acid achieved a greater rate of loss, although the exact amount is not given in the report.

Dosage Levels at Which Effects Occur
Weight loss: May occur within the usual dosage range of 10–20mg. daily.

Remedies
Weight loss: Not applicable.

How Long It Takes Till Reversal of Drug Effects
Half the dose of nicotinic acid is eliminated from the blood in about 45 minutes.

Source
Stein, P.M., et al. "Predicting weight loss success among obese clients at a hospital nutrition clinic." *American Journal of Clinical Nutrition*, 1981, 34(10): 2039–44.

PHENYLALANINE

Brand Names
U.S.A.: *†Aminolete (Tyson), *†Aminomine (Tyson), *†Amino-

---

*Combination drug.
†Denotes over-the-counter availability in the U.S.A.

plex (Tyson), *†Aminosine (Tyson), *†Aminostasis (Tyson), *†Aminotate (Tyson), *†Endorphan (Tyson), †Endorphenyl (Tyson), *†Saave (Matrix Technologies).
Canada: None.
Great Britain: None.

What This Drug Does
Amino acid.

How This Drug Works
Phenylalanine, when given by intravenous infusion, may promote a rise in the plasma level of human growth hormone. Human growth hormone is a substance associated with decreased fat storage in the body.

Government-Approved Uses for This Drug
As a dietary supplement.

Unofficial Uses
To treat depression; to treat some symptoms of Parkinson's disease.

When Not to Use This Drug
In phenylketonuria (a birth defect that prevents the body from utilizing phenylalanine); if allergic to this substance or to any related substance.

Side Effects From Use of This Drug
Headache; vertigo.

Effects on Appetite and Body Weight as Disclosed by the Drug's Manufacturer
None.

Detailed Effects on Appetite and Body Weight
Growth hormone release: Phenylalanine may promote the secretion of human growth hormone. Levels of these secretions in the body usually decrease after age 30. This may result in increased fat accumulation. Phenylalanine, by stimulating growth

*Combination drug.
†Denotes over-the-counter availability in the U.S.A.

hormone secretions, may decrease fat storage, resulting in leaner body mass.

Five normal, healthy male volunteers all within 10% of their ideal body weight were given an intravenous infusion of phenylalanine the morning after an overnight fast. All subjects experienced a significant rise in growth hormone release.

In another study of 6 healthy young adults given intravenous phenylalanine, the amino acid consistently induced increased levels of growth hormone release.

Dosage Levels at Which Effects Occur
Growth hormone release: Occurred at a dose of 20–30 grams by intravenous infusion over 30 minutes.

Remedies
Growth hormone release: Not applicable.

How Long It Takes Till Reversal of Drug Effects
Unknown.

Sources
Bratusch-Marrain, P., Waldhäusl, W. "The influences of amino acids and somatostatin on prolactin and growth hormone release in man." *Acta Endocrinologica* (Copenhagen), 1979, 90: 403–8.

Knopf, R.F., et al. "Plasma growth hormone response to intravenous administration of amino acids." *Journal of Clinical Endocrinology and Metabolism*, 1965, 25, 1140–44.

PYRIDOXINE (VITAMIN B₆)

Brand Names
U.S.A.: ‡Beesix (Forest), ‡Hexa-Betalin (Lilly), †Nestrex (Fielding), ‡Pyroxine (Kay).
Canada: Hexa-Betalin (Lilly).
Great Britain: Benadon (Roche), Compliment (Napp).

What This Drug Does
Vitamin.

‡Denotes prescription-only status in the U.S.A.
†Denotes over-the-counter availability in the U.S.A.

How This Drug Affects Body Weight

Increased pyridoxine levels may result in higher serotonin levels. Serotonin, a chemical messenger in the body, is thought to be an appetite suppressant.

Government-Approved Uses for This Drug

To treat pyridoxine deficiency.

Unofficial Uses

To treat hydrazine poisoning; to treat premenstrual syndrome (PMS); to treat high levels of oxylate in the urine and oxylate kidney stones.

When Not to Use This Drug

If allergic to this vitamin or to any related substance.

Side Effects From Use of This Drug

Numbness and tingling sensations; decreased sensation of touch, temperature, and vibration; drowsiness; unstable gait; reduced blood levels of folic acid.

Effects on Appetite and Body Weight as Disclosed by the Drug's Manufacturer

None.

Detailed Effects on Appetite and Body Weight

Weight loss: Vitamin B_6 has been included in many weight control programs, even though evidence of its efficacy is lacking. It is given based on the theory that increased pyridoxine levels result in elevated serotonin concentrations. Serotonin is thought to act as a natural appetite suppressant.

Dosage Levels at Which Effects Occur

Weight loss: Pyridoxine has been included in various weight control programs at a dosage of 1,000–7,500% of RDA (recommended daily allowance). Since the RDA for B_6 is 2mg., this translates to a range of 20–150mg. daily.

Caution: Daily doses of 500–2,000mg. have resulted in possibly irreversible nerve damage to the hands and feet. This may continue even after the withdrawal of the vitamin.

Remedies

Weight loss: Not applicable.

How Long It Takes Till Reversal of Drug Effects
It may take as long as 15–20 days for half the dose of pyridoxine to be cleared from the blood.

Sources
Covington, T.R. "Vitamins: Part I—Common myths." *Facts and Comparisons Drug Newsletter*, 1987, 6(7): 54–55.
"Vitamin B$_6$ therapy in PMS [letter]." *Pharmacy Times*, 1988, 54(5): 120.

L-TRYPTOPHAN

Brand Names
U.S.A.: *†Aminolete (Tyson), *†Aminomine (Tyson), *†Aminoplex (Tyson), *†Aminosine (Tyson), *†Aminostasis (Tyson), *†Aminotate (Tyson), †L-Tryptophane (Rugby), †Trofan (Upsher-Smith), †Tryptacin (Arther Inc.).
Canada: None.
Great Britain: Optimax (E. Merck), Pacitron (Berk).

What This Drug Does
Amino acid.

How This Drug Affects Body Weight
L-tryptophan is a precursor of the neurotransmitter (chemical messenger) serotonin. Serotonin may inhibit eating behavior, and some reports claim loss of appetite to be accompanied by low blood levels of L-tryptophan. It may also selectively decrease craving for carbohydrate foods while leaving protein consumption unimpaired.

Government-Approved Uses for This Drug
For oral amino acid therapy.

Unofficial Uses
As a sleeping aid; as an antidepressant.

*Combination drug.
†Denotes over-the-counter availability in the U.S.A.

When Not to Use This Drug

If taking or have taken within the last 14 days any monoamine oxidase inhibitor drug; if allergic to this drug or to any related drug.

Side Effects From Use of This Drug

None.

Effects on Appetite and Body Weight as Disclosed by the Drug's Manufacturer

None.

Detailed Effects on Appetite and Body Weight

Decreased appetite: Three of 8 obese subjects given L-tryptophan showed a significant decrease in preference for carbohydrate foods. As part of the syndrome of obesity, many of these individuals report intense, frequent cravings for carbohydrate-rich foods.

In a study of 16 healthy males given L-tryptophan, selective appetite suppression was achieved. Total carbohydrate intake was markedly decreased, whereas protein intake was much less affected.

In a 5-day trial involving 11 volunteers, administration of L-tryptophan decreased carbohydrate consumption in 18% of participants by 50% or more, and by 10–50% in 27% of subjects.

In a series of studies involving 32 males, all within 10% of their ideal body weight, total food consumption was decreased 18–20% by administration of L-tryptophan in doses above 2 grams daily. Much of this reduction came at the expense of carbohydrate foods.

In a study of 16 males given L-tryptophan before eating a meal, a 10% decrease in total caloric consumption was seen at the highest dose (2 grams daily).

Treatment of anorexia nervosa: A case report details the treatment of an emaciated, depressed female with a combination of L-tryptophan and clomipramine (an antidepressant). Her weight was reported to have increased from about 66 pounds to 198 pounds in 7 months. Although dosage information for L-tryptophan was not given, the author suggests that priming the patient with L-tryptophan is advisable before initiating the use of antidepressants.

Treatment of bulimia: A 21-year-old female bulimic with a 5-

year history of nightly binging followed by self-induced vomiting was given L-tryptophan for 6 weeks. Within 1 week there was a marked decrease in the bingeing urge. Within 2 weeks binge frequency decreased to twice weekly with less food (20% the caloric intake) consumed per episode. During the last 3 weeks of the study, binging ceased entirely. Withdrawal of L-tryptophan resulted in a rapid reemergence of bulimic behavior. When the patient was restarted on L-tryptophan, binging activity was again suppressed.

Dosage Levels at Which Effects Occur
Decreased appetite: Reported as low as 2 grams daily.
Treatment of anorexia nervosa: May be effective within the usual daily dosage range of 500mg.–2 grams.
Treatment of bulimia: Reported effective at 1 gram daily.

Remedies
Decreased appetite: Not applicable.
Treatment of anorexia nervosa; treatment of bulimia: Not applicable.

How Long It Takes Till Reversal of Drug Effects
Half the dose of L-tryptophan is cleared from the blood in about 16 hours.

Sources
Cole, W., Lapierre, Y.D. "The use of tryptophan in normal-weight bulimia." *Canadian Journal of Psychiatry*, 1986, 31(8): 755–56.

Hrboticky, N., et al. "Effects of l-tryptophan on short-term food intake in lean men." *Nutrition Research*, 1985, 5: 595–607.

Katz, J.L., Walsh, B.T. "Depression in anorexia nervosa." *American Journal of Psychiatry*, 1978, 135: 507.

Silverstone, T., Goodall, E. "The clinical pharmacology of appetite suppressant drugs." *International Journal of Obesity*, 1984, 8(suppl. 1): 23–33.

Silverstone, T., Goodall, E. "Serotonergic mechanisms in human feedings: The pharmacological evidence." *Appetite*, 1986, 7(suppl.): 85–97.

Wurtman, J.J., et al. "Carbohydrate craving in obese people: Suppression by treatments affecting serotonergic transmission." *International Journal of Eating Disorders*, 1981, 1: 2–15.

Wurtman, J.J., Wurtman, R.J. "Suppression of carbohydrate consumption as snacks and at mealtime by dl-fenfluramine or tryptophan." In S. Garattani and R. Samanin, eds., *Anorectic Agents: Mechanisms of Action and Tolerance*. New York: Raven Press, 1981.

VITAMIN A

Brand Names
U.S.A.: †Aquasol A (Armour), ‡Del-Vi-A (Del-Ray).
Canada: Aquasol A (USV).
Great Britain: Ro-A-Vit (Roche).

What This Drug Does
Vitamin.

How This Drug Affects Body Weight
Unknown. Vitamin A is essential to new cell growth and healthy tissue. It is also needed to maintain normal vision in dim light.

Government-Approved Uses for This Drug
To treat vitamin A deficiency.

Unofficial Uses
None.

When Not to Use This Drug
If one has taken in abnormally large amounts of vitamin A; when taken orally to treat malabsorption syndrome; by intravenous injection; if allergic to this substance or to any related substance.

Side Effects From Use of This Drug
Adverse reactions from vitamin A use stem from chronic overuse and overdosing. Among these are: fatigue; malaise; night sweating; abdominal discomfort; vomiting; slowed growth; joint and bone pain; irritability; headache; vertigo; drying and cracking of the skin; lip fissures; hair loss; various skin reactions; inflammation of the tongue, lips, and gums; inhibited menstruation; enlarged liver and spleen; jaundice; excessive thirst; excessive urination; high blood calcium levels.

†Denotes over-the-counter availability in the U.S.A.
‡Denotes prescription-only status in the U.S.A.

Effects on Appetite and Body Weight as Disclosed by the Drug's Manufacturer

Adverse reactions from vitamin A use stem from chronic over-use and overdosing. Among these are: anorexia; water retention in the lower extremities.

Detailed Effects on Appetite and Body Weight

Loss of appetite; weight loss: A case report describes a 25-year-old Mexican man who took megadoses of vitamin A for about 2 months. He ingested this in the form of vitamin A capsules, as well as multivitamins containing additional vitamin A. When finally seen by a physician, a 10-pound weight loss was noted and, among other symptoms, loss of appetite was evident. The patient responded rapidly to withdrawal of vitamin A.

A 52-year-old woman is described by her physician as taking daily doses of vitamin A that were about 25 times the recommended daily requirement (RDA). Over a period of 4 years, vitamin A abuse resulted in a loss of over 30 pounds, as well as myriad other symptoms including loss of appetite. Withdrawal of vitamin A resulted in progressive improvement of her symptoms until almost all were reversed.

Dosage Levels at Which Effects Occur

Loss of appetite; weight loss: In one report cited above, this occurred within a daily dosage range of 200,000–275,000 I.U. (international units) over a period of 2 months. In the other case, a daily dosage of 100,000 I.U. for 4 years was taken.

Remedies

Loss of appetite; weight loss: A decrease in daily dosage could help alleviate vitamin A's effects on appetite and body weight. But this must be carefully balanced against maintaining adequate therapeutic blood levels.

How Long It Takes Till Reversal of Drug Effects

Loss of appetite; weight loss: In one case, appetite and body weight returned to normal within 2 months after withdrawal of vitamin A; in the other report, this took 6 months.

Sources

Bifulco, E. "Vitamin A intoxication: Report of a case in an adult." *New England Journal of Medicine*, 1953, 248: 690–92.

Shaw, E.W., Niccol, J.Z. "Hypervitaminosis A: Report of a case in an adult male." *Annals of Internal Medicine*, 1953, 39: 131–34.

ZINC

Brand Names
U.S.A.: †Medizinc (U.S. Chemical), †Orazinc (Mericon), †Scrip Zinc (Scrip), †Verazinc (Forest), †Zinc 15 (Mericon), †Zinc-220 (Alto), †Zincaps-220 (Ortega), ‡Zincate (Paddock), †ZNG (Western Research), *†Z-Pro-C (Person & Covey).
Canada: Egozinc (Pharmascience).
Great Britain: Zincomed (Medo Chem).

What This Drug Does
Mineral supplement.

How This Drug Affects Body Weight
Zinc plays a role in the synthesis of nucleic acids and proteins. It may be needed to prevent the rapid degradation of RNA (ribonucleic acid). Zinc deficiency has been linked to alterations in taste, and nutritional supplementation with this element has been successful in treating this condition.

Government-Approved Uses for This Drug
As a dietary supplement; to treat zinc deficiency.

Unofficial Uses
To treat acrodermatitis enteropathica (an inherited disorder of the skin and bowels); to treat delayed wound-healing associated with zinc deficiency; to treat rheumatoid arthritis; to delay onset of genetically linked dementia (deterioration of mental function); to improve the immune response in older persons; to treat Wilson's disease (a liver disease causing abnormal copper metabolism).

When Not to Use This Drug
If allergic to this substance or to any related substance.

† Denotes over-the-counter availability in the U.S.A.
‡ Denotes prescription-only status in the U.S.A.
*Combination drug.

Side Effects From Use of This Drug
Nausea; vomiting; gastric upset, irritation, or ulceration.

Effects on Appetite and Body Weight as Disclosed by the Drug's Manufacturer
None.

Detailed Effects on Appetite and Body Weight
Treatment of altered taste: Several researchers have reported a possible link between zinc levels in the body and taste sensation. They suggest that taste acuity may be an indicator of the functional availability of this element. In patients suffering from anorexia nervosa, a condition that has been shown to deplete zinc levels in the body, most report impaired ability to distinguish bitter and sour foods. Salt sensation was less often affected and sweet taste was the least disturbed of all.

In a study of 103 patients complaining of decreased taste acuity, their average blood zinc concentration was 23% lower than in a normal control group. Oral zinc supplements were given in a low- and high-dose regimen. The low-dose subjects reported slight improvement, while 50% of those receiving high-dose zinc reported a return to normal taste sensation.

Treatment of anorexia nervosa: A report of a 24-year-old female diagnosed as suffering from anorexia nervosa reveals that, after 8 months of unsuccessful treatment, oral zinc sulfate was added to the diet. This resulted in a gradual weight gain in which the patient went from 94.6 pounds to 120 pounds in 1 year.

Another report describes a 13-year-old girl with anorexia nervosa whose weight had dropped to 69.3 pounds. A zinc supplement was begun and after 4 months her weight increased 28.6 pounds to 98 pounds. When zinc was withdrawn after 10 months, her weight began to fall and only when zinc was reintroduced did she regain the lost weight.

Treatment of anorexia, poor growth, and altered taste in children: In a study of 388 subjects, most of whom were children, 10 children who were 4 years old or more had low zinc levels as measured by its concentration in the hair. Seven of these 10 children had a history of poor appetite and were in the lowest 10% height category for their age group. In 6 of these children tested for taste acuity, 5 showed some loss of taste sensation.

When zinc was added to their diet, all subjects regained normal taste sensation and their hair zinc levels increased.

Dosage Levels at Which Effects Occur

Treatment of altered taste: Taste changes result from zinc deficiency. An oral zinc supplement of 100mg. daily successfully restored normal taste in 50% of cases according to one report.

Treatment of anorexia nervosa: Reported effective within a daily dosage range of 45–150mg. zinc sulfate.

Treatment of anorexia, poor growth, and altered taste in children: Reported effective at 1–2mg. zinc sulfate per kilogram of body weight per 24 hours. In the study cited above, this regimen was given for 1–3 months.

Remedies

Not applicable.

How Long It Takes Till Reversal of Drug Effects

Not applicable.

Sources

Bryce-Smith, D., Simpson, R.I. "Case of anorexia nervosa responding to zinc sulfate." *Lancet*, 1984, 2(8398): 350.

Casper, R.C., et al. "An evaluation of trace metals, vitamins, and taste function in anorexia nervosa." *Annals of Clinical Nutrition*, 1980, 33: 1801–8.

Hambidge, K.M., et al. "Low levels of zinc in hair, anorexia, poor growth and hypogeusia in children." *Pediatric Research*, 1972, 6: 868–73.

Russell, R.M., et al. "Zinc and the special senses." *Annals of Internal Medicine*, 1983, 99: 227–39.

Safai-Kutti, S., Kutti, J. "Zinc and anorexia nervosa." *Annals of Internal Medicine*, 1984, 100(2): 317–18.

THE DIETER'S PHARMACY GLOSSARY

DRUGS CAUSING INCREASED APPETITE:

Astemizole
Bupropion
Chlorpromazine
Clofibrate
Cyproheptadine
Estrogen
Fluoxetine

Insulin
Marijuana
Methadone
Perphenazine
Pimozine
Prednisolone
Prednisone

Prochlorperazine
Terfenadine
Trazodone
Triamcinolone
Trifluoperazine
Triflupromazine
Valproic Acid

DRUGS CAUSING DECREASED APPETITE:

Acetazolamide
Albuterol
Amitriptyline
Amphetamine
Atenolol
Bumetanide
Bupropion
Captopril
Carbamazepine
Cefaclor
Cefadroxil
Cephalexin
Chenodiol
Chlortetracycline
Chlorothiazide
Chlorpromazine

Cholestyramine
Clomipramine
Clonidine
Colestipol
Cyclobenzaprine
Cyproheptadine
Desipramine
Dextrothyroxine
Diazepam
Digoxin
Diltiazem
Doxepine
Ephedrine
Erythromycin
Estrogen
Fluoxetine

Flurazepam
Furosemide
Haloperidol
Hydrochlorothiazide
Ibuprofen
Imipramine
Indapamide
Interferon
Isocarboxazid
Levodopa
L-Histidine
Lorazepam
L-Tryptophan
Maprotiline
Marijuana
Methadone

Methazolamide
Methotrexate
Metronidazole
Metoprolol
Molindone
Naltrexone
Nicotine
Nitrazepam
Nortriptyline
Oxytetracycline
Pimozine

Piroxicam
Penicillamine
Perphenazine
Phenelzine
Phenformin
Probucol
Propranolol
Scopolamine
Sulindac
Temazepam

Tetracycline
Theophylline
Timolol
Trazodone
Triamcinolone
Triazolam
Trifluoperazine
Triflupromazine
Valproic Acid
Vitamin A

DRUGS CAUSING WEIGHT GAIN:

Alprazolam
Amitriptyline
Astemizole
Bupropion
Carbamazepine
Chlorpromazine
Chlorpropamide
Clofibrate
Clomipramine
Clonidine
Cyproheptadine
Danazol
Desipramine
Diltiazem
Doxepin
Estrogen
Fluoxetine
Imipramine
Insulin

Labetalol
Levodopa
Lithium
Maprotiline
Marijuana
Methadone
Methandrostenolone
Methyldopa
Methysergide
Molindone
Naltrexone
Nandrolone
Nitrazepam
Norethandrolone
Nortriptyline
Oral Contraceptives
Oxandrolone
Perphenazine

Phenytoin
Pimozine
Pindolol
Prazosin
Prednisolone
Prednisone
Prochlorperazine
Propranolol
Terazosin
Terfenadine
Testosterone
Tetracycline
Tolbutamide
Trazodone
Triamcinolone
Trifluoperazine
Triflupromazine
Valproic Acid

DRUGS CAUSING WEIGHT LOSS:

Acetazolamide
Alcohol
Alprazolam
Amitriptyline

Amphetamine
Arginine
Belladonna
Benzocaine

Bupropion
Chlorothiazide
Clomipramine
Desipramine

Dextrothyroxine
Diethylpropion
Enalapril
Ephedrine
Estrogen
Evening Primrose Oil
Fenfluramine
Fluoxetine
Gemfibrozil
Glucomannan
Guarana
Guar Gum
Haloperidol
Hydrochlorothiazide
Imipramine
Indapamide

Interferon
Levodopa
Levothyroxine
L-Histidine
Liothyronine
Maprotiline
Mazindol
Methylcellulose
Methyldopa
Mineral Oil
Molindone
Naltrexone
Nicotinic Acid
 (Niacin)
Nitrazepam

Oral Contraceptives
Perphenazine
Phendimetrazine
Phenmetrazine
Phenylpropanolamine
Pimozide
Propranolol
Pyridoxine (Vitamin
 B_6)
Scopolamine
Tetracycline
Thyroid
Trazodone
Triamcinolone
Vitamin A

DRUGS CAUSING WATER RETENTION:

Alprazolam
Amitriptyline
Atenolol
Bupropion
Captopril
Carbamazepine
Chlorpromazine
Chlorpropamide
Cholestyramine
Clonidine
Cyclobenzaprine
Cyproheptadine
Danazol
Dextrothyroxine
Diazepam
Diltiazem
Estrogen
Furosemide
Gemfibrozil
HCG (Human
 Chorionic
 Gonadotropin)

Human Growth
 Hormone
Ibuprofen
Insulin
Interferon
Isocarboxazid
Labetalol
Levodopa
Lithium
Lorazepam
Marijuana
Methadone
Methandrostenolone
Methimazole
Methyldopa
Methysergide
Metoprolol
Naltrexone
Nandrolone
Naproxen

Nifedipine
Nitrazepam
Norethandrolone
Oral Contraceptives
Oxandrolone
Penicillamine
Phenelzine
Phenytoin
Pindolol
Piroxicam
Prazosin
Prednisolone
Prednisone
Probucol
Sulindac
Timolol
Testosterone
Trazodone
Triamcinolone
Vitamin A

DRUGS CAUSING TASTE CHANGES:

Albuterol
Amitriptyline
Amphetamine
Ampicillin
Belladonna
Bupropion
Captopril
Carbamazepine
Chlorhexidine
Chlorothiazide
Chlorphentermine
Cyclobenzaprine
Desipramine
Diethylpropion
Diltiazem
Doxepin
Enalapril

Etidronate
Fenfluramine
Fluoxetine
Flurazepam
Gemfibrozil
Griseofulvin
Hydrochlorothiazide
Imipramine
Indapamide
Interferon
Labetalol
Levodopa
L-Histidine
Lithium
Maprotiline
Marijuana
Mazindol

Methimazole
Metronidazole
Nicotine
Nifedipine
Penicillamine
Phendimetrazine
Phenformin
Phenmetrazine
Phentermine
Pimozide
Probucol
Sulindac
Temazepam
Tolbutamide
Trazodone
Triazolam

ANTIARTHRITIC DRUGS CAUSING WATER RETENTION:

Ibuprofen
Naproxen

Penicillamine
Piroxicam

Sulindac

ANTIBIOTICS CAUSING TASTE CHANGES:

Ampicillin
Chlorhexidine

Griseofulvin

Metronidazole

ANTIDEPRESSANTS CAUSING WEIGHT GAIN:

Amitriptyline
Bupropion
Clomipramine
Desipramine

Doxepin
Fluoxetine
Imipramine

Maprotiline
Nortriptyline
Trazodone

ANTIDEPRESSANTS CAUSING WATER RETENTION:

Amitriptyline	Isocarboxazid	Trazodone
Bupropion	Phenelzine	

ANTIDEPRESSANTS CAUSING TASTE CHANGES:

Amitriptyline	Doxepin	Maprotiline
Bupropion	Fluoxetine	Trazodone
Desipramine	Imipramine	

ANTIDIABETIC DRUGS CAUSING WEIGHT GAIN:

Chlorpropamide	Insulin	Tolbutamide

ANTIEPILEPTIC DRUGS CAUSING WEIGHT GAIN:

Carbamazepine	Phenytoin	Valproic Acid

ANTIHISTAMINES CAUSING INCREASED APPETITE:

Astemizole	Cyproheptadine	Terfenadine

ANTIHISTAMINES CAUSING WEIGHT GAIN:

Astemizole	Cyproheptadine	Terfenadine

ANTIOBESITY DRUGS CAUSING TASTE CHANGES:

Amphetamine	Mazindol	Phenmetrazine
Chlorphentermine	Phendimetrazine	Phentermine
Diethylpropion		

ANTIPSYCHOTIC DRUGS CAUSING INCREASED APPETITE:

Chlorpromazine   Pimozine   Trifluoperazine
Perphenazine   Prochlorperazine   Triflupromazine

ANTIPSYCHOTIC DRUGS CAUSING WEIGHT GAIN:

Chlorpromazine   Perphenazine   Trifluoperazine
Lithium   Pimozide   Triflupromazine
Molindone   Prochlorperazine

DIURETIC DRUGS CAUSING DECREASED APPETITE:

Acetazolamide   Furosemide   Indapamide
Bumetanide   Hydrochlorothiazide   Methazolamide
Chlorothiazide

HIGH-BLOOD-PRESSURE DRUGS CAUSING DECREASED APPETITE:

Atenolol   Diltiazem   Propranolol
Captopril   Metoprolol   Timolol
Clonidine

HIGH-BLOOD-PRESSURE DRUGS CAUSING WEIGHT GAIN:

Clonidine   Pindolol   Propranolol
Diltiazem   Prazosin   Terazosin
Labetalol

HIGH-BLOOD-PRESSURE DRUGS CAUSING WATER RETENTION:

Atenolol   Labetalol   Pindolol
Captopril   Metoprolol   Prazosin
Clonidine   Nifedipine   Timolol
Diltiazem

HIGH-BLOOD-PRESSURE DRUGS CAUSING TASTE CHANGES:

Captopril   Enalapril   Nifedipine
Diltiazem   Labetalol

HORMONES CAUSING WATER RETENTION:

Danazol   Chorionic   Hormone
Estrogen   Gonadotropin)   Methimazole
HCG (Human   Human Growth   Oral Contraceptives

TRANQUILIZERS/SLEEP AIDS CAUSING DECREASED APPETITE:

Diazepam   Lorazepam   Temazepam
Flurazepam   Nitrazepam   Triazolam

TRANQUILIZERS/SLEEP AIDS CAUSING WATER RETENTION:

Alprazolam   Lorazepam   Nitrazepam
Diazepam

TRANQUILIZERS/SLEEP AIDS CAUSING TASTE CHANGES:

Flurazepam   Temazepam   Triazolam

VITAMINS/NUTRITIONALS CAUSING WEIGHT LOSS:

Arginine   L-Histidine   Pyridoxine (Vitamin
Evening Primrose Oil   Nicotinic Acid B_6)
Glucomannan   (Niacin)   Vitamin A

SOURCES

Blackburn, G.L., et al. "Fad reducing diets: Separating fads from facts." *ASDC Journal of Dentistry for Children*, 1984, 51(5), 382–5.

Bray, G.A. "Treating obesity with drugs." *Drug Therapy*, 1984, 14(7), 93–100.

Bray, G.A., Greenway, F.L. "Pharmacological approaches to treating the obese patient." *Clinics in Endocrinology and Metabolism*, 1976, 5(2), 455–75.

Carruba, M.O., and Blundell, J.E., eds. *Pharmacolgy of Eating Disorders*. New York: Raven Press, 1986, 141–50.

Carson, J.A.S., et al. "Disease-medication relationships in altered taste sensitivity." *Journal of the American Dietetic Association*, 1976, 68, 550–53.

Covington, T.R. "Vitamins: Part I—Common myths." *Facts and Comparisons Drug Newsletter*, 1987, 6(7), 54–5.

Covington, T.R. "Obesity: Health implications and approaches to management." *Facts and Comparisons Drug Newsletter*, 1987, 6(9), 65–7.

D'Arcy, P., Griffen, J.P. *Iatrogenic Diseases*. New York: Oxford Press, 1986.

Douglas, J.G., Munro, J.F. "Drug treatment and obesity." *Pharmacology and Therapeutics*, 1982, 18, 351.

Fisher, M.C., et al. "Nutrition evaluation of published weight reducing fads." *Journal of the American Dietetic Association*, 1985, 85(4), 450–4.

Galloway, S. Mc.L., et al. "The current status of antiobesity drugs." *Postgraduate Medical Journal*, 1984, 60(suppl. 3), 19–26.

Gossel, T.A. "High fiber diet products." *U.S. Pharmacist*, 12(7), 1987.

Gottfries, C.G. "Influence of depression and antidepressants on weight." *Acta Psychiatrica Scandinavica*, 1981, 63(suppl. 290), 353–6.

Lamy, P.R. "Effects of diet and nutrition in drug therapy." *Journal of the American Geriatric Society*, 1982, 30, S99–112.

March, D.C. *Handbook: Interactions of Selected Drugs with Nutritional Status in Man (2nd edition)*. The American Dietetic Association, 1978.

Maslakowski, C.J. "Drug-nutrient interactions/interrelationships." *Nutritional Support Services*, 1981, 1(7), 14–17.

Olin, B. R. (ed.) *Facts and Comparisons*. St. Louis: Facts and Comparisons, 1988.

Physicians' Desk Reference. Oradell, NJ: Medical Economics, 1988.

Pope, H.G., Hudson, J.I. "Antidepressant drug therapy of bulimia: Current status." *Journal of Clinical Psychiatry*, 1986, 47, 339–45.

Rockwell, W.J., et al. "Psychotropic drugs promoting weight gain: Health risks and treatment implications." *Southern Medical Journal*, 1983, 76(11), 1407–12.

Roe, D.A. "Nutrient and drug interactions." *Nutrition Review*, 1984, 42, 141–53.

Roe, D.A., ed. *Drugs and Nutrients: The Interactive Effects*. New York: Dekker, 1984.

Reynolds, James E.F., ed. *Martindale the Extra Pharmacopoeia*. London: The Pharmaceutical Press, 1982.

Schwartz, H. *Never Satisfied: A Cultural History of Diets, Fantasies and Fat*. New York: Free Press, 1986.

Shaban, H.M., Galizia, V.J. "(Part II) Obesity: Drug treatment." *Pharmacy Times*, 1988, 54(6), 134–43.

Smith, C.H., Bidlock, W.R. "Dietary concerns associated with the use of medications." *Journal of the American Dietetic Association*, 1984, 84, 901–14.

Starr, C. "Feast or famine: Research takes on eating disorders." *Drug Topics*, 1988, 132(20), 24–6.

Sullivan, A.C., et al. "Novel anti-obesity agents whose primary site of action is in the gastro-intestinal tract." In *Recent Advances in Obesity Research: III*. London: John Libbey, 1981, 199–207.

Sullivan, A.C., Gruen, R.K. "Mechanisms of appetite modulation by drugs." *Federation Proceedings*, 1985, 44 (Pt. 1), 139–44.

Uretsky, S.D. "A pharmacists' guide to quack weight products." *American Pharmacy*, 1985, NS25(2), 104–109.

USP DI. Rockville, MD: The United States Pharmacopeial Convention, Inc., 1989.

White, J.P. "New pharmaceuticals joining fight against fat." *Drug Topics*, 131(5), 1987.

INDEX